**Combined Movement Theory**

*Commissioning Editor: Rita Demetriou-Swanwick*
*Development Editor: Veronika Watkins*
*Project Manager: Frances Affleck*
*Designer: Kirsteen Wright*
*Illustration Manager: Gillian Richards*
*Illustrator: Jennifer Rose*

# Combined Movement Theory

## Rational Mobilization and Manipulation of the Vertebral Column

Chris McCarthy PhD MCSP MMACP

Fellow in Spinal Orthopaedics,
Imperial College Healthcare, London, UK

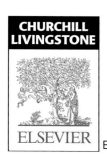

CHURCHILL
LIVINGSTONE

ELSEVIER

Edinburgh   London   New York   Oxford   Philadelphia   St Louis   Sydney   Toronto   2010

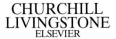

First published 2010, © Elsevier Limited. All rights reserved.

ISBN 978-0-443-06857-7

**British Library Cataloguing in Publication Data**
A catalogue record for this book is available from the British Library

**Library of Congress Cataloguing in Publication Data**
A catalogue record for this book is available from the Library of Congress

**Notices**
Knowledge and best practice in this field are constantly changing. As new research and experience broaden our understanding, changes in research methods, professional practices, or medical treatment may become necessary.

Practitioners and researchers must always rely on their own experience and knowledge in evaluating and using any information, methods, compounds, or experiments described herein. In using such information or methods they should be mindful of their own safety and the safety of others, including parties for whom they have a professional responsibility.

With respect to any drug or pharmaceutical products identified, readers are advised to check the most current information provided (i) on procedures featured or (ii) by the manufacturer of each product to be administered, to verify the recommended dose or formula, the method and duration of administration, and contraindications. It is the responsibility of practitioners, relying on their own experience and knowledge of their patients, to make diagnoses, to determine dosages and the best treatment for each individual patient, and to take all appropriate safety precautions.

To the fullest extent of the law, neither the Publisher nor the authors, contributors, or editors, assume any liability for any injury and/or damage to persons or property as a matter of products liability, negligence or otherwise, or from any use or operation of any methods, products, instructions, or ideas contained in the material herein.

*The Publisher*

 your source for books, journals and multimedia in the health sciences
**www.elsevierhealth.com**

Working together to grow
libraries in developing countries

www.elsevier.com | www.bookaid.org | www.sabre.org

ELSEVIER   BOOK AID International   Sabre Foundation

The Publisher's policy is to use paper manufactured from sustainable forests

Printed in China

# Contents

# Contributors

**Gail Forrester** MSc MMACP MCSP PgCertEd
Senior Lecturer in Physiotherapy, Department of
Physiotherapy, Faculty of Health & Life Sciences,
Coventry University, UK

**Roger Kerry** MSc MMACP MCSP PGCHE
Associate Professor, MSc Course Director, Division of
Physiotherapy Education, University of Nottingham,
Nottingham, UK

**Chris McCarthy** PhD MCSP MMACP
Fellow in Spinal Orthopaedics, Imperial College
Healthcare, London, UK

**Ioannis Paneris** BSc MCSP MMACP
Extended Scope Practitioner, Clinical Specialist,
Manchester Community Health, Manchester, UK

**Louise Potter** BSc Osteopathy PhD
Registered Osteopath, Medical School, University of
Leicester, Leicester, UK

**Alan J. Taylor** MSc MCSP
Lead Physiotherapist, Nuffield Health and Wellbeing
Centre, Nottingham, UK

# Dedication

To B.G.

*Who so loves, believes the impossible.*
(Elizabeth Barrett-Browning)

To move is to change place, position or posture. Thus, the positions at the initiation and cessation of movement are integral to the analysis of movement. Combined movement theory (CMT) offers the investigator a framework to examine the influence of starting and finishing positions on movement impairment and use these positions to intervene therapeutically. This book is structured in two parts. The first part of the book details the theoretical concepts underpinning the combined movement approach, whilst the second part describes the practical application of the concept for each region of the spine. Significant contributions have been made by manipulative therapy colleagues and it was our intention to ensure that the book is a practical reference for those undertaking combined movement treatment as well as a resource for musculoskeletal practitioners generally.

## Aims

The aims of this book are to provide readers with grounding in the principles of a method of spinal dysfunction assessment and treatment that facilitates:

- The recognition of when to consider combined movements theory in the management of spinal impairment and pain
- The expansion of the subjective and objective examination to more sensitively classify spinal impairment
- The management of spinal impairment with passive and active movements
- The management of spinal impairment with positioned muscular contractions
- The progression and regression of treatment based on position and grade of passive movement
- Selecting and applying manipulative techniques
- An understanding of spinal biomechanics, the physiological basis of manual therapy and clinical reasoning.

Dr Chris McCarthy
London 2009

# Acknowledgements

My eternal thanks to the late Dr Brian Edwards for showing me that combinations of movement could offer speedy return of spinal function. His teaching, at the beginning of my career, has guided my practice for nearly 20 years. Many thanks to my contributing experts and to Heidi Allen, publisher, who, in addition to initiating this project, modelled for the pictures and video clips.

# ELSEVIER DVD-ROM LICENCE AGREEMENT

# Section 1

## Combined Movement Theory

# Chapter One

# Introduction to combined movement theory

Chris McCarthy

## CHAPTER CONTENTS

To move is to change place, position or posture. Thus, the positions at the initiation and cessation of movement are integral to the analysis of movement. The spinal positions we adopt to allow full function are three-dimensional and continuously adapting to the functional demands placed on us. Naturally, the spinal system cannot always immediately accommodate to these demands and consequently short- and long-term impairment can result. In a system that continuously changes position and demands the acquisition of new and challenging positions the integrated control of movement can be compromised. Combined movement theory (CMT) offers the investigator a framework to examine the influence of starting and finishing positions on movement impairment and use these positions to intervene therapeutically.

Spinal dysfunction is a complex situation that must be considered in a biopsychosocial context. Our spines are continuously moving from one starting position of movement to another. The point at which this process becomes dysfunctional is dependent on the schema of the individual. The psychological perspective of the individual and societal influences have a huge bearing on just when function is considered to have become dysfunctional. For some, the spine has become dysfunctional only as they await the anaesthesia prior to surgery and others when they develop an inkling that 'something is not quite right in their back'. Thus, the presentation of spinal dysfunction is incredibly variable. Within this group of presentations are patterns of dysfunction that have become recognizable to healthcare practitioners. With the development of taxonomy of spinal dysfunctions, specific therapeutic interventions such as manual therapy have been developed; however there is no panacea for spinal dysfunction. There will never be one intervention that optimally matches all spinal dysfunctions. Thus, the search for efficacious interventions for specific presentations of dysfunction is the greatest test of our ingenuity in the short and long term.

Patients are people undergoing treatment for a problem they are perceiving. Patients do not generally attend for treatment for a problem they are not perceiving. Thus, all patients have a perception that something is problematical. If we accept this stance then we must assess patients from a biopsychosocial perspective. Each patient will present with a biopsychosocial profile that will need to be interpreted to allow the successful tailoring of intervention to optimally influence the patient's perception of their problem. In other words, we cannot afford to look at a patient from only one perspective. Tailoring an approach to management that only considers the biomedical or psychosocial factors influencing the patient's perception of their problem is not appropriate. For example, a patient with specific low back pain, for example a fractured coccyx, will be approached in a manner that matches their schema of the problem. Thus, whilst all patients with such a fracture would benefit from education and advice on the prognosis, timescales and options for management, the addition of a rehabilitation programme will depend on the psychological profile of the patient. Some patients would require a formal rehabilitation programme whilst others will manage by themselves. Some patients might develop compensatory, mechanical low back pain whilst others might not need this complication addressed formally. The strength of our examination to predict likely outcomes, discriminate different conditions and to correlate with objective tests of dysfunction is vital for our practice.

There are some presentations of spinal dysfunction that suggest a mechanically-focused intervention may be the optimal strategy for treatment. There are some spinal presentations that suggest the dysfunction has a strong relationship to the positions the spine is held or moved into. There are some presentations of dysfunction that appear to be more dominantly influenced by mechanical factors than the psychosocial influences underpinning them. Indeed, some presentations of spinal dysfunction lead individuals to consult manual therapists for their assessment and treatment rather than a psychologist, cognitive behavioural therapist or faith healer. The quest to identify who is most suited to manual therapy as opposed to other conservative therapies is currently being undertaken by clinicians and researchers around the world; however, we are at the beginning of this journey with its end being some way over the horizon.

In the muddy waters of spinal pain it is clear that when it appears appropriate to intervene with therapeutic spinal movement, be it with muscle contractions, passive mobilization or manipulative thrust techniques, the starting and ending positions of these movements are crucial. The underlying hypotheses of these interventions is that the position in which these movements are undertaken has a superior

effect on reducing dysfunction than inducing movement in a random fashion. Thus if we believe that, for certain presentations of spinal pain, the painful position of the spine is related to the patient's dysfunction, then interventions that take this relationship into consideration may be more effective than invoking random movement or generic exercise.

This simple assumption leads the quest for appropriate treatment into the realm of specific assessment and induction of spinal motion in spinal dysfunction. Thus, the examination and treatment of spinal dysfunction in presentations where positions and postures are important in its aetiology and maintenance must include a three-dimensional assessment of motion. In addition, therapeutic strategies must include a consideration for starting and finishing positions. CMT fulfils these requirements and thus has considerable clinical utility. It is a system of examination that emphasizes the expansion of the musculoskeletal examination to fully evaluate the active and passive combinations of physiological and accessory movement of the vertebral column and offers the investigator greater scope for identification and treatment of dysfunction.

The concept of 'combined movements' examination and treatment was developed by Dr Brian Edwards, a specialist manipulative physiotherapist from Perth, Western Australia. The work of Brian Edwards (1987) was incorporated into the seminal writings of Geoff Maitland and is seen as an important corollary of the 'Maitland Concept' (Maitland, 1986). Having been taught the principles of CMT by Dr Edwards and subsequently corresponded with him over its development I hope this book provides you with a reference that shows that CMT has developed into a comprehensive approach to the management of specific types of spinal dysfunction.

# Essential components of combined movement theory

CMT is defined by a number of essential components.

## Starting positions

CMT encourages the consideration of starting positions in the choice of therapeutic treatments. Whilst even the most ardent follower of the CMT concept may occasionally treat the patient in a relatively neutral position, the vast majority of treatments require the careful consideration of the position the treatment is conducted in. The consideration of starting positions starts during the patient interview, continues through the initial examination and throughout the progression of treatment. Home exercise and discharge programmes will continue to emphasize the value of the positions to the patient.

The simple addition of 'In' and 'Did' into the process of note-taking during treatment will encourage a consideration of the starting position in practice. This attention to the recording of position and treatment technique has been recently recommended by the fellows of the American Academy of Orthopaedic Manual Physical Therapists (2006).

For example:

IN: supine, mid-cervical extension, right side flexion.

DID: antero-posterior pressure on the right C6 transverse process, Grade III+, 1 × 1 minute.

## Biomechanical basis

CMT follows a model of spinal biomechanics based on the arthrology and myology of the spine. In other words CMT is aimed at influencing the active and passive, physiological and accessory movements of the intervertebral disc, zygapophyseal and interbody joints and surrounding paravertebral muscles. The intervertebral foramen will also be influenced in the extremes of combined positioning. The influence that movement can have on the contents of the intervertebral foramen should be carefully observed during positioning and treatment with combined positioning of the spine resulting in 'opening' or 'closing' of the intervertebral space.

## 'High-dose' movement

One of the major advantages of this method of applying movement is the ability to use high-dose movement in conditions that are very severely painful. By utilizing starting positions that are biomechanically derived to be painless, greater therapeutic movement can be induced. High-dose movements, in the context of manual therapy, mean that a large therapeutic effect is likely to be elicited from the movement. This therapeutic effect will influence mechanical and neurological mechanisms and should have an immediate effect on movement patterns.

More detail on the theoretical mechanisms of combined movement is discussed in Chapter 2.

## Treatment in resistance

When performing a passive movement of a joint there is typically a range of movement that has imperceptible resistance to that movement. As the joint is moved towards the end of its range the peri-articular structures and joint capsule will come under increasing stretch. Consequently, a perception of resistance to movement develops. The use of therapeutic movement in this 'resistance' range has a number of therapeutic advantages over treating in the earlier part of joint and muscle range. The mechanisms are described in Chapter 2; however, CMT encourages the use of this resistance range of movement during assessment and treatment.

## Mini-treatment during assessment

During the assessment of movement dysfunction, an assessment of passive movement is undertaken at several functional spinal units. Typically, the manual therapist is seeking information on the position, pain, perception of resistance and the relationship between position, pain and resistance. In addition, they will make comparisons between segments to establish the primary source of movement dysfunction. CMT encourages the addition of another component to this investigative process. In addition to gathering the information above, the effect of briefly treating the dysfunctional spinal units with movement or muscle contractions are assessed. Thus, by influencing afferent information from the dysfunctional segment and then assessing the effect of this 'mini-treatment' on dysfunction the importance of the movement findings can be interpreted. This is detailed in Chapter 3; however, this process ensures that the most influential treatments are applied at all times.

## The incorporation of mobilization and manipulation

Having evaluated the positions that result in dysfunction the manual therapist can utilize combined starting positions to mobilize (slow, oscillatory, passive movements), manipulate (slow or fast movements that induce cavitations) or induce isometric muscle contractions (muscle contraction that alters muscle activity post contraction) to treat. Indications for each modality are detailed in Chapter 3. The decision to mobilize, manipulate or use muscle work is governed predominantly by the perceptions gained from skilful palpation and the relative effect of mini-treatments. The strongest indication for considering a manipulative thrust requires an accurate passive assessment of segmental physiological movement; thus, the manual therapist's accuracy in passive physiological assessment must be high. In Chapter 2, a case will be made for the use of manipulative technique (Grade IV−) as a precursor to mobilization technique, rather than as the last choice of treatment (Grade V).

## Inhibition of muscle with isometric muscle contraction

Changes in static spinal muscle activity can be evoked in response to isometric contraction of the muscle or its antagonist. It has been suggested that contraction of an agonist muscle will evoke a Golgi tendon mediated inhibition of muscle activity and result in a reduction in hypertonicity. In addition, contraction of the antagonist muscle group will reciprocally inhibit the agonist. The starting positions utilized within the CMT concept place the spinal muscles in ideal positions to effectively evoke these reflex responses. Thus, with an understanding of CMT the clinician is afforded a choice of specific, localized treatment options.

## Palpation

Cues, used to decide on treatment selection, are gathered from palpation. Palpation of soft tissue, muscle and joint feel during movement are integral to deciding which passive or active treatment technique is adopted. Changes in soft tissues and muscle tone can give reliable guidance in identifying the spinal level of greatest dysfunction and the proportion of the dysfunction that is arthrogenic or myogenic. Whilst palpating the quality of a joint end feel during physiological movement, strong guidance with regard to the suitability of mobilization or manipulation is gained. Palpation is a vital skill within CMT and is used in decisions regarding type, location, duration and dosage of treatment. Intra-examiner reliability will only be adequate with repetition and practice.

## Patterns of movement: regular and irregular patterns of movement

Differentially diagnosing spinal dysfunction is notoriously difficult; however, there is a strong contention that there exist patients who present with typical patterns of movement dysfunction. Patients may present with pain produced with combinations of movements that match the normal coupling of the spine, suggesting that they have a mechanical pattern of presentation. In contrast, patients occasionally reproduce their pain with movements that do not follow the normal coupled movement of the spine. The first situation can be described as a 'regular pattern' of movements suggesting a mechanical presentation, whilst the second scenario is an 'irregular pattern' with movement characteristics that do not as clearly suggest a predominantly mechanical pattern. The initial management of these two patterns is very different.

Patients presenting with regular patterns of movement will fall into one of two categories. These categories are beginning to demonstrate some evidence for their usefulness in categorizing subgroups of patients within the non-specific low back pain group (Fritz et al, 2007). These patterns have been variously described as 'closing down', 'compression', and 'anterior stretch' patterns or the alternative pattern of 'opening up', 'stretch' or 'posterior stretch'. Essentially, the former represents a dysfunction associated with ipsilateral movement of the superior segment towards the side of pain, whilst the latter is associated with contralateral movement away from the side of pain.

Patients presenting with irregular patterns demonstrate patterns of dysfunction that do not follow the normal mechanics of the spinal region. For example, pain reproduced with ipsilateral sideflexion and contralateral rotation would not follow a simple model of nociceptive pain induced by progressively increasing the stretch on hypomobile structures. Increasing the stretch on hypomobile structures using movements following the mechanics of the region will progressively increase afferent nociceptive input. This relationship of stretch and pain is much less regular if the source of pain is emanating from hypermobile or inflamed/sensitized structures. Irregular patterns of pain production make the use of CMT less appropriate and other methods of treatment are more appropriate (rest, TENS, anti-inflammatory modalities). As patients with irregular patterns of spinal impairment resolve, and the inflammatory nature of their condition reduces, presentations often becomes more regular and thus appropriate for management with CMT.

## Progression of treatment by change of position

Treatment that takes into account the starting position requires a consideration of where treatment will need to go in order to resolve the dysfunction, the position it is acceptable to start in and the mechanism of effect the treatment is using to affect dysfunction. Thus, one of the most important priorities in the use of CMT is the change of treatment position in response to change in pain and movement dysfunction. The position in which we are able to start treatment will range from a position diametrically opposite to the position of dysfunction to the very position of dysfunction itself. In a situation where it is not appropriate to reproduce symptoms (severe pain presentations or in light of other cautions), treatment will be applied in the position of least dysfunction and using movement that most safely evokes descending pain mechanisms, shown to reduce nociceptive pain perception (see Ch. 2). As a dysfunction resolves and it becomes more acceptable to treat in positions closer to the position of dysfunction the mechanism of treatment will incorporate elements of 'tissue stretching' to influence afferent nociceptive information from the region.

Initial treatment is a matter of deciding on the mechanism the therapist wishes to use to evoke pain relief. In a dysfunction with severe pain, movement evoking high-threshold mechano-receptive afferent information in a position that does not reproduce pain will be the most appropriate choice. As the severity of the pain reduces, positions can be selected that, in addition to this mechanism, reduce afferent nociceptive barrage by physically lengthening hypomobile, nociceptively active tissues. In reality, this involves a progression of starting position from the quadrant opposite to the dysfunction to the quadrant of dysfunction itself.

## Aims

The aims of this book are to provide readers with a grounding in the principles of a method of spinal

dysfunction assessment and treatment that facilitates:

- The recognition of when to consider CMT in the management of spinal impairment and pain
- The expansion of the subjective and objective examination to more sensitively classify spinal impairment
- The management of spinal impairment with passive and active movements
- The management of spinal impairment with positioned muscular contractions
- The progression and regression of treatment based on position and grade of passive movement
- The selection and application of manipulative techniques
- An understanding of the theoretical and pathophysiological mechanisms underpinning the concept.

## Summary

- Manual therapy is suitable for specific presentations of spinal impairment. CMT facilitates the identification of these specific spinal dysfunctions.
- Manual therapy's strongest paradigm is the contention that specific movement will elicit normal function faster than generic movement or other methods of regaining function.
- CMT incorporates awareness of spinal biomechanics, considerations of dosage, mini-treatments during assessment, mobilization, manipulation and isometric muscle techniques.
- Patterns of movement dysfunction are used to assess and treat spinal dysfunction.
- The starting and finishing positions of movement are vital in the management of specific spinal dysfunction.
- Progression and regression of treatment can be by change of starting position.
- Progression involves evoking pain relief in pain-free positions and moves to add in stretching of restricted tissues.
- The CMT concept requires a strong appreciation of spinal biomechanics, the physiological basis of manual therapy and clinical reasoning.

## QUESTIONS

**1. Are all presentations of spinal dysfunction suitable for management with manual therapy?**

    A. Yes

    B. No

**2. What would lead you to consider a patient suitable for CMT during the patient interview?**

    A. An irritable condition with pain in all positions

    B. A mechanical presentation of dysfunction

**3. Is it important to interpret presentations of dysfunction in terms of positions and likely biomechanical sources of symptoms when undertaking a CMT examination?**

    A. Yes

    B. No

**4. Which patterns of presentation will you be identifying in patients suitable for CMT management?**

    A. Irregular patterns

    B. Regular patterns

    C. Anterior stretch patterns (also called compression patterns)

    D. Posterior stretch patterns (also called stretch patterns)

**5. Which techniques will you be using to treat using CMT?**

    A. Mobilization of spinal articulations in the 'resistance range'

    B. Manipulation of spinal articulations

    C. Isometric muscle contractions

**6. Who was the physiotherapist who originally developed combined movements?**

    A. Mr Geoff Maitland

    B. Dr Chris McCarthy

    C. Dr Brian Edwards

**7. When treating a dysfunction in a position diametrically opposite to the position of pain reproduction, what is the predominant mechanism of effecting a change?**

    A. Stimulation of mechanoreceptors leading to a decrease in perception of nociceptive pain

    B. Stretch of tissues (capsule peri-articular structures, muscle) in the direction of restriction

**Answers: 1** B; **2** B; **3** A; **4** A,B,C,D; **5** A,B,C; **6** C; **7** A

# References

Edwards, B., 1987. Clinical assessment: the use of combined movements. In: Twomey, J., Taylor, J. (Eds.), Physical therapy of the low back. Churchill Livingstone, Melbourne.

Fritz, J.M., Lindsay, W., Matheson, J.W., et al., 2007. Is there a subgroup of patients with low back pain likely to benefit from mechanical traction? Results of a randomized clinical trial and subgrouping analysis. Spine 32 (26), E793–E800.

Maitland, G., 1986. Vertebral manipulation. Elsevier Health Sciences, Sydney.

# Chapter Two

2

# Theoretical basis of combined movement theory

Chris McCarthy, Louise Potter

## CHAPTER CONTENTS

## Introduction

The physiological and psychological mechanisms of a treatment approach as diverse as 'manual therapy' are extraordinarily complex. An individual receiving manual therapy will be presenting for this treatment with a profile of characteristics (anxious, in pain, moving abnormally, experiencing some hypertonicity and associated muscle inhibition) that will be a representation of an infinite number of combinations of mechanisms. The influence of manual therapy on some of these mechanisms is understood whilst others have been insufficiently researched. The skill of the manual therapist is to interpret the profile of the individual patient and target manual therapy treatment towards the predominant mechanism of dysfunction. Some patients will have restricted movement due to joint stiffness or to muscle hypertonicity, others will be fearful of specific movements, whilst others may not be aware or concerned about how they excessively move a region of their spines.

This chapter details some of the underlying evidence to support the use of manual therapy and, in particular, the use of specific movement in the treatment of spinal pain. The mechanisms discussed below are by no means exclusive to, although they are particularly relevant to, the CMT approach. There is a certain mystique surrounding spinal manual therapy that does not follow manual treatment on the periphery. Attending for manual therapy to increase mobility and reduce pain following a fractured radius is not considered to be controversial, whilst attending for spinal manual therapy is often the source of considerable discussion.

Some of the reasons for this controversy are:

- Lack of clarity regarding effects
- Lack of clarity regarding effectiveness
- Lack of clarity of terminology.

We are still developing a body of evidence to establish the physiological and psychological effects of manual therapy. Ultimately, manual therapy is a method of intervention for musculoskeletal dysfunction that encourages accelerated recovery. In light of this we must consider how we are measuring our effectiveness. The measurement of manual therapy against other treatments when judged in terms of change in disability, and reported 12 months after our intervention, may not be a sensitive method of capturing our effect (McCarthy & Cairns, 2005).

### Clinical relevance

When discussing the risks and benefits of manual therapy with our patients we must convey the uncertainty of the available evidence. We cannot give our patients complete information about their personal odds for short- and long-term benefit or their personal odds for risk. It is important to highlight the uncertainty of the evidence during the consent process.

## Spinal manipulation

Whilst there is considerable difference in individual practitioners' approaches to manipulation there are some common features that define manipulation and mobilization. Some difference in practice may be professionally driven or by schools of thought within professions. It is worth considering that, even within the small world of manipulative therapy, we may mean very different things by the same terminology. A synopsis of the multi-disciplinary groups practising manual therapy leads us to a number of common features in a definition of manipulation:

- A small amplitude, high velocity thrust, applied to a spinal joint
- Extends beyond a restriction in range
- Occurs at the end of range
- Occurs at the beginning of resistance
- Results in a popping sound/cavitation.

Whilst there is huge debate about where in the range of movement a technique is performed the two features that are common to many definitions of manipulation are: (1) reference to motion at one functional spinal unit and (2) mention of an audible 'popping' sound.

### The effects of manipulation?

- Tearing adhesions in the capsule
- Lengthening of the joint capsule
- Freeing trapped menisci or loose synovium
- Reducing the tone in hypertonic paraspinal muscle.

Above are four of the main hypotheses suggested as possible effects of spinal manipulative techniques. Let us address these points individually and then draw some conclusions on the likely effects of manipulative therapy technique.

## Tearing adhesions in the capsule or stretching joints?

Imagine a scenario where your patient has attended with pain at three quarters range, right rotation, depicted in the top line of Figure 2.1. You feel a manipulative technique will be potentially of value in your management programme. The starting position you would adopt for the manipulative thrust would be formed by a combination of three physiological movements. In extension, ipsilateral flexion and contra-lateral flexion, the amount of rotation developed will be much less than the amount of rotation required to stretch or 'tear' an adhesion. Thus, it is unlikely that we are aiming to lengthen or tear tissue with our manipulative thrusts, whereas we feel we are aiming to lengthen tissues with our mobilization/stretching techniques.

Is the thrust element of the technique applied at end of range? Physiotherapists familiar with the Maitland Concept will be used to the nomenclature of grades of movement as described by Geoff Maitland (Maitland, 1986). Grades I and II refer to passive movement (of small and large amplitude respectively) performed in the early part of the range. In this range the therapist will not perceive resistance to movement. Grades III and IV are (large and small amplitude) movements conducted in a range where resistance is detected by the therapist. Small amplitude movement in early ranges of resistance are noted as IV− whilst movement at end of range as IV+. Manipulative thrusts techniques have been notated as Grade V, suggesting that the technique is conducted beyond the end of range and indeed some therapists may perform a

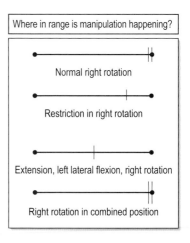

Where in range is manipulation happening?

Normal right rotation

Restriction in right rotation

Extension, left lateral flexion, right rotation

Right rotation in combined position

**Figure 2.1** • Range at which manipulation can occur.

high velocity thrust at the end of passive range. In common with many other manual therapists and osteopaths we feel there are disadvantages to performing manipulative thrusts at the end of passive range and numerous advantages to avoiding this starting position (Evans & Breen, 2006). This assertion is based on an understanding of the effects of passive manipulation and mobilization and represent an individual viewpoint on the objectives of the technique. However, there are many views on the objectives of manipulative technique and some manual therapists may feel they should conduct a manipulation as an end-of-range technique in order to stretch tissue.

One of the aims of manual therapy is to elongate soft tissue. In the process of stretching connective tissue a stress/strain curve has been identified that represents the behaviour of the tissue. Figure 2.2 depicts the relationship between the application of a strain on tissue and its resultant change in length. The relationship is speed specific with changes in the speed of application resulting in differing lengthening characteristics (Lederman, 2005).

Connective tissue that is loaded quickly will deform less than tissue loaded slowly, with the same amount of force. This is an important factor when considering manipulative thrusts and lengthening tissue. Figure 2.3 illustrates the fact that greater force is required to elongate tissue if applied quickly rather than slowly. Less force is required to lengthen hypomobile soft tissue if applied slowly, and as quick, forceful movements have greater potential to evoke nociceptive afferent barrage, the

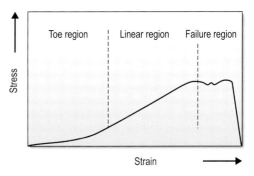

**Figure 2.2** • Stress–strain curve for soft tissue. Distinct areas: 'the toe', 'the linear/elastic region' and the 'area of plastic deformation'. The toe area of the curve represents the initial stage of deformation where the crimping of bunches of collagen fibres occurs. The linear region of the curve represents deformation without micro-failure of collagen. The area after approximately 3–5% deformation represents micro-failure of collagen fibres and plastic deformation. At around 8% deformation there is macro-failure. Stress = force applied; Strain = deformation. (Threlkeld, 1992)

therapist should consider carefully the use of thrust techniques when deliberately trying to reduce hypomobility, particularly in the presence of pain.

## Clinical relevance

If we want to comfortably stretch tightened soft tissue we can use less force by stretching slowly rather than quickly.

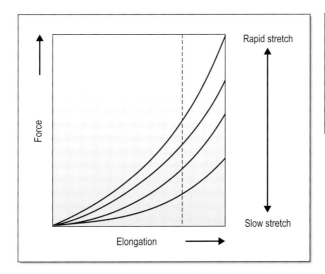

**Figure 2.3** • Relationship between speed and elongation.

## What about the pop/cavitation?

In the 1970s, Sandoz conducted a series of experiments looking at distraction of finger joints. He noted that if cavitation occurred during distraction (signified by an audible popping sound), there was a gain of 5–10° in the range of passive movement of the metacarpophalangeal joint in all directions and the active range of movement was also increased, but to a lesser extent. Sandoz also noted that regardless of the direction of the distraction to the metacarpophalangeal joint, the refractory period remained the same and a radiolucent space appeared on the X-ray film. Sandoz (1976) went on to review what was known about the mechanical effects of joint cavitation at the time and produced a summary diagram (Fig. 2.4).

In Figure 2.4, two important features of the effects of distraction on a synovial joint can be identified. Firstly, the phenomenon of cavitation does not occur at the end of the joint's distraction range but rather in the middle of range. Secondly, there is a change in the profile of resistance to movement exhibited in the range preceding cavitation and immediately following it. Post cavitation there is a reduction in the force required to distract the joint; it is less resistant to movement.

This leaves the question of whether cavitations at the finger joints are the same as those that occurred at the facet joint. Méal and Scott (1986) and Conway *et al* (1993) conducted studies examining the sound signals created by distractions of the fingers and those produced by spinal manipulation. Observing that the sound signals had similar acoustic nature led them to postulate that a similar mechanism was occurring and that joint gapping resulting in an increased range of movement was likely. Since then Cramer *et al* (2000) and Cramer *et al* (2002) have examined the effect of manipulation on the zygapophysial (facet) joints using magnetic resonance imaging (MRI). Following a successful pilot study on 16 healthy subjects they went on to randomize 64 healthy volunteers into four groups (Cramer *et al*, 2002). All participants had their initial scan whilst lying supine, then group one were placed in a side-lying posture and re-scanned. The second group had a manipulation and then were re-scanned in a supine position. The third group received a manipulation and were then placed in a side-lying position and re-scanned and finally, the fourth group were turned onto their side briefly and then re-scanned in a supine position. The second scan was conducted within 15–20 minutes of the intervention.

The authors demonstrated that the average change in joint separation following manipulation noted between the three radiologists blinded to the groups (intra and inter-rater reliability reported to be high with ICCs; 0.97 and 0.95 respectively) for the third group was +1.32 mm (manipulated then re-scanned in side-lying position), whereas for the second group (manipulated then re-scanned in a supine position), the average change was only +0.01 mm. In the final group the subjects were just

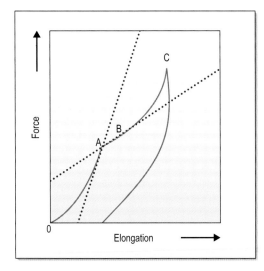

- A–B 'crack'

- B–C = range for post-manipulation mobilization

**Figure 2.4** • Profile of resistance to movement before and after cavitation.

placed in a side-lying posture and the change was −0.01 mm. They concluded that the results are consistent with the hypothesis that chiropractic manipulations gap the facet joint.

## Clinical relevance

Following cavitation, there is a palpable change in the resistance profile of the passive movement. What was perceived as a short sharp build-up in resistance can immediately be perceived to change to a longer range of resistance, starting at the same point in range, but extending further into passive range. This perception can be depicted using movement diagrams (Fig. 2.5), as described by Maitland (1986).

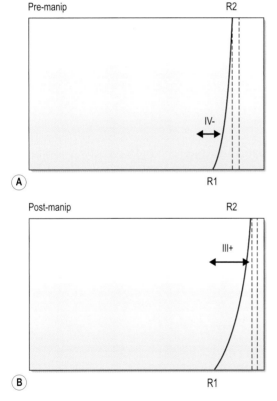

**Figure 2.5 •** Depiction of the perception of resistance felt during a passive movement. Using right lateral flexion of C4/C5 as an example, (**A**) shows the resistance profile towards the end of the range of movement. (**B**) shows the profile perceived after cavitation. The short resistance profile in (A) would indicate that a grade IV mobilization would be an appropriate mobilization to treat in resistance, whilst the longer profile in (B) suggests a grade III would be indicated. For more detail on the selection of grades see Maitland (1986).

The phenomenon of cavitation is more commonly described in engineering and bioengineering fields. Cavitation is the phenomenon of gas bubble formation and collapse within fluids. The phenomenon occurs in response to reductions in pressure with fluids to levels below the vapour pressure for that fluid. At this point, gas bubbles are formed and quickly collapse, often resulting in an audible popping (two pops within milliseconds of each other) (Brennen, 1995).

Any movement that increases the volume within a synovial joint and consequently drops the intra-articular pressure will have the potential to evoke a cavitation response. However, movements that encourage the natural sliding of one joint surface on another are unlikely to increase joint volumes enough to drop intra-articular pressures to below the vapour pressure. Movements that incorporate an element of distraction that gap one joint surface from the other typically result in cavitation. Patients often describe manoeuvres they perform themselves, that when analyzed in detail, mimic the manipulative thrust starting positions used by clinicians. These positions universally position the joint to facilitate gapping of one joint surface from another, be it without a high velocity thrust, using a high velocity thrust or during the relaxation of paraspinal muscles around joints after a muscular contraction.

### The physiology of synovial cavitation

- Rapid formation and collapse of gas bubbles in response to a reduction in pressure below vapour pressure
- Reduction in viscosity and surface tension that leads to a change in mechanical compliance
- Temporary effect as gas is reabsorbed over approximately an hour

A review of the many manipulative therapy texts published by physiotherapists, osteopaths and chiropractors reveals a common feature to manipulative technique. Spinal joints are positioned in such a manner that during their positioning, or as a result of a high velocity thrust performed in that position, one joint surface is gapped from its partner. This may involve gapping the whole surface from its partner using techniques that utilize an obvious element of distraction (Fig. 2.6) or by distracting one edge of the joint from its partner using positioning that opens one 'side' of the joint (Fig. 2.7).

There is some good evidence that spinal manipulation does create gapping of the facet joints. It is

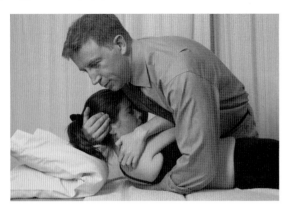

**Figure 2.6 •** An antero-posterior, cephalad distraction thrust technique is shown. With this technique the therapist fixes the inferior level and using pressure transmitted through the sternum and ribs distracts the superior level superiorly and in an antero-posterior direction. The thrust is perpendicular to the plane of the facet joint and is likely to gap one surface directly from another, resulting in cavitation.

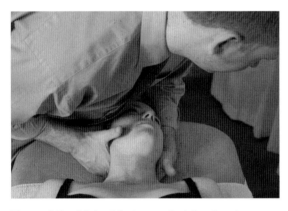

**Figure 2.7 •** A lateral flexion manipulative thrust technique that has positioned C4/C5 in extension, right lateral flexion and left rotation, is shown. In this position the superior facet cannot slide naturally down its partner. Whether encouraged to distract by the positioning, a high velocity thrust or during the relaxation following an isometric contraction, one edge of the C4/C5 facet may distract from its partner and cavitation may occur.

theoretically possible that gapping a facet joint may release a trapped menisci or section of loose synovium (another commonly cited theory for therapeutic benefit), however, it may be impossible to establish if this has occurred. It is possible that

improving joint range of movement may create a window of opportunity to allow the patient to exercise and rehabilitate. It may be that gapping joints stimulates muscle or joint sensory afferents, which might be responsible for initiating analgesic responses within the central nervous system (CNS). Cavitation, whether initiated by the application of a thrust or by other low-velocity methods, has an influence on joint biomechanics that complements more traditional methods of stretching soft-tissues.

## Clinical relevance

Cavitation produces a mechanical effect, induced in a starting position that is not end of range, that mimics the effects of end of range of stretches, i.e. an increase in range of movement and reduction in paraspinal hypertonicity.

## The neurophysiological effects of manipulation and mobilization

Wyke (1975) identified the existence of four types of synovial joint receptors. Types **I, II** and **III** are classified as mechanoreceptors which function to convert mechanical stimuli into electrical energy. Mechanoreceptors offer positional and kinaesthetic information from the joint to the CNS. Type **IV** receptors are nociceptors responsible for signalling pain. Wyke proposed that these receptors are only activated in the presence of inflammatory sensitizers. Based on the classic gate theory of Melzack and Wall (1965), Wyke proposed that the information produced in the larger diameter joint afferents would impede the afferent passage of information conveyed by joint nociceptors at the level of the spinal cord. It has been shown that the majority of large diameter fibres are stimulated by mainly end-of-range movements and that excitation is not selective. A significant proportion of small diameter afferents are excited at the same time (Schaible & Schmidt, 1983). In inflamed joints, movement prior to resistance can stimulate sensitized small diameter joint nociceptors (Type IV). The simple gate theory of pain modulation is therefore not adequate in explaining the pain modulation observed with mobilization. The understanding of the influence of movement on perception and generation of pain has progressed with the development of our understanding of descending pain mechanisms.

## Descending pain inhibitory systems

The periaqueductal grey area (PAG) of the brain stem has been shown to be an important component of the CNS with regard to post-mobilization/manipulation hypoalgesia. There are distinct areas within the PAG that provide two forms of analgesia: the dorsal PAG and the ventral PAG. The ventral PAG elicits recuperative behaviour and a reduction in general mobility response and is an opioid-mediated reaction. The sympathetic system is temporarily inhibited. This response is observed 20–45 minutes post treatment (acupuncture, manipulation). The dorsal PAG elicits a fight-or-flight reaction, with sympatho-excitation. The onset of analgesia is rapid and a non-opioid-mediated reaction. The noradrenergic system particularly mediates nociceptive pain, rather than thermal pain, with inhibition of substance P release at the source of pain (Sterling *et al*, 2001; Wright, 1995). Passive movement that stimulates high threshold mechanoreceptors, by moving joints towards end of range, has been shown to have a sympatho-exitatory effect on the autonomic nervous system (Chiu & Wright, 1996; Petersen *et al*, 1993; Vincenzino *et al*, 1994; Wright 1995; Zusman, 1994), with increased adrenal sympathetic activity (Zusman, 1994). Slater *et al* (1994) have demonstrated an increase in skin conduction in the upper limb following 'sympathetic slump' techniques. In addition, there is some evidence that the magnitude of effect of manual therapy on sympathetic responses is related to the side of application (Perry & Green, 2008). This evidence would suggest that the specific application of manual therapy techniques would be more effective than evoking general movement in patients, an underpinning concept of manual therapy. See Figure 2.8.

Altered patterns of muscle recruitment have also been shown with spinal manipulation by Sterling *et al* (2001), i.e. there is a decrease in activity of superficial neck flexor muscles, indicating an increase in deep flexor muscle activity. The authors suggest this improvement in muscle function could be due to an increase in activity of alpha motor neurons (bringing the deep cervical flexors closer to threshold firing via activation of descending pathways) as it occurred concurrently with hypoalgesia and sympatho-excitation. The authors also suggest that it may be due to improved hypoalgesia. Colloca and Keller (2001) have demonstrated an immediate reflex effect on spinal segmental muscle activity.

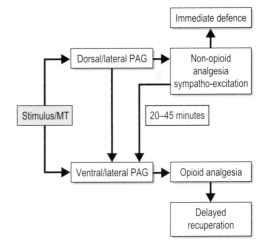

**Figure 2.8** • The theoretical model of descending pain inhibition. Manual therapy (MT) (adapted from Wright, 1995)

## Effect of thrust techniques on muscle

Another theory describing a potential mechanism of effect for manual therapy is the reflexogenic response to spinal manipulation. This is the theory that manipulative thrust techniques cause a reflexogenic reduction in pain, reduction of hypertonicity in muscles and improvement in functional ability (Herzog, 2000). Theoretically, reflex responses may be elicited from a variety of receptors, including facet joint mechanoreceptors located in the capsule (type $A\beta$ fibres), nociceptors (type $A\delta$ and C fibres), cutaneous receptors ($A\alpha$ and $A\beta$ fibres) and proprioceptors in the skeletal muscles (type $A\alpha$ from the Golgi tendon organ and muscle spindle primary; $A\beta$ from muscle spindle secondary fibres).

Dishman and Bulbulian (2000) conducted an experiment on 17 young asymptomatic subjects. They were randomized into two groups: one group received a spinal manipulation with thrust, and the other group received a spinal mobilization without a thrust and then an hour later a manipulation with thrust. The results showed that a short-term attenuation of $\alpha$-motoneuronal activity was seen after spinal manipulation. The results from the second group showed that mobilization, in combination with manipulation, exerted a greater inhibitory effect on $\alpha$-motoneuronal activity than a single manipulation. The results also showed a similarity in magnitude of attenuation of motoneuronal activity between manipulation and mobilization. The authors suggested that these results supported previous evidence that the results from manipulation are the same, even without an audible response, and that the force and velocity may not be the most important factor in altering α-motoneuronal activity. However, these results were collected from a small sample of subjects, who were free from back pain and so should be interpreted with caution.

Lehman and McGill (2001) performed an experiment on 19 patients with low back pain. In this study the authors recorded the normalized electromyograph (EMG), Oswestry low back pain disability scores and spinal movements pre and post manipulation. The active movements tested were flexion, extension, lateral bend and axial twist. They were measured immediately before and after the manipulative thrusts and again 20 minutes later. The authors found very small or no changes in superficial EMG post manipulation and small changes in the range of movement. The greatest changes were seen in those subjects who had the highest pain levels. Changes in range of movement tended to be small whilst EMG changes tended to decrease. Thus, the available evidence does not make it clear whether performing a thrust technique, in itself, reduces hypertonicity or reduces pain.

## Summary

It is not surprising that the effectiveness of mobilization and manipulation are equivocal. Both will produce afferent information that will evoke descending pain inhibitory mechanisms. In patients who have a nociceptive 'driver' to their spinal dysfunction, manual therapy will effectively reduce pain. Mobilization, when performed in a position that is comfortable and allows movement into resistance towards the end of range, will evoke the appropriate afferent stimulus for immediate reduction in perception of nociceptive pain. Thus, treating in the opposite corner to a patient's dysfunction will be predominantly a neurophysiologically-mediated, pain-relieving treatment. Stretching non-severe movement dysfunction into the direction of movement loss will evoke similar neurophysiological mechanisms as well as mechanical effects on hypomobile tissue.

Manipulation techniques, inducing cavitation and stretching local muscles will give a temporary window of opportunity. In the hour post manipulation the motion segment will be more compliant to movement and have reduced local hypertonicity. It is in this window that more successful mobilization or motor control training will be achieved. The short-term reductions in pain and improvements in movement evoked by manipulation and mobilization are strong methods of educating patients about the specific mechanical faults they experience. It is important that the immediate effects experienced are related to the physiology and explained to the patient in order for them to be educated as to the importance of the patient's active participation in using the window of opportunity to self-manage the problem. Patients should be given the message that manual therapy is not in itself a cure; it is simply a specific way of dealing with specific mechanical dysfunctions.

Manual therapy is an excellent method of educating certain patients that their dysfunction is not dangerous and that with specific movement their function can be regained. Manual therapy can be viewed as a shortcut to educating suitable patients back to functional motor control.

## QUESTIONS

**1. At what point in range is the least force required to cause cavitation?**

A. Before resistance is perceived

B. At end of range of movement

**2. If the joint cavitates during your process of establishing the starting position for application of a manipulative thrust, what should you do next?**

A. Perform a thrust regardless

B. Reassess the resistance profile to see if the joint has cavitated

**3. What is the predominant mechanism for improvement in function following the application of passive movement in the quadrant opposite to the quadrant of dysfunction?**

A. Stimulation of mechanoreceptive afferents that induce descending pain inhibition

B. Stretch of the hypomobile tissue which is likely to be the source of the patient's nociceptive pain

**4. Which is the phenomenon that distinguishes manipulation from mobilization?**

A. Cavitation

B. Stimulation of the dPAG

C. Reduction in paraspinal hypertonicity

D. Increase in passive, segmental mobility

**5. According to the Maitland Grading system how would you notate the method of inducing cavitation suggested by the chapter above?**

A. Grade V thrust

B. Grade IV+ thrust

C. Grade IV thrust

D. Grade IV− thrust

E. Grade I+ thrust

F. Grade I thrust

**Answers: 1 A; 2 B; 3 A; 4 A; 5 D**

## References

Brennen, C.E., 1995. Cavitation and bubble dynamics. Oxford University Press, Oxford.

Chiu, T., Wright, A., 1996. To compare the effects of different rates of application of a cervical mobilisation technique on sympathetic outflow to the upper limb in normal subjects. Man. Ther. 1 (4), 198–203.

Colloca, C.J., Keller, T.S., 2001. Electromyographic reflex responses to mechanical force, manually assisted spinal manipulative therapy. Spine 26 (10), 1117–1124.

Conway, P.J., Herzog, W., Zhang, Y., et al., 1993. Forces required to cause cavitation during spinal manipulation of the thoracic spine. Clin. Biomech. 8, 210–214.

Cramer, G.D., Tuck, N.R. Jr, Knudsen, J.T., 2000. Effects of side posture positioning and side posture adjusting on the lumbar

zygapophysial joints as evaluated by magnetic resonance imaging: a before and after study with randomization. J. Manipulative Physiol. Ther. 23 (6), 380–394.

Cramer, G.D., Fournier, J.T., Henderson, C.N., et al., 2002. The effects of side posture positioning and spinal adjusting on the lumbar Z joints. Spine 27 (22), 2459–2466.

Dishman, J.D., Bulbulian, R., 2000. Spinal reflex attenuation associated with spinal manipulation. Spine 25 (19), 2519–2524 discussion 2525.

Evans, D.W., Breen, A.C., 2006. a biomechanical model for mechanically efficient cavitation production during spinal manipulation: prethrust position and the neutral zone. J. Manipulative Physiol. Ther. 29, 72–82.

Herzog, W., 2000. Clinical biomechanics of spinal manipulation. Churchill Livingstone, Philadelphia.

Lederman, E., 2005. The science and practice of manual therapy. Elsevier Health Sciences, London.

Lehman, G.J., McGill, S.M., 2001. Spinal manipulation causes variable spine kinematic and trunk muscle electromyographic responses. Clin. Biomech. 16 (4), 293–299.

McCarthy, C.J., Cairns, M., 2005. Editorial: Why is the recent research regarding non-specific pain so non-specific? Man. Ther. 4 (10), 239–241.

Maitland, G., 1986. Vertebral manipulation. Elsevier Health Sciences, Sydney.

Méal, G.M., Scott, R.A., 1986. Analysis of the joint crack by simultaneous recordings of the sound and tension. J. Manipulative Physiol. Ther. 9 (3), 189–195.

Melzack, R., Wall, P.D., 1965. Pain mechanisms: A new theory. Science 150 (3699), 971–979.

Perry, J., Green, A., 2008. An investigation into the effects of a unilaterally applied lumbar mobilisation technique on peripheral sympathetic nervous system activity in the lower limbs. Man. Ther. 13 (6), 492–499.

Petersen, N., Vincenzino, B., Wright, A., 1993. The effects of a cervical mobilisation technique on sympathetic outflow to the upper limb in normal subjects. Physiother. Theory Pract. 9 (3), 149–156.

Sandoz, R., 1976. Some physical mechanisms and effects of spinal adjustments. Ann. Swiss Chiro. Assoc. 6, 91–141.

Schaible, H.G., Schmidt, R.F., 1983. Activation of groups III and IV sensory units in medial articular nerve by local mechanical stimulation of the knee joint. J. Neurophysiol. 49, 35–44.

Slater, H., Vincenzino, B., Wright, A., 1994. Sympathetic slump: the effects of a novel manual therapy technique on peripheral sympathetic nervous system function. Journal of Manual and Manipulative Therapy 2 (4), 156–162.

Sterling, M., Jull, G., Wright, A., 2001. Cervical mobilisation: concurrent effects on pain, sympathetic nervous system activity and motor activity. Man. Ther. 6 (2), 72–81.

Threlkeld, A.J., 1992. The effects of manual therapy on connective tissue. Phys. Ther. 72 (12), 893–902.

Vincenzino, B., Collins, D., Wright, A., 1994. Sudomotor changes induced by neural mobilisation techniques in asymptomatic subjects. J. Manipulative Physiol. Ther. 2, 66–74.

Wright, A., 1995. Hypoalgesia post manipulative therapy: a review of a potential neurophysiological mechanism. Man. Ther. 1, 11–16.

Wyke, B., 1975. The neurology of the joints. Clin. Rheum. Dis. 7 (1), 223–239.

Zusman, M., 1986. Spinal manipulative therapy: Review of some proposed mechanisms and a new hypothesis. Austr. J. Physiother. 32 (2), 89–99.

Zusman, M., 1994. What does manipulation do? The need for basic research. In: Boyling, J., Palastanga, N. (eds.), Grieve's modern manual therapy. second ed. Churchill Livingstone, Edinburgh, pp. 651–660.

# Chapter Three

## The theory of clinical reasoning in combined movement therapy

3

Roger Kerry

### CHAPTER CONTENTS

## Introduction

This chapter introduces and discusses the clinical reasoning processes required to make the best decisions when assessing and managing patients with spinal pain syndromes. There is an increasing amount of attention given towards clinical reasoning in physiotherapy and manual therapy literature, which is an indication of the importance these processes can have on the progression of practice. The practical basis for considering clinical reasoning is simple: some clinicians get more people better, and quicker, than other clinicians. We call these people *experts*. These experts display characteristically different methods of assessing and managing patients than clinicians who do not have such high levels of success (Case *et al*, 2000; Doody & McAteer, 2003; James 2001; Jensen *et al*, 2000, 2007; King & Bithell, 1998; Resnik & Hart, 2003; Robertson, 1996; Roskell & Cross, 2001). The

cognitive differences recognized in clinical practice are supported by decades of work in the psychology of expertise (Chase & Simon, 1973; Craik & Lockart, 1972; DeGroot, 1965; DeGroot & Gobet, 1996; Gobet & Simon, 1998, 2000; Gobet & Wood, 1999; Neisser, 1998). It would therefore be advantageous for all of us to try and behave like experts. Expertise is not simply proficiency in the physical application of technical skills. Of course, this excellence in technique is of vital importance in treating patients with a combined movement approach, but it is equally important to know precisely *when*, *how*, and with *which* patients to apply these techniques. This knowing, or cognitive level of the clinical process can be what we mean when we say 'clinical reasoning'. Thus, it is the balance of thought and technique that produce excellence in practice:

> Manual skills are the hallmark of the therapy clinician;
> combining the intellectual process of clinical
> reasoning and manual dexterity
>
> (Singer, 2000)

Clinical reasoning has been defined as the cognitive process that incorporates thinking skills and knowledge (facts, procedures, concepts, principles and patterns) used to make clinical decisions and judgements through the evaluation, diagnosis and management of a patient problem (Jones, 1994). Models and definitions largely based on descriptions of clinical reasoning in medicine (Barrows & Feltovitch, 1987; Elstein *et al*, 1978; Feltovitch & Barrows, 1984; Groen & Patel, 1985) have been utilized and adapted to the physiotherapy process in a number of texts, e.g. Higgs & Jones (2000) and Jones (1994, 1995, 1997a, 1997b, 1997c). Additionally, alternative reasoning approaches to medicine-based modelling have been proposed from within the therapy professions, e.g. Bradnam (2002), Edwards *et al* (2006), Edwards *et al* (2004), Gifford (1998), Jette *et al* (2003), Ladyshewsky (2002), Rothstein *et al* (2003) and Steiner *et al* (2002). These authors, among many others authors, state quite convincingly that a meaningful appreciation of the cognitive processes underlying our decision-making is critical to the quality of our practice. This appreciation can, however, be difficult due to the complexity and unfamiliarity of the literature (Kempanien *et al*, 2003). With this in mind, this chapter attempts to discuss the complexities of clinical reasoning in a practical, meaningful and context-related way in relation to combined movement therapy (CMT).

In order for us to understand what makes for good clinical reasoning, let us put ourselves on the other side of the process and at the mercy of the 'reasoner'. Imagine you are driving your car when you suddenly hear a rattle and clunking sound and then feel a juddering sensation through the steering wheel. You quite wisely pull onto the hard-shoulder and call for roadside assistance, explaining to the phone operator what has happened. The scenario has two alternative endings – one as a result of Mechanic A attending, and the other as a result of Mechanic B attending.

### Mechanic A scenario
* *Diagnosis* – a broken steering column
* *Outcome* – the car is towed to garage where the diagnosis is confirmed. The car is repaired. You drive trouble-free for the next 3 years and then you change your car.

### Mechanic B scenario
* *Diagnosis* – a dirty fuel tank
* *Outcome* – you are advised to add injector cleaner to the full tank of fuel and drive fast at high revs to clean out the system, which you do. You then crash because the steering column was broken.

It is clear that in this case, Mechanic A made the better decisions. Let us see what each mechanic has to say about their actions.

### Mechanic A's experience
I have 10 years roadside experience and work for a large, national roadside assistance organization for which I receive a salary and performance bonuses based on quality of work and maintaining and updating my skills. When I got the call for this car, I had a number of

thoughts about what could be wrong. These are fairly common descriptions of various mechanical problems ranging from oil and fuel problems to damage to mechanical structures of the engine, steering column, chassis, or wheels. When I arrived on the scene, the age of the vehicle (10 years old), type (estate), and state (used) made me think that I should consider the fact that something could well be mechanically broken. The guy reported a type of juddering that I have only come across a few times, but it sounded different to the more gentle shuddering which people with fuel problems tend to report. Considering this, and also the consequences of continuing driving if there was mechanical damage, I thought I would check out the most accessible possible structure – the steering column – first. There seemed to be an awful lot of play in it which indicated to me that it was quite likely broken in its shaft. The only way to really know this though is to strip the platform and have a good old look. There was no way this guy was driving the car so I got him towed to the garage. I rang the garage a week later to complete my log book and they said it was fixed now.

### Mechanic B's experience
I've got 10 years experience as a mechanic and I work with my mate. We do all sorts really – servicing, repairs, bit of body work. Work can be good, but you do get slack periods. Roadsides can be good work – quick and pricy! Sounded like this bloke was having some fuel problems. You get this all the time – I've seen this loads. People running on nearly empty, trying to get the most out of their tank. You're supposed to add an injection cleaner every few tank fills, but nobody ever does – I carry a load of bottles around with me in the van – get everyone to buy some. Anyway, typical, this guy's driving along, shuddering starts, panics, pulls over, rings me – good job as well! I'd got him sorted in 5 minutes – £70 and a bottle of injection cleaner. –Not heard from him since – job done!

Based on the above two accounts, we can consider the following questions:
* Is there a difference in experience between Mechanic A and Mechanic B?
* Is there a difference in knowledge of cars between Mechanic A and Mechanic B?
* Is there a difference in the way that each mechanic inquired about what had happened on the motorway?
* Is there a difference in the way in which each mechanic inspected your car?
* Is there a difference in the way each mechanic interpreted the information gained from the two points above?
* Is there a motivational difference between the two mechanics?

Their areas of inquiry are quite logical, and they may be the sort of questions you would instinctively want to ask – particularly if you had been unfortunate enough to have the experience of being assisted by Mechanic B! As well as being instinctive and logical, they also reflect a number of core principles of clinical reasoning. The similarity between the above scenario and clinical reasoning in manual therapy is not, however, due to chance – clinical reasoning is quite simply based in logic. It is made up of the sort of things that we naturally want to ask about when trying to work out what is happening in a given situation. Clinical reasoning has been meaningfully linked to, and often referred to as, 'wise' action (Butler, 2000). In the above scenario then, which mechanic displayed the wisest actions? The answer in this case is straightforward. It is now a matter of what constitutes this wise action and where this 'wisdom' comes from.

As stated already, the points above – asking about differences between the two mechanics – reflect an understanding of the underpinning principles of clinical reasoning. Higgs & Jones (2000) present a well-recognized and oft-quoted framework of clinical reasoning which we can use as a basis for considering how the clinical reasoning process can be harnessed in CMT. Figure 3.1 illustrates this framework.

The core components of the client's input, environment, clinical problem, knowledge, cognition, and metacognition are inter-dependent and each factor is influenced and enriched by a variety of considerations. These components represent the foundation of the reasoning process, i.e. the parts of our interactive thought process required to produce sound reasoning. It is obvious, however, that within this framework there is still scope for varying degrees of reasoning quality. When analyzing a situation for the quality of the reasoning process, it is helpful to keep this framework in mind as a structure in which to set about the analysis.

This chapter continues with attention to the various models and processes of clinical reasoning, the use of which determines the nature and quality of an individual's reasoning. The intention of this chapter is not to provide a comprehensive analysis of clinical reasoning in its entirety – the reader is instead referred throughout this chapter to existing texts which already do this. Rather, an overview of contemporary thought in clinical reasoning and its relevance to combined movement and manual therapy is provided. A simple case study is used throughout as a vehicle to highlight the different aspects of clinical reasoning.

## Stages of reasoning in combined movement theory

Within the following analysis we can see how different models, or strategies, of reasoning can be utilized to facilitate making the best decisions at different points within the assessment and management process. The reasoning process has been broken down into stages to represent, in chronological order, the different decision-making challenges that the manual therapist is faced with during the assessment and management of a patient with spinal pain. Although artificial in as much as these decision-making mechanisms often invariably run in parallel and are in reality inseparable, this is a useful way of analyzing the flowing process to explore contemporary thought on clinical reasoning. The following stages of decision-making are presented and examined in turn:

• Early differential diagnosis (pattern recognition)
• Decision-making during the history-taking: what questions to ask and why (hypothetico-deductive reasoning)
• What do we know and how do we know it (the theory of knowledge)?

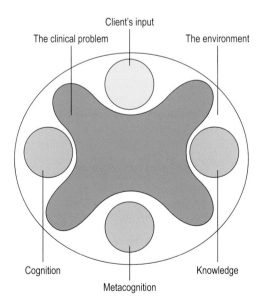

Client's input
The clinical problem
The environment
Cognition
Knowledge
Metacognition

**Figure 3.1** • Client-centred clinical reasoning. This framework represents the core components and the interactive thought process required for good reasoning. (Higgs & Jones, 2000)

- Diagnostic testing (probability theory)
- Treatment decisions (interpretive reasoning).

## Stage 1: Pattern recognition

Below is a piece of information from our case example of a patient with spinal pain who has sought treatment from the manual therapist. Further information will be revealed as we pass through the assessment chronologically.

> 38-year-old male complaining of left-sided mid to upper cervical pain and headache.

This is the first piece of information obtained. It may be written on your referral note for example. Research has demonstrated that expert practitioners begin the cognitive process of solving the problem from a very early stage of assessment and are able to recognize clinical *patterns* even at this early point (Barrows & Feltovitch, 1987; Jensen *et al* 2000; King & Bithell, 1998; Schon, 1991). The information above might not be much to go on, but it is arguably enough for the expert clinician to start to organize their thoughts and knowledge in order to make the next few minutes of the assessment more efficient and productive. Efficient organization of knowledge is a trait associated with expert practice (Rivett & Jones, 2004).

The brief information given above includes:

- Gender of patient
- Age of patient
- Site of pain.

With this information, it is possible to begin organization of knowledge into potentially meaningful patterns in relation to what the cause of the problem could be, for example:

- Benign, neuromusculoskeletal (NMS)
- Cervicogenic headache and local somatic neck pain
- Possible structural causes, e.g. facet joint, peri-articular structures, local muscular causes, disc
- Inflammatory or degenerative disease
- Intracranial space occupying lesion (tumour)
- Intracranial vascular dysfunction (aneurysm, haemorrhage)
- Extracranial space-occupying lesion (tumour; arterial aneurysm)
- Non-neuromusculoskeletal tissue trauma (arterial dissection)

- Spinal cord/meningeal involvement
- Infection
- Upper cervical instability.

Of course, it is far too early to exclude or further support the majority of the above possibilities, but two cognitive processes may take place:

1. The patterns are now 'set up' in the clinician's mind ready and waiting to be *tested*
2. The patterns may be *prioritized*, or at least the beginnings of the prioritization process may be in sight.

The second point relates to the clinician's judgement of which of the above possibilities (patterns) are *most likely* and which are *least likely* to be the cause of the problem, given the information at hand. Detailed attention is given to this concept of probability later in the chapter, but for now, the clinician's mind should be considering prioritization. In this case, the clinician might think: 'I have experience of many male patients in this age group with unilateral pain such as this, and in my experience, most turn out to be treatable, benign NMS conditions, not many in this age group have had inflammatory or degenerative disease, and very rarely has this presentation been something serious'. Therefore, based on this clinician's *experience*, the diagnosis is *more likely* to be a treatable NMS condition, and *least likely* (but not impossible) to be serious pathology or a red flag. The above is an example of how, at this stage, clinicians rely predominantly on their own experiences and observation to formulate potentially meaningful patterns (Elstein & Schwarz, 2000; Jones, 1999). Thus, the pattern recognition model of reasoning is reliant on experience (Simon, 1980). The value of this early recognition of patterns is predominantly the fact that it makes the process of 'diagnosing' quick and efficient. However, there are a few caveats with placing too much value and reliance on this model that should be considered before we proceed:

### Clinical relevance

- Pattern recognition is the domain of the expert practitioner and we are not all expert practitioners!
- Although it is reliant on experience, experience alone is not the sole basis for good pattern recognition.
- There is significant potential for error in this reasoning process.
- The logical basis of this model is fundamentally flawed.

The first point in the box above speaks for itself! We shall, therefore, pick up on the last three points.

## Experience

Cognitive psychologists have suggested that it takes 10 years experience to become 'expert' in a discipline (Gobet & Wood, 1999). However, as others have pointed out (Rivett & Jones, 2004), simply gaining experience (as measured in time) is not enough. In order to display true proficiency, there must be other factors influencing the clinician's development:

> ... there are clinicians who have had 20 years experience in 20 years of clinical practice, there are others who have 20 years of experience in one year of clinical practice. The latter has reasoned, learned, experimented with management techniques, remained open, been aware of the outcomes movement, and has read widely
>
> (Butler, 2000, p. 139)

The differentiator in terms of whether a clinician progresses to expertise or not is therefore multi-factorial and not a simple matter of accumulating 'patient mileage' – it is what is *done* with that experience that counts. It is important therefore, that clinicians engage in a framework of reasoning and reflective practice at all stages of their career progression.

Using clinical experience and prior observation is prone to bias. This will be discussed in a psychological context below. However, on a very practical basis, it is important to consider that experiential observation can be influenced by biases of natural recovery, statistical regression, politeness of patients, placebo response and recall (Herbert, 2005).

## Error

Some authors have highlighted the potential for error in the reasoning process (Rivett & Jones, 2004; Scott, 2000). The patterns that are recognized in this first stage will, in the majority of situations, later develop (generate) into testable hypotheses and it is this collection of hypotheses which will form the shape of the remaining assessment and examination process. Therefore, the whole diagnostic and decision-making procedure is reliant on the quality and accuracy of these early patterns. In respect of early pattern recognition, potential errors may take the form of developing the wrong initial concept of the problem; over-emphasis on favoured hypotheses, misinterpreting early information, making assumptions (this

should be carefully considered as being very different to pattern recognition), considering too few (narrow range of) patterns (or hypotheses), making hypotheses too vague, and failing to detect early cues for serious pathology. There is equal potential for reasoning errors throughout the whole assessment procedure, but it is problems within the hypothesis generation stage that will misdirect the subsequent procedure. Hence utmost attention should be given to the potential for error at this stage.

The concept of error in pattern recognition is paradoxical: pattern recognition relies on experience yet it is that very experience which is the most likely cause of error in pattern recognition. Common errors, as stated above, include narrowness of hypotheses, misinterpreting information, and failure to recognize early signs of serious pathology. These errors are *products* of experience which have not been subject to the scrutiny of careful thought (cognition), reflection, critical analysis or self-monitoring (metacognition). In the absence of careful cognitive and metacognitive processing, external (to the clinician) experience may be internally (to the clinician) mis-interpreted. This is the psychological phenomenon of *perception*. The interpretation of any experience is subjective and specific to the individual. All external experiences are filtered through our own, personal *schemata*, which is itself developed by experiences. Thus, if we have psychological schemata which are built of aberrant/limited/biased interpretations of *previous* experiences, all *future* experiences are going to be interpreted within these skewed schemata. A good way of demonstrating this concept is with the use of an optical illusion (Fig. 3.2).

The image in Figure 3.2 has two interpretations: (1) an old woman and (2) a young girl. Now that you know this information, you should be able to see both interpretations (although some will still find this harder than others). However, if you did not know that there are two interpretations, you will probably only see one and be satisfied that this is a nice picture of *either* an old woman *or* a young girl. Each subsequent time you see the picture, you will automatically interpret the image you are familiar with, because your personal schemata has been 'set up' with this first experience. Additionally, each subsequent time that you see the image, your interpretation of whatever that early experience was will be reinforced. Therefore, you could coast through life *believing* that this picture has only a single interpretation and this belief would

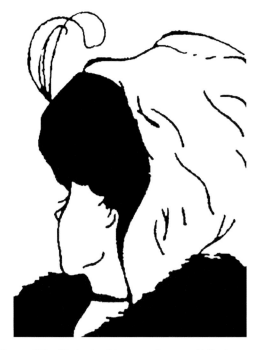

**Figure 3.2** • Boring's old woman/young girl illusion as adapted by cartoonist W. E. Hill in 1915. This classic pictographic illusion is an example of the problems associated with individual perception. (Source: http://www. grand-illusions.com/woman.htm)

continue to get stronger and stronger, eventually becoming almost impossible to break away from. However, the critical reasoner would want to question their early experience of interpreting the picture. In this case, you could perhaps spend longer examining the image to see for yourself if there really was another interpretation. Or you could spend time thinking about whether there at least *could* be an alternative. Or you could challenge your own perception of the image and re-examine it. Or you could ask another viewer if they see the same thing as you. Better still, ask a number of other viewers to see what their interpretations are – the more viewers you ask, the more likely it would be that you would come across someone who has seen the alternative interpretation, thereby challenging your belief. These later activities are part of the cognitive/metacognitive process associated with good reasoning and are more likely to reveal something closer to reality than just accepting the first interpretation. The continual inclusion of the reflective cognition/metacognition process is imperative in determining the quality of pattern recognition and hypothesis generation.

## Clinical relevance

Pattern recognition has been recognized for its many values, e.g. efficiency in dealing with a problem quickly without the need to clarify and re-check, efficiency in dealing with uncertainty, imprecise data, or limited premises (Albert *et al*, 1988). However, effective and efficient pattern recognition is reliant on the following three conditions being met:

1. You are an expert
2. The clinical problem is not complex
3. You are very familiar with the clinical problem.

If all three of these conditions are not in place, the process is prone to error (as discussed above) and the limitations of the logical basis of pattern recognition are exposed. The logical basis of pattern recognition is known as *induction*. Hence, pattern recognition is also referred to as 'inductive reasoning' (Higgs & Jones, 2000, p. 6). The basis of induction is one of making inferences about something from prior experience or observation(s) of a similar event. For example, I have switched my kettle on 200 times and it has never exploded, therefore I affirm that when I switch it on now (the 201st time), it will again not explode. This seems quite a reasonable assumption, and this logical process is largely what drives us to make all sorts of decisions and choices on a daily basis throughout our lives. However, there is a strong philosophical argument which challenges reliance on inductive reasoning and questions its logical basis. Consider the following inference:

**Premise A:** I have seen 20 patients this week whose headache was caused by upper cervical facet dysfunction.

**Premise B:** Upper cervical facet dysfunction causes headaches.

**Conclusion:** My next (21st) patient that I see with headache will have upper cervical facet dysfunction as the cause.

This is a simple logical inference of which the third statement (conclusion) is a product of the first two statements (premises A and B). It is an example of inductive reasoning. However, its logic is fundamentally flawed: despite the fact that both premises A and B are true, it does not necessarily follow that the conclusion drawn is also true, i.e. even if upper cervical dysfunction can produce headache and all the previous 20 patients had cervicogenic headache, it does not guarantee that the 21st, or indeed any future, patient will also have cervicogenic headache – for we know that there are many other causes of headache.

A counter-argument in support of induction logic is often made using the concept of probability to strengthen the assertion that the conclusion is a reliable product of the premise. For example, we might think: 'well, surely the more times I observe something, then the *more likely* it is that the subsequent event can be predicted based on my observations', i.e. likelihood is directly proportionate to number of times observed. Clinically, this could be reflected as: 'actually, I have been practising for 20 years and I have seen 3000 patients who have presented with this type of headache and it has always been caused by upper cervical dysfunction. Surely, with this number of experiences, it is *very likely* that future patients will have upper cervical facet dysfunction?'

Even if we ignore the errors of perception and experience as discussed above, and if it *is* true that *all* the 3000 previous patients had upper cervical facet dysfunction, the assertion that future similar patients will have the same cause is still flawed. The attempt at using probability ('the more I have seen, the *more likely* it is that I can predict future events) does not strengthen the case for inductive logic. Let us explore the logical basis a little further. Essentially, with induction we are stating a *general law* (e.g. all headache of this type is cervicogenic) from *particular observations* (e.g. *I* have observed a number of individual occurrences of cervicogenic headache) with the implication that the general law is true (e.g. it is true that this type of headache is cervicogenic). The general law transcends the individual; in other words the statement we are making is intended to be applied to *all* headaches of this type – in the past, the present, and the future, and in the whole world. The simple way in which this logic fails is, of course, by the single discovery that, in the past (by someone else), in the present (by anyone), in the future (by anyone), anywhere in the world, this type of headache is not cervicogenic. In an attempt to counteract this flaw, induction dictates that we should aim to make statements (general laws) with *maximal probability*. So, rather than stating that 'all headaches of this type are cervicogenic' which possesses the above probability flaw, we should say 'either this type of headache is cervicogenic or it is not', or 'headaches are caused by a number of things', i.e. these statements have *maximized* the *probability* of the law being true. Of course, these statements *are* true,

but have *minimal informative content*, i.e. they do not actually tell us anything informative about understanding the nature of the headache. This is analogous to saying 'it will either rain or it will not'. This is true, but it does not help me decide whether to wear my raincoat or not. Thus, the unquestioned accumulation of personal experience to inform future decisions should be judged with great caution in the intellectual clinical reasoning approach.

Consideration of the problems of induction is nothing new. The argument against inductivism was highlighted in the work of an eminent 20th century philosopher called Karl Popper. His claim was that adherence to an inductivist approach is erroneous and limited and that in order for a more accurate approximation to what is correct to be made, a *deductive* approach should be taken (Popper, 1980). Luckily, for us manual therapists, this has already been given some thought and forms the next stage in our reasoning process.

## Stage 2: Hypothetico-deductive reasoning

Now that patterns have been recognized, the clinician has two choices:

1. Accept the most likely pattern as the diagnosis and begin treatment
2. Use these patterns to generate a number of hypotheses which can then be tested for their validity.

Option one would be an extreme form of expert practice and is totally reliant on the pattern recognition model. As stated above, this can be very quick and efficient. However, also as stated above, it will only work if certain conditions are met, and the model is prone to error and logical limitation. Therefore, for most people at most times, option two would be the most reasonable option. For the clinical reasoner, the rest of the history-taking is not a random, or even pre-structured, list of questions but a reasoned, hypothesis-driven process of inquiry. This process is referred to as a hypothetico-deductive model of reasoning, and is written about extensively in both general clinical reasoning (e.g. Barrows & Tamblyn, 1980; Elstein *et al*, 1978) and manual therapy specific clinical reasoning literature (e.g. Higgs & Jones, 1995; Jones, 1995; Rivett & Jones, 2004). The hypothetico-deductive model describes a process of data collection, hypothesis generation, interpretation and hypothesis testing. As stated earlier, in reality, a combination of various reasoning models will be operationalized, e.g. simply because we have now stated that the predominant process has evolved to a hypothetico-deductive structure does not mean that future patterns will not be recognized, and subsequently tested as hypotheses, and so on. However, for clarity, at this point we shall focus our attention on hypothetico-deductive reasoning.

It was suggested above that superior, efficient organization of knowledge was a cognitive ability commonly attributed to the expert practitioner. This process can be clearly demonstrated at this stage of the assessment process. A natural cognitive link between the early *recognition* of patterns and the subsequent *testing* of those patterns is the organization, or *encapsulation*, of the clinician's existing knowledge in the form of 'packaged' lists of characteristics/information regarding what actually constitutes each pattern. These packages of pattern-specific information have been referred to as 'illness scripts' (Feltovich & Barrows, 1984). More recent work has identified this theoretical notion as an integral component of efficient reasoning (Boshuizen & Schmidt, 2000; Rivett & Jones, 2004; Sefton *et al*, 2000). Figure 3.3 demonstrates the temporal operationalization between the early recognition of patterns, the instantaneous formulation of illness scripts, and the subsequent guiding of hypothesis-driven questioning.

In the middle box representing the illness script in Figure 3.3, you will notice that the 'script' is separated into three distinct components, i.e. potential diagnosis A is conditional of (1) there being a specific type of trauma, (2) that specific tissues have been affected, and (3) that the manifestation of (1) and (2) are a specific set of signs and symptoms. Boshuizen and Schmidt (2000) refer to these three components as:

**1.** The enabling condition
**2.** The fault
**3.** The consequences of the fault.

The *enabling conditions* are the conditions under which the problem/disease may occur, and considers such information as social history, hereditary conditioning, medical or environmental background, etc. The *fault* refers to the actual pathophysiological process taking place for this problem/disease. The *consequences of the fault* are therefore those clinically observable signs and symptoms considered to be associated with the specific problem/disease. For our case

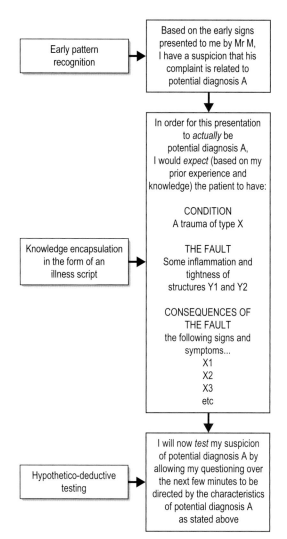

**Figure 3.3** • Example of the chronological thought process associated with the transition from early pattern recognition, illness script recall, and hypothesis driven questioning.

study we can construct examples of possible illness scripts which may be associated with the patterns recognized early on for our 38-year-old male with neck and head pain. Table 3.1 shows three patterns (for illustrative purposes, only three patterns have been used in this example – of course, it is probable that, in reality, there would be more than three potential diagnoses) and the associated illness scripts which *could* be potential diagnoses for this patient.

The clinician's structuring and prioritization of questioning within this part of the assessment procedure is now directly governed by consideration of

**Table 3.1  Example of three patterns and associated illness scripts related to the case study of upper cervical neck pain and headache**

| | Patterns | | |
|---|---|---|---|
| | **Treatable** | **Non-treatable (with manual therapy)** | |
| | *Cervicogenic neck pain and headache (upper cervical spine motion segment dysfunction)* | *Cervical arterial dysfunction* | *Upper cervical instability* |
| **Illness scripts** | | | |
| **Enabling conditions** | History of mild to moderate trauma<br>History of sustained postural activities<br>History of repeated aberrant movement patterns<br>Poor sleeping postures | History of moderate to severe trauma, or repeated trauma<br>Atherosclerotic risk factors (including family history) | History of moderate to severe trauma<br>Underlying congenital syndrome (e.g. Down's, Marfan's, Ehlers-Danlos)<br>Inflammatory disease (e.g. rheumatoid arthritis) |
| **The fault** | Specific motion segment dysfunction (affecting articular/peri-articular structures of upper cervical facet joints)<br>Associated muscular response (tightness, inactivity) | Possible intimal dissection event in vertebral or internal carotid arterial vessels<br>Traumatic (haemodynamic) localized atherosclerotic plaque development<br>Genetically compromised endothelial status/fibrodysplasia | Loss of integrity of specific upper cervical ligamentous structures<br>Excessive posterior translation of the dens articularis<br>Possible impingement of the spinal cord |
| **Consequences of the fault** | Pain consistently related to specific movements/directions/combinations of functional movement<br>Clinically identified movement pattern associated with segmental dysfunction<br>Clinically identified muscular irregularity | Atypical head/neck pain<br>Cranial nerve palsies<br>Partial Horner's syndrome<br>Symptoms of hind-brain ischaemia<br>Hypertension | Inability to maintain prolonged postures<br>Need to support head<br>Specific peri-oral/intra-oral neurological symptomology<br>Specific non-dermatomal distal limb sensation changes<br>Possible clinically identified increased upper cervical joint motion |

these factors. Hence, hypotheses are generated and then tested for their validity by specific, hypothesis-driven interrogation – thus the hypothetico-deductive process evolves. This 'testing' procedure derives its logic from, as the name of this model suggests, deduction. Unlike the inductivist logic of pattern recognition, this logical form is considered in many ways to be a more robust process of inquiry. However, compared to a true pattern recognition dominant approach, it is arguably a more time-consuming and thus less efficient model. The 'robustness' of deductive reasoning can also be examined in a philosophical context. The following logical progression is an example of deductive logic:

**Premise A:** all treatable cervicogenic headache and neck pain is differentially characterized by features X, Y and Z (as encapsulated in the specific illness script).

**Premise B:** Mr M has features X, Y, and Z.

**Conclusion:** Mr M has treatable cervicogenic headache and neck pain.

Unlike inductive inference, deductive logic dictates that if premises A and B are true, then the conclusion must also be true. In other words if it *is* true that features X, Y, and Z are differentially characteristic of cervicogenic headache and neck pain, and if it *is* true that Mr M demonstrates these precise features, then it follows that Mr M has cervicogenic headache and neck pain. Thus the premises entail the conclusion. Clinically, we can harness and exploit this process to take us closer to what the actual problem might be. The process is effectively a test of strength, and only the strongest hypotheses (i.e. those that survive the directed and rigorous questioning) will make it to the next stage of assessment – the physical examination. In reality, it is likely that only in the most straightforward of situations, only one surviving hypothesis will be considered for testing in the physical examination. Most commonly, there will still be a number of competing hypotheses to refute during the physical examination – hence the hypothetico-deductive model continues. Additionally, with one primary hypotheses (e.g. upper cervical motion segment dysfunction) there will be a number of secondary hypotheses (e.g. left-sided C1 on C2 posterior-anterior hypermobility relating to a regular movement pattern X versus C2 on C3 anterior-posterior hypermobility; alternative hypotheses regarding the SIN status of the patient's condition) contending for survival.

Although the logic of this inference is philosophically robust, it is obvious that the 'truthfulness' of the conclusion is dependent on the 'truthfulness' of both premises. This 'truthfulness' is a different matter altogether and is dependent on the *quality of the knowledge sources* from which the clinician has (a) constructed the illness script, and (b) assessed the patient. Thus, *knowledge* and its integration into the reasoning process must also be explored.

## Stage 3: What do we know and how do we know it? Knowledge

Knowledge is a key component in the framework of clinical reasoning (see Fig. 3.1). As stated above, the validity of the deductive logical inference is dependent on the quality of knowledge which supports its premises. If our reasoning is reliant on our knowledge, we must consider the *nature* and *quality* of our knowledge, and question where it comes from.

If you were a patient concerned with receiving the best care, what would your reaction be if, following you asking your therapist what he thinks is wrong with you and how he knew that his diagnosis was as accurate as possible, the reply was something along the lines of: 'Your pain is caused by evil spirits possessing your upper cervical spine and I know this because I went on a course by a Mongolian shaman and he said that this is what causes neck pain'. I suspect (and hope!) that you would immediately question the logic of this knowledge. If so, you would come to the conclusions that:

- The type of knowledge (i.e. pain related to upper cervical evil spirits) is not valid
- The source of this knowledge (i.e. knowledge acquired from the shaman) is also not valid.

It may be the case that if you were in some other period of history, or another part of the world, you would accept this type of explanation. However, in our modern, thoughtful, and accountable society, this kind of justification for decisions involving other people is neither substantiated nor acceptable. We therefore need to consider what types and what sources of knowledge are considered substantiated and acceptable. Uncomfortably, this area of study is akin to having that annoying, pedantic companion who continually retorts to everything you say with the question 'but *how* do you know that'! However, as responsible reasoners we must be happy to go through this process.

Let us continue with our clinical scenario: to summarize at this point, we have established the following details:

- *Age of patient:* 38
- *Gender:* male
- *Pain site:* left-sided mid to upper cervical pain and parietal headache
- *Possible causes:* for our selected examples – the three hypotheses in Table 3.1.

Embedded within this summary are a number of 'facts', the source of which can be subjected to scrutiny. The first two summary points (age and gender of patient) are fairly robust statements based on reliable and valid knowledge sources, i.e. date of birth (verified by birth certificate if needed), and chromosomal and physical characteristics of being male (verified by DNA analysis and physical examination if needed). The third point (pain site), is reliant upon the patient's report (to which we shall return below). It is the fourth point however, which is of most interest to us as this opens up a variety of knowledge, and therefore reasoning issues, which may directly influence the accuracy of our clinical decisions, i.e. if our knowledge is not correct, then our subsequent clinical decision may not be correct.

Table 3.1 suggests a number of characteristics (in the form of illness scripts) suggestive of each proposed hypothesis. We can now question the quality of this information and examine *where* this information comes from, i.e. *how* do we know that characteristics X, Y, Z equate to diagnosis A.

The formal theoretical study of knowledge is called *epistemology*. The substantial, underpinning detail of this branch of philosophy is beyond the scope of both this book, and, I imagine, the desire of many readers to go into in any great detail! However, it is quite accurate to say that we are all now undertaking an *epistemological review* of our clinical practice.

## Types of knowledge

Types, or forms, of knowledge have been discussed and presented in a number of therapy-specific texts and publications, e.g. Higgs *et al* (2004), Higgs and Titchen (2000), Jones (1995), Resnik and Hart (2003), Resnik and Jensen (2003) and Swisher (2002). Classically, types of knowledge have been sub-divided into the categories which are shown in Figure 3.4.

The interested reader is referred to Higgs and Titchen (2000) and Higgs *et al* (2004) for detailed information regarding this classification. In summary, propositional knowledge is knowledge about propositions! Propositions are the assertion that something is the case, e.g. the sun is the centre of our universe. In manual therapy, propositional knowledge refers to theoretical or scientific knowledge derived through scientific study and accessed through publicly available information sources such as peer-reviewed journal articles and books. Thus propositional knowledge is *know-that* knowledge. Professional craft knowledge

is that which relates to actual practice skills, information, and competencies required of clinicians and is acquired through experience and is often tacit or 'sub-conscious'. Personal knowledge is similarly gained through social (clinical) experiences but refers to that reflective, more conscious component of practice which forms our individualized frames of references, values and beliefs. Professional craft knowledge could, for example, include the manual skill needed to assess upper cervical passive physiological movement dysfunction as learnt on a post-graduate course and practised over a period of time. Personal knowledge, however, would be that independent, unique appreciation of what 'stiffness' actually feels like, or where 'resistance' begins, etc. Professional and personal knowledge are forms of 'non-propositional' knowledge and are related to *ability*, i.e. I am *able* to accurately assess resistance on this regular combined movement pattern and am *able* to make judgement on the degree of stiffness. Thus, these types of knowledge are often referred to as *know-how* knowledge.

The importance of attempting to understand types of knowledge is to make a judgement, as inferred above, on the *quality* of that knowledge. An expert practitioner will not only have more knowledge, but will utilize *different* knowledge types (compared to a novice), in turn from a variety of logically valid sources (Boshuizen & Schmidt, 2000; Gobet, 1998; Gobet & Wood, 1999; Jensen *et al*, 2000; King & Bithell, 1998).

## Sources of knowledge

### Personal experience

As stated, non-propositional sources rely on experience. Earlier in the chapter, we considered the limitations of individual experience as the dominant basis for reasoning. Therefore, significant reliance on personal experience can be erroneous in the reasoning process and it has been demonstrated in study that experience alone is not enough to form the basis of expert practice (e.g. King & Bithell, 1998). However, there are strong arguments for continued attention towards the importance of non-propositional knowledge in clinical reasoning (Higgs *et al*, 2004; Higgs & Titchen, 2000). The mechanism for ensuring that perception of personal experience is not distorted and misinterpreted is to devise mechanisms of continual *reflection* of practice. This is, of course, the advantage that personal knowledge has over professional craft knowledge.

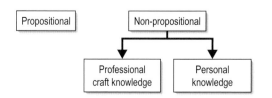

**Figure 3.4** • Types of knowledge. Propositional *know-that* knowledge and non-propositional *know-how* knowledge.

Without this component of reflection, experience is arguably the simple collection of data which is then used to inform the next judgement and as such is prone to the logical limitations of inductive logic. Reflective practice, therefore, should be considered the backbone to the reasoning process, and the interested reader is directed to the work of Donald Schon (1991) for further detail regarding reflective practice.

## Research

The word 'research' is used here to refer to the many methods that are capable of generating information and that are considered logically robust enough to be accepted (philosophically) valid sources of knowledge. To be consistent with previous therapy literature in this area (especially Higgs & Titchen, 2000), the term 'paradigm' (meaning a framework characterizing the nature of the research activity) is used, as is the categorization system shown in Figure 3.5.

Knowledge derived from the three research paradigms in Figure 3.5 contributes to that category of knowledge we now understand as propositional knowledge, although there is inevitable overlap and diffusion of information into non-propositional knowledge types. The main purpose of referring to this system of source categorization here is to highlight the variety of research activities which are capable of producing philosophically valid information.

The empirico-analytical paradigm refers to the predominantly experimental activity of reductionist, medical-model science. We have considered above the logical strengths of experimentation, i.e deductive logic. Although this was considered in the context of the independent reasoning process (i.e. utilization of the hypothetico-deductive model during clinical assessment), conceptually the argument is the same in the wider world of public research activity. Indeed, some would suggest that

due to its logical strengths, experimentation is the only valid source of knowledge!

> The test of all knowledge is experiment. Experiment is the sole judge of scientific 'truth'
>
> (Feynman, 1995, p. 2)

The use of experiment in the health sciences has, however, been under much debate and discussion (e.g. Bouter *et al*, 1998; Robertson, 1996). It has been proposed that within the health sciences, relying on knowledge generated within the reductionist experimental paradigm (in particular, experiment in the form of controlled trials) will result in the exclusion of equally valid knowledge sources which may actually be more meaningful to our practice. Furthermore, some authors have suggested that perhaps the nature of healthcare practice lends itself better to methods of inquiry other than experimental designs (e.g. Parry, 1997; Richardson, 1993). Without going into full discussion here, it is suggested that to dismiss the experimental approach would be short-sighted and destructive to the profession's knowledge base. However, there are also a number of other methods which have sound utility. These fall under the categories of the interpretive paradigm, and the critical paradigm.

The interpretive paradigm refers to investigation which, rather than searching for a cause–effect relationship, seeks to understand social phenomena in a meaningful context through the interpretation of, for example, structured observation of behaviour within that social situation. Although it is not entirely accurate to attribute this activity to the more commonly recognized 'qualitative' category of research, some of the methodologies, such as interviews, questionnaires, etc, are familiar designs within this paradigm. Knowledge underpinning contemporary thought on the bio-psychosocial aspects of pain or the relationship between physiotherapy practice and evidence is an example of knowledge derived from this paradigm.

The critical paradigm is, as the title suggests, centred on critical debate. As a source of knowledge, this is considered valuable, valid, and important (Higgs & Titchen, 2000). Knowledge referred to as *emancipatory knowledge* is the product of this activity. This knowledge can facilitate the clinician from 'freeing' themselves from existing thoughts and beliefs by *understanding* how these thoughts and beliefs are socially and historically constructed and how these structures themselves can limit change and progression (Schnelker, 2006).

With the above information in mind, it is now possible to return to our illness scripts, analyze the

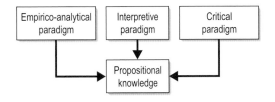

**Figure 3.5** • Sources of knowledge. Examples of research paradigms that contribute to propositional knowledge in the health sciences.

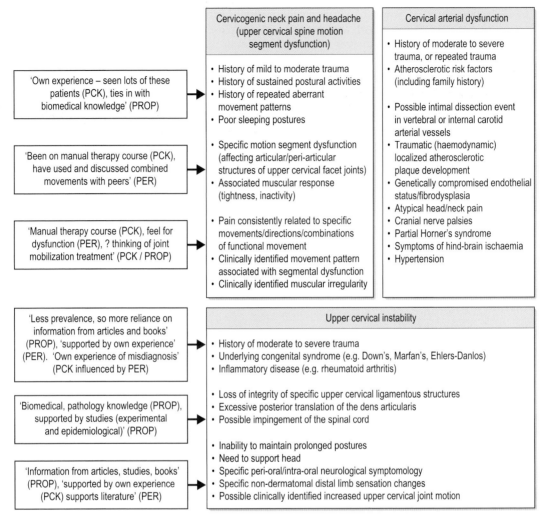

**Figure 3.6** • Example of illness script analysis with respect to the potential sources of knowledge. PCK – Professional craft knowledge; PROP – Propositional; PER – Personal.

knowledge types and sources within these scripts, and pass judgement on whether the assumptions made in the scripts hold any validity or not. Figure 3.6 shows how we can deconstruct our assumptions by considering what we now know about knowledge:

The analysis of our illness scripts shows a balance of the three knowledge types discussed above. In hypothesis one, non-propositional knowledge was arguably the dominant type. This may be because this benign neuromusculoskeletal explanation for neck and head pain is actually more common than the two competing hypotheses, and therefore there is the chance to be exposed through experience to the features suggestive of this explanation. The

important factor is, however, that despite the fact that the clinician probably sees this kind of presentation many times per week, it has still not been left to experience alone to develop the illness script. The accumulation of experiential, patient mileage derived *'know-how'* information (professional craft knowledge) has been continually scrutinized by *reflection* upon this experience (personal knowledge), and reference to external sources of information regarding this presentation (propositional knowledge). The converse is also apparent in the remaining two hypotheses. Due to the relatively low prevalence of these causes of neck and head pain, it is unlikely that the clinician is building up their professional craft base on a weekly basis.

Therefore, a more directed attempt to continually analyze practice (personal knowledge), and stronger reliance on external information sources resulting from appropriate forms of study (propositional knowledge), is apparent.

Overall, there is a balance of different valid knowledge types which in turn have been derived from the relevant valid sources (i.e. propositional from an appropriate research paradigm, non-proposition from (a) experience and tuition (professional craft knowledge), and (b) reflective practice on experience (personal knowledge)). Nowhere in this analysis is there evidence of an illogical and unsubstantiated assumption (e.g. upper cervical evil spirits) which has been derived from an illogical and unsubstantiated source (e.g. a shaman).

## Stage 4: Diagnostic testing: probability theory

Let us now assume that we have taken a well-reasoned and informative history which in itself, through its judicious use of inductive and deductive reasoning, has been a source of valid knowledge, i.e. a more accurate estimation of the nature of the problem. We are now undertaking the physical examination, which in line with hypothetico-deductive reasoning, has been formed and sculpted to suit this patient and to test the remaining hypotheses. We shall use this stage of the assessment process to highlight further components of clinical reasoning: probability, the further inclusion of evidence-based information into the reasoning process, and the utilization of probability analysis in decision-making.

There are two important points necessary to remember in clinical practice:

**1.** Nothing is ever 100% certain (in terms of our clinical diagnosis)

**2.** No diagnostic test or examination procedure is 100% valid.

Therefore, we work in an environment of *uncertainty*. As it happens, it is not just the manual therapy environment that is uncertain, but the physical world in general! Interested readers should refer to Heisenberg's Principle of Uncertainty, or the indeterminacy principle (Heisenberg, 1983) whereby, since the realization that sub-atomic particles influence their own behaviour, nothing could ever be certain or controlled in a truly objective manner. We must, therefore, accept and embrace this uncertainty,

working with it to make sense of our clinical presentations (West & West, 2002). And this is quite possible.

Let us then imagine that we now have the following information regarding our patient:

- *Age of patient:* 38
- *Gender:* male
- *Pain site:* left-sided mid to upper cervical pain and parietal headache
- *Possible causes:* for our selected examples: the three hypotheses in Table 3.1
- *Following subjective examination:*
  1. Hypothesis 3 (upper cervical instability) refuted
  2. Among other information, patient reports dizziness related to head movement
- *Possible causes:*
  1. Hypothesis 1 – benign NMS dysfunction
  2. Hypothesis 2 – cervical arterial dysfunction.

Hypothesis one and two have 'survived' the history-taking and will therefore be considered in the physical examination. Seeing as one of our surviving hypotheses is cervical arterial dysfunction, the example of 'testing' for the presence or absence of vertebrobasilar insufficiency (VBI) can be used to demonstrate how clinically we can utilize available information (evidence) in our reasoning process. At a superficial level, our reasoning process could be as shown in Figure 3.7.

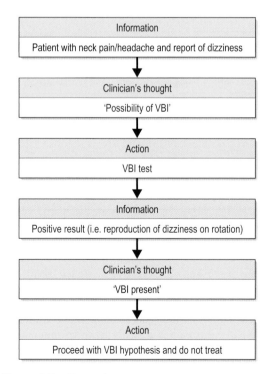

**Figure 3.7** • Reasoning process.

However, this process can now be analyzed in a little more depth. The crux of the clinical decision (and therefore management action) in this case has been the result of the VBI test. If we are relying on a test to directly influence our decisions like this, we would want that test to be useful, i.e. it does what it is intended to do. By using the test in clinical practice, we are hoping that the test will separate those *with* the condition of VBI from those *without* the condition of VBI. In the above scenario, there has been the assumption that a positive test equals presence of VBI.

## To test or not to test: using the evidence base to calculate how useful a test is

Like everything else, diagnosis is never definitive. At best, the clinician considers the *level* of certainty to which they judge a condition to exist. Thus, words such as possibly, probably, likely, unlikely, etc are often used to describe this level of certainty (Gilbert *et al*, 2001b). Although these words are often used as casual adjectives during clinical conversation, they do have a more specific, mathematical meaning to them which can assist in judging the usefulness of a test. It is with this mathematical concept in mind that the *clinical utility* of the VBI positional tests can be analyzed.

Straus *et al* (2005) define a model which can be used to assess the clinical usefulness of diagnostic tests by considering relevant published data relating to the accuracy of that test. This model of *diagnostic utility* is used extensively in medicine to assist the clinician in evidence-based decision-making and there is a wealth of available information demonstrating the pragmatic value of such an approach (e.g. Altman & Bland, 1994a, 1994b; Deeks & Altman, 2004; Elstein & Schwarz, 2002a, 2002b; Gilbert *et al*, 2001a, 2001b; Johnson *et al*, 2001; Knottnerus *et al*, 2002; Round, 2001; Sackett & Haynes, 2002). Despite being subject to potential criticism on the basis of being too quantitative for healthcare decisions (Downing & Hunter, 2003), such data-driven modelling is encouraged and supported in a number of 'human' activities (Chae *et al*, 2003; Fang *et al*, 2003a, 2003b; Kopelman *et al*, 1999; Niskanen, 1999; Tien, 2003). A number of physiotherapy-specific papers have been published which have utilized the concept of this model related to, for example, shoulder labral tests (Stratford, 2001), and the VBI rotational test (Gross *et al*, 2005; Ritcher & Reinking, 2005). Information provided by the latter two papers, plus other published data, can now be used to enhance the clinical appreciation of

both the clinical utility of the VBI test, and the concept of probability analysis in relation to clinical practice.

As mentioned above, there are certain key words which need to be considered when assessing the diagnostic role of a test. The conceptual mathematical meaning of these words needs to be appreciated in order to understand how assessment of the diagnostic test works. Davidson (2002) provides a thorough overview of these concepts and as such the detail presented here will be brief and relevant to the VBI test. Table 3.2 provides simple definitions

**Table 3.2 Summary of key terms associated with diagnostic utility analysis**

| Term | Definition |
| --- | --- |
| Probability | This is expressed as a number within the range 0.1 to 1.0 (1 to 100%) which reflects the clinician's estimate of how likely it is that the condition exists. Pre-test probability is this estimate before a diagnostic test is undertaken, and post-test probability is the estimate after the test has been performed |
| Sensitivity | The 'true positive rate'. The sensitivity of a test refers to that proportion of people who actually have the condition being correctly identified by the test. A negative result from a highly sensitive test will confidently rule the presence of the condition out |
| Specificity | The 'true negative rate'. The specificity of a test refers to that proportion of people who do not have the condition being correctly identified by the test as not having it. A positive result from a highly specific test will confidently rule the condition in. Sensitivity and specificity are expressed numerically as a percentage between 0 and 100 |
| Prevalence | The proportion of people within a given sample or population who actually have the condition. This again is expressed as a percentage and is synonymous with the pre-test probability |
| Likelihood ratio (LR) | The ratio between getting a true result and getting a false result. The LR is expressed as a number between 0.001 and 1000. The further the LR is away from 1 (above 1 for LR positive; below 1 for LR negative), the better the test is at separating those with the condition from those without it. The LR represents the *valve* of a test for increasing the certainty about a diagnosis. |

of the terms needed to be understood when determining the diagnostic utility of a test.

The presence of a condition existing in a patient can also be referred to in terms of *odds*, e.g. 'have the odds of this condition actually existing changed since the test was performed?'. Odds are different, but intrinsically related to, probability. Odds are an expression of probability divided by 1 minus probability.

All the above information can be calculated by using data from available studies that have focused on the diagnostic accuracy of a test. In terms of the VBI test, this means studies that have used blood flow analysis of a high calibre or 'Gold Standard'/'near Gold Standard' (i.e. either magnetic resonance angiography (MRA) or Doppler ultrasound insonation) to examine the effect of the position used in the VBI test (e.g. cervical rotation) on blood flow in the vertebrobasilar system (seeing as the underlying principle of the VBI test is that blood flow is affected by this position). Clinically, a positive test is defined as one where the patient reports the onset of symptoms during this sustained position. Valid studies would, therefore, be those which report on both changes in blood flow and the onset of symptoms during examination of the subjects. For a test to be useful, it would be necessary for these two factors to correlate, i.e. those people who demonstrate reduced blood flow also report the onset of symptoms during the time of this change, and equally, those people who do not demonstrate a reduction in blood flow report no onset of symptoms.

So, we can extract data from a number of studies to input into our utility calculation. For the purpose of this illustration, we can use the data reported in the two existing VBI test utility studies (i.e. Gross *et al*, 2005; Ritcher & Reinking, 2005). This data (the number representing the number of subjects) can then be separated into four different categories:

A – Those with a positive flow result and positive VBI test

B – Those with a negative flow result and positive VBI test

C – Those with a positive flow result and negative VBI test

D – Those with a negative flow result and negative VBI test

Common sense would tell us that in order for a test to be good, most subjects should fall into categories A or D, but we can use some simple calculations to robustly establish factors which allow us to judge more accurately the utility of the test.[1] The basis for such calculations (e.g. specificity, sensitivity, likelihood ratios) is a 'two-by-two table'. For our example, the results are presented in Table 3.3.

The results of this analysis show that most subjects fall into categories B and C, which is the opposite of what we would hope for! The subsequent

Table 3.3 Two by two table for the VBI test. Data from two sources (Gross *et al*, 2005; Ritcher & Reinking, 2005) is collated in cells A to D. The number represents number of individual subjects

| Rotation test | | MRA/doppler US | |
| --- | --- | --- | --- |
| | | Positive | Negative |
| Rotation test | Positive | A 20 | B 112 |
| | Negative | C 173 | D 89 |
| | | | |
| Sensitivity a/(a+c) | | 10% | |
| Specificity d/(b+d) | | 44% | |
| Pre-test probability ('prevalence') (a+c)/(a+b+c+d) | | 49% | |
| Likelihood ratio + sensitivity/(1-specificity) | | 0.19 | |
| Likelihood ratio − (1-sensitivity)/specificity | | 2.02 | |

calculations result in a poor sensitivity, moderate specificity, and very poor likelihood ratios.[1]

We shall consider the 'prevalence' result later. In clinical terms, this means that the VBI test will not be very useful in informing us that the condition is absent if it is negative, might be informative if it is positive, but overall unlikely to change our clinical decision.

So, did the clinician in the flowchart in Figure 3.7 make the correct decision? There is some conflict now between the moderate specificity which *might* suggest that the condition is present, and the very low likelihood ratios which suggest that whatever the result of the test, our clinical decision will not be altered. Mathematically, the likelihood ratios are better indicators of a test's value than either the sensitivity or specificity values in isolation (Deeks & Altman, 2004; Gilbert *et al*, 2001b). Therefore we could say that we will go with the likelihood ratios and not let the result of the test change our clinical decision. Based on this, we could argue a case for not incorporating this test in our clinical investigation. However, we have not considered the complete picture. To help us further, we need to continue our exploration of probability.

It is inferred above that there is an estimation of how *likely* VBI exists in this patient *before* the test is performed. In basic clinical terms, there must be some suspicion of the condition being present or otherwise the test would not have been performed. It is important to establish this estimation – known as the *pre-test probability* – as it actually influences the impact a test will have on the clinical decision, i.e. the interpretation of a test result is not only reliant on the calculation in Table 3.3, but also the pre-test probability. In the ideal world, we would have used better quality data to input into our utility calculation – this is not a criticism of the study reports from which our data was taken, but rather a comment on the lack of specific utility studies done in this field. The calculation is therefore skewed by a *spectrum bias* (Pewsner *et al*, 2004). In the absence of studies on patients, we have relied on studies on normal subjects with the chance reporting of symptom reproduction.

This has resulted in a chance finding that perhaps the subjects who reported symptoms during the rotation test and also had positive flow results, did not actually have pathological VBI. It may be that blood flow reduces in normal individuals anyway (see Ch. 6). This has resulted in an unexpectedly high 'prevalence', or 'pre-test probability' figure of 49%. Ordinarily, this figure would be used, literally, as the sole basis of our pre-test probability estimation, i.e. the 38-year-old male with left-sided neck pain and headache has a 49% (almost 1 in 2) chance of having VBI. This is extremely incongruous with other information we have about VBI. More formally, because the studies used in the calculation were not carried out on 38-year-old males with unilateral neck and head pain, we cannot make this assumption. We must therefore use other information to inform our pre-test probability.

Firstly, let us briefly clarify *how* pre-test probability estimation has the potential to affect the impact a test has on post-test clinical judgement. The simplest way to demonstrate this is by use of a *likelihood ratio nomogram* (Fig. 3.8): The nomogram works by plotting a straight line joining the known integers of pre-test probability and likelihood ratio of the test. The straight line continues towards the right where it intersects the last line marked 'post-test probability'. The nomogram immediately illustrates that there is a direct relationship between pre-test probability and post-test probability (being swayed in the middle by the test's likelihood ratio).

Using the nomogram we can calculate the post-test probabilities of the condition existing in the event of a positive or negative test. The results are presented in Table 3.4 which uses two examples of different pre-test probability judgements: scenario A, a low pre-test probability judgement (10%) of the condition existing, and scenario B, a high pre-test probability judgement (90%) of the condition existing.

As stated earlier, the *greater* than 1 a LR+ is, the better the test is at ruling the condition in, whilst the *lower* than 1 a LR– is, the better the test at ruling the condition out. The VBI test actually has LR+ *less* than 1, and a LR– *greater* than 1! We are therefore getting aberrant results, e.g. scenario B suggests that with a 90% pre-test probability, if we get a positive test result, the post-test probability actually reduces! This, of course, is illogical. This concept occurs in all the above scenarios. Because of the obvious poor utility of this test, mathematically we could argue the case for not using it to directly inform our clinical decision.

---

[1]The mathematics of these calculations will not be presented here. Readers are referred to Strauss *et al* (2005) for further information. If you do this, you will see that it is possible (and easier) to use an online programme to perform all the necessary calculations for establishing the diagnostic utility of a test.

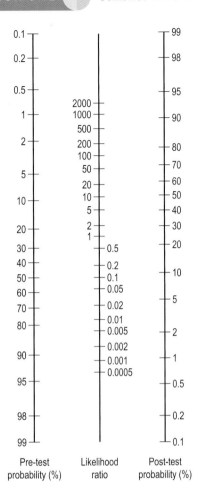

Pre-test probability (%)    Likelihood ratio    Post-test probability (%)

**Figure 3.8 •** Likelihood ratio nomogram. If the pre-test probability and likelihood ratio are known, a straight line can be drawn to read-off the post-test probability. (Source: http://www.cebm.net/likelihood_ratios.asp)

Now let us imagine we have another test which is actually very good (LR+ 15; LR– 0.5). The results for this test are presented in Table 3.5.

The results of this analysis demonstrate that if there is low pre-test probability, a good positive test will significantly affect the clinical decision (scenario A – probability changed from 10% to 60% chance of the condition existing). However, if the pre-test probability is high, the difference between pre- and post-test judgement is *not* significantly affected (scenario B – 90% to 99% chance of the condition existing); in other words, it was quite certain that the condition might exist and the positive result from the (good) test simply supports that suspicion but does not alter judgement.

With a good LR– test, if the pre-test probability is low and the test is negative, judgement will be supported towards the fact that it is unlikely that the condition exists. If the pre-test probability is high and the test is negative, the probability will change (in the case of scenario D, by 30%), *but* there is still a 60% chance that the condition exists!

In summary, with the exception of a very good LR+ test being used in the presence of low pre-test probability (which is an unusual scenario), even good tests have limited influence on pre-test probability.

## Clinical relevance

In light of the above it is the responsibility of the therapist to do their utmost to make the best judgement on the probability of a problem existing *prior* to performing any physical tests. In other words, the physical examination should only be entered into with a good estimation of what is wrong – this is good clinical reasoning!

**Table 3.4 Results of nomogram calculations for existing VBI test showing post-test probabilities for A: a positive likelihood ratio, and B: a negative likelihood ratio**

| A | Pre-test probability % | + Likelihood ratio | Post-test probability % |
|---|---|---|---|
| Scenario A | 10 | 0.19 | 4 |
| Scenario B | 90 | 0.19 | 50 |
| B | Pre-test probability % | – Likelihood ratio | Post-test probability % |
| Scenario A | 10 | 2.02 | 35 |
| Scenario B | 90 | 2.02 | 95 |

**Table 3.5** Results of nomogram calculations for hypothetical improved VBI test showing post-test probabilities for A: a positive likelihood ratio, and B: a negative likelihood ratio

| A | Pre-test probability % | + Likelihood ratio | Post-test probability % |
|---|---|---|---|
| Scenario A | 10 | 15 | 60 |
| Scenario B | 90 | 15 | 99 |

| B | Pre-test probability % | − Likelihood ratio | Post-test probability % |
|---|---|---|---|
| Scenario A | 10 | 0.2 | 2 |
| Scenario B | 90 | 0.2 | 60 |

## Estimating pre-test probability

In the absence of established patient group diagnostic utility data, other information should be used to estimate pre-test probability (Davidson, 2002; Elstein & Schwarz, 2002b). This information can be derived from other published literature (i.e. other than specific diagnostic utility studies), subjective impression, and personal experience (subject to the provisos of this as discussed earlier). Ideally, the clinician should attempt to quantify this is as a percentage, and this is acceptable despite it not being mathematically formulated. As an example of this, let us return to our case scenario:

Utilizing contemporary information about cervical arterial dysfunction (see Ch. 6), we can reasonably estimate the probability of posterior cervical arterial dysfunction (VBI) being present for the two following versions of our case:

**VERSION 1**

38-year-old male, with 3-month history of intermittent left-sided mid to upper cervical pain, temporal/crown headache. Episodic over 3 years, related to sustained posture (involving combined neck position – use of phone, etc) at work; responds well to manual therapy. This episode similar to previous. Movement related dizziness. No previous trauma. Fit and well otherwise. No own or family history of cancer or cardiovascular disease. Pain responds positively to analgesia.

**VERSION 2**

38-year-old male with 5-day history of constant left-sided, mid upper cervical pain, occipital headache. Not experienced pain like this before. Twisted head violently to right 5 days ago (related to onset). History of 3 road traffic accidents in past 2 years. Experiencing nausea, hoarseness of voice, and tingling in left side of face. Known hypertension and hypercholesterolemia. Family history of stroke and heart disease.

Although at a very superficial level (i.e. at first referral) both of these versions appear similar (i.e. a 38-year-old male with head and neck pain), there are, of course, obvious differences which allow to develop different estimation of the probability of certain pathologies being present. As stated above, we can use our existing knowledge formed by a combination of published literature, experience, tuition, and reflective practice to inform our estimate.

Version 1 conforms well to the illness script in hypothesis one (Table 3.1) and there is little evidence of risk factors or signs and symptoms of cervical arterial dysfunction. Therefore, it would be reasonable to suggest a high (say 80% +) probability of the pain being related to a benign, treatable facet movement dysfunction, and a low (say < 10%) chance of there being evidence of arterial dissection.

Conversely, version 2 demonstrates a number of risk factors for, and signs/symptoms of, arterial dissection, and conforms well to the illness script of hypothesis two in Table 3.1. Therefore, it would be reasonable to assign a high (say 80% +) pre-test probability of arterial dissection.

This whole concept of estimating probability based on particular sets of information during the analysis of a situation is referred to as *conditional probability*. It is based on the premise that the accumulating evidence related to a proposition (in this case a particular diagnosis) contributes towards the continual re-estimation of the probability of the proposition being present.

In Table 3.6, we can see that by the end stage of the accumulation of information, we have made the estimation of 80% probability of the condition of VBI existing. There are two important points to note here:

**1.** Each point of re-estimation is influenced by prior information, e.g. at stage 4 'History of 2 road traffic accidents', the probability estimation is

**Table 3.6** Demonstration of conditional probability progression. Each re-estimation of the probability is influenced by the preceding information

| Information | Clinician's thoughts | Probability estimation |
|---|---|---|
| 38-year-old male | Although this is within the age range in which most arterial dissections occur, the overall prevalence of VBI is reportedly very low | < 5% |
| 5-day history of constant left-sided, mid-upper cervical pain, occipital headache | Common site for vertebral artery induced pain, but there are also many other sources for pain in this site | 10% |
| Not experienced pain like this before | Commonly quoted pain description for arterial pain | 20% |
| Twisted head violently to right 5 days ago (related to onset) | Typical mechanism for potential dissection event | 30% |
| History of three road traffic accidents in previous 2 years | Strong history of repeated trauma – impact of endothelial dysfunction | 40% |
| Experiencing nausea, hoarseness of voice, and tingling in left side of face | Typical presenting characteristics of VA dissection | 60% |
| Known hypertension and hypercholesterolemia | Supported pre-disposing factors for endothelial dysfunction | 70% |
| Family history of stroke and heart disease | Supporting risk factors from genetically pre-disposed endothelial dysfunction | 80% |

40%. This *does not* mean that if someone has had two road traffic accidents they are at a 40% risk of having VBI! It *does* mean that in this clinician's informed estimation for this patient at this time,

the history of this particular repeated trauma has raised the clinician's suspicion of the presence of VBI by 10% from the last piece of information. In other words, '40% probability' at this point is based on the age of the patient, the type and site of pain, the mechanism of injury, and the history of previous trauma.

2. In the absence of strong, well-researched data, each additional piece of information is likely to make only a small adjustment to the probability estimation. In the presence of good quality data, larger, more confident, adjustments may be made.

The notion of conditional probability, and the impact that new information has on the revised probability, is based on Bayes' Theorem (Harbison, 2006; Marlow, 2006). This is a mathematical theorem used to calculate precise probability estimates in the presence of imprecise data sources. It is imperative to reiterate a fundamentally important point here. We are inputting subjective judgement into our conceptual Bayes' Theorem, and coming out with a number. Therefore, this whole process is prone to criticism, i.e. 'how can a number be attributed to a subjective judgement?' It must be remembered that the number is not an attempt to absolutely quantify our judgement, it is a tool to help us direct our decision-making. It is a mechanism of taking a judgement of 'very unlikely'/'moderately likely'/'very likely' to a numerical level facilitating the deeper assessment of the impact of a clinical test, as discussed above. The accuracy of the resultant numerical representation of our subjective judgement of probability is only ever going to be as good as the information that goes into the process. Thus, the GIGO principle (Garbage In Garbage Out) (Dawkins, 2006) is highly applicable here! We must be constantly aware of doing our utmost to ensure, in the absence of good published data, that the information input is *reasonable* (i.e. from valid sources, logically robust), and as repeatedly stated throughout this chapter, this relies on our basic reasoning skills and use of appropriate knowledge, cognition and metacognition – this is our quality assurance mechanism. Dawkins (2006) refers to the ridiculously aberrant use of Bayes' Theorem in estimating the probability of the existence of God in a recently published text (Unwin, 2003). It is of great importance that, as responsible accountable healthcare practitioners, we do not fall into this trap of the erroneous use of unreasonable information and knowledge. With this caveat in mind, the careful and judicious use of conditional probability can be an important and informative mechanism of analysis in manual therapy clinical reasoning process.

Up to this point, we have focused on reasoning processes used to work out 'what the problem is', and have focused on structural explanations for our examples. This chapter now concludes with a review of narrative reasoning, which encompasses non-diagnostic matters, and its place with manual therapy practice.

## Stage 5: Interpretative reasoning

Many of the reasoning strategies focused on so far (i.e. pattern recognition, hypothetico-deduction, diagnostic utility) have been referred to as 'diagnostic' reasoning (e.g. Edwards *et al*, 2004; Rivett & Jones, 2004). However, the use of these strategies alone is artificial, and contemporary studies have demonstrated the use of integrated approaches incorporating non-diagnostic strategies in expert reasoning (Edwards *et al*, 2004; Kaminker *et al*, 2004; Smart & Doody, 2006). Effective clinical reasoning necessitates a rich, transcending, interpretive dimension in order to make the patient's problem fully understood and meaningful. The modern manual therapist is evolving rapidly as a responsible, informed, and conscientious healthcare practitioner, and there are several factors for this:

- Advances in our understanding of pain (pain theory)
- Advances in our understanding of people, e.g. patients and therapists (psychology)
- Exponential growth of information, some of which may challenge our beliefs in the effectiveness of what we do (research evidence)
- The continual, intelligent, pragmatic exploration of the quality of what we do (reflective practice).

In turn, these factors have informed recent thought and inquiry into clinical reasoning processes. As such, recent propositions have been made which extend the reasoning process beyond that of biophysical diagnosis. These approaches embrace and exploit understanding regarding the cognitive, psychological, social and intellectual components of both the patient's and the therapist's understanding of the pain episode. It is sometimes difficult for the manual therapist to appreciate how these complex cognitive components are congruous with existing management approaches of benign, neuromusculoskeletal

dysfunctions. This might seem especially incongruous as part of a book focusing specifically on the seemingly biophysical, technical concept of CMT. However, it is proposed herewith that the clinical reasoning process cannot be complete or effective if these components are not considered with all patients. Hence, this final section focuses on the broad arena of which we shall refer to as *interpretive reasoning*[2]. It is not the intention of this section to provide a fully informed critical discussion on this topic, but rather to suggest how this modern thinking can be incorporated into our CMT. The reader is strongly encouraged to supplement their reading of this chapter with sources of far more detailed analysis of interpretive reasoning approaches (e.g. Higgs *et al*, 2004; Jensen *et al*, 2007; Jones & Edwards, 2006; Pincus, 2004).

There are two areas of concern that have been recognized when attempting to embrace non-biological concepts into the manual therapy reasoning process. Firstly, the apparent over-simplified, superficial, or even aberrant attempts by therapists to include, for example, cognitive-behavioural strategies into their practice (Edwards *et al*, 2006), Secondly, the unreasonable dismissal of manual therapeutic techniques on the grounds that they are passive, and therefore deconstructive, in a psychosocial model. It must be said that these concerns are not necessarily the fault of individual clinicians – they are rather a sign of the state of our early understanding of complex issues which are only just beginning to impact on clinical and academic practice. We do, however, contend that neither of these actions are well reasoned or form part of an intelligent, informed practice approach.

Although we are considering our final models of reasoning at the end of the assessment process, i.e. incorporating the treatment decision, it is necessary to appreciate that, like the other models, this process is utilized throughout the whole period of patient assessment and management. It is also

---

[2]It is appreciated that there are many synonyms for the reasoning concepts which are considered in this section. It is also appreciated that it is not accurate to use the term *interpretative reasoning* as the umbrella heading for these strategies. However, we have chosen here to use this term for two reasons: (1) to refer to the broad range of reasoning strategies concerned with the cognitive process related to working out or understanding a given patient-orientated problem – thus 'interpreting' the information derived from the patient–therapists interaction in a deep, meaningful context, and (2) to provide an analogous link with what we already know about research paradigms, and highlight by way of a title that the sources of knowledge we are referring to are philosophically removed from the empirico-analytical sources considered in diagnostic reasoning strategies.

important to understand that these interpretive reasoning strategies are not 'additional', or 'alternatives', or even run in parallel, to the diagnostic models already discussed. This level of reasoning should be integral to the therapist's thought process and therefore inseparable from other forms of cognitive reasoning. The importance of intertwining this process within the cognitive network of the manual therapist's reasoning cannot be overstated.

A fundamental strategy that facilitates access to components of the social (patient–therapist) interaction required for developing deep and meaningful appreciation of the problem is *narrative reasoning*. Narrative reasoning describes the notion of encapsulating information from a number of sources (e.g. own experience, the patient, the patient's carers, other professionals) into 'stories' – the word 'narrative' literally meaning story or tale – through which the therapist can interpret and understand the patient's problem (Fleming & Mattingly, 2000; Jones & Edwards; 2006, Mattingly, 1998). Narrative reasoning has been reported to exist in the reasoning strategies employed by expert healthcare clinicians (e.g. Crowe & O'Malley, 2006; Edwards *et al*, 2006; Gevitz, 2006; Wiitavaara *et al*, 2006; Zhou *et al*, 2005). It has recently been reported that the narrative interpretation of events by the patient influences their understanding of the problem and the outcome of interventions in a number of settings (Brannstrom *et al*, 2006; Chapple *et al*, 2006; Jones *et al*, 2006; Weaver *et al*, 2006).

Let us assume we have now come to the diagnostic decision that our patient's physical problem is related to a treatable mechanical vertebral articular dysfunction in the upper cervical spine. We are therefore at the stage to make some decisions regarding best management of the patient. In line with the basis of diagnostic reasoning we can draw, if the evidence allows, from the empirico-analytical knowledge source to inform our decision, e.g. are there any good randomized control trials which would direct our decision-making? This forms *part* of good evidence-based practice. And it is only part, which is in line with the literal definition of evidence-based practice (Strauss *et al*, 2005), i.e. evidence-based practice being the integration of:

• The best of research evidence
• The best of clinical expertise
• Patient values and patient circumstances.

We still have three remaining components to include in our decision-making process.

Through our reflective experience, which has contributed to our expertise plus the information which the patient holds, we can build stories that help us to understand the *contextual reality* of the situation. As per the interpretive research paradigm, narrative reasoning relies on the assumption that truth is a socially constructed concept, and not a pre-existing positivistic objective reality simply waiting to be discovered. Therefore, what the therapist considers truthful might not be what the patient, or indeed another therapist, considers it to be, because 'the truth' *has* to come from within the individual patient–therapist interaction, i.e. 'the truth' is *the product* of that interaction.

We can break our case analysis down as follows: we have some biomedical knowledge which has allowed us, through reasoned assessment, to come to the conclusion that there is a biophysical dysfunction which should be treatable by the application of a good, well-practised physical technique (e.g. a combined movement technique). But this is still therapist-centred logic. Of course, information from the patient has been used in coming to this conclusion, e.g. information about the pain, how it affects them (activity-wise), severity of pain, physical impairments. However, the conclusion is fundamentally based on the biomedical/biophysical understanding of the problem – information *contained within the therapist*. Reasoning could be enhanced further by supporting the conclusion with more knowledge, e.g. treatment options supported by research trials, previous use of these techniques to good effect, course tutor advocated use of these treatments. However, therapist-centred logic is still the driving force. The reasoning process is not complete. We need to explore information *constructed from the interaction*.

The question which should now be concerning the narrative reasoner is: 'how do the ideas I now have regarding (in this instance) treatment relate to the patient's understanding of their problem?' Going back to our case, we find that the patient offered the following information as a result of the assessment:

As you know, this pain began about 12 weeks ago. It's much worse than previous episodes of neck pain that I have had. The first physiotherapist I saw a week after the pain advised some exercises and used a machine to help the pain. I didn't do the exercises for long. I only went for three sessions, then stopped attending. I saw a chiropractor 5 weeks ago and was attending three times a week until a few days ago. He gave me a thorough explanation of what was wrong. I didn't quite understand what he was talking about – he kept going on about 'rotated segments' and things being out of place – but he obviously knew his stuff. He said that there were all sorts of things to work on, which is why I needed to go fairly frequently. I used to feel a bit better for a short while after I had treatment, but things haven't really got any better. My GP referred me here because he thought you might be able to help.

A number of aberrant conclusions could be made based on this script if it is either (a) analyzed too superficially and/or (b) the concept of interpretative reasoning and non-biological components to pain are misunderstood, e.g.:

'The patient has 'psychosocial' issues and manual therapy isn't appropriate.'

'The first two clinicians had a good go, but my techniques are better, so we will proceed with manual therapy.'

Thoughts along the above two lines are missing the point of interpretive reasoning and consideration of non-biological factors. The script offers a potentially rich source of narration which could lead to informing the therapist, not only what treatment intervention to use, but whether that intervention is, even with it being biophysically justified, permissible.

There are a number of themes emerging from within the script which require further examination, e.g.:

- Evidence of failed treatment
- Patient's perception of cause of the pain
- Patient's behaviour during the 12-week pain episode
- Patient's expectations of their interaction with you
- Patient's needs/wishes.

Let us explore one of these themes from a narrative perspective: the patient's perception of cause of pain. This, of course, may well impact on the other themes, e.g. failed treatment, patient's behaviour and expectations, so it is an important consideration. This theme leads to a number of potential hypotheses, which require some form of validation e.g.:

- H1 – patient thinks that the cause is not musculoskeletal
- H2 – patient thinks that nobody knows what is causing the pain
- H3 – patient thinks that the cause is serious and will get worse
- H4 – patient thinks that this pain is caused by something different to previous pain episodes, etc.

These hypotheses can, of course, be tested for validity by further questioning. This hypothesis falsification process is in line with the deductive reasoning discussed earlier, and is considered an *instrumental* approach to problem solving (Jones & Edwards, 2006). Suppose, for example, we pursued the hypotheses above by asking the opening (and open) question 'what do *you* think is the cause of your pain?' and the patient's response is:

Well, I have been rather worried. I know that my GP sent me to see you, but I have been concerned that it may be cancer. You see, my uncle had a brain tumour which began with headache. Because this headache feels different to previous pain, and that no one seems to be able to help, I have been getting quite stressed about it. My aunt lent me some information about cancer, and I did some looking on the internet, and it seems to be true that you can have these tumours in your head and they cause pain.

If we pause our reasoning progression for a moment and review the information we have, we can see evidence of conflict between the knowledge and beliefs of the clinician and the patient – this is summarized in Table 3.7.

The instrumental, deductive inquiry has got us this far. If we curtailed our reasoning at this point

**Table 3.7 Differences in beliefs and knowledge sources between clinician and patient**

| | Most likely cause of pain | Underpinning knowledge sources and reasoning |
|---|---|---|
| *Clinician* | Benign, treatable, upper cervical musculoskeletal motion dysfunction | Biomedical knowledge Biophysical knowledge Careful differential diagnosis by: Subjective examination Physical examination |
| *Patient* | Cancer | Two episodes of failed treatment Pain not familiar Uncle had brain tumour Read about headache and cancer Internet searches |

we are in danger of still making incomplete, superficial, or erroneous judgements. For example, one
instinctive line of thinking in response to the above
situation might be 'OK, you think it's cancer, I think
it isn't. I am an expert in this area with sound
knowledge and experience. You are a patient with
limited and questionable experience and knowledge. I can therefore reassure you that it is not cancer and we can get on with treatment'. Although we
might consider that we have 'explored the patient's
beliefs' about their pain, this is still far too inadequate, and hence the above thought process holds
a number of limitations.

Although the clinician might think they are being
helpful by reassuring the patient that they do not
have cancer, they have not taken into account the
fact that the patient has already, in the space of
12 weeks, been let down by three independent
'experts' (physiotherapist, chiropractor, then GP).
The sources of knowledge the patient quotes (aunt,
internet, own experience of uncle's illness) are val-
ued more by the patient than any information previously dispensed by the experts, i.e. the patient has
overridden the experts' opinions. The clinician has
reinforced the expert's position of authority by dis-
missing the patient's thoughts and enforcing their
own (albeit with the intention of being helpful).
There was already conflict with authority figures.
By attempting to help the patient, the clinician has
in fact reinforced the existing conflict between their
own and the patient's beliefs. What is required is a
process to develop *consensus* in decision-making
between two individuals in the presence of inconsistent knowledge (Guo *et al*, 2002).

Narrative reasoning requires that our inquiry goes
a significant stage further, utilizing what Jones and
Edwards (2006) refer to as a *communicative* process. It has been stated (Mezirow, 2000) that this
is about understanding what someone *means* (at a
deep level) when they say something. The patient's
statement above tells us what they think, or even
believe, but it is still missing a dimension of *meaningfulness* without which clinical progress is limited.
In other words, we need to understand *why* the
patient has made some inferences from failed treatment to cancer, from the experience of the uncle's
illness to suspicion of own cancer, from reading
about cancer to suspicion of own cancer, etc. What
has influenced *this* patient to make these links?
What social, cultural, personal, or psychological
factors have played a role in determining the

interpretation of events for this patient? A model
of 'schema enmeshment' has been proposed to
help explain the information processing in patients
(Pincus & Morley, 2001). Although this model is
based on experiences of chronic pain patients, the
concept of personal schema is relevant to all individuals (as per the discussion earlier on in this
chapter). Hence, through collation of experiences,
the patient will develop their own cognitive network through which all future experiences are
filtered.

This schema and the interrelated meaningfulness
of experiences, is not necessarily readily available in
the subject's consciousness and therefore cannot be
readily accessed by the process of deductive questioning. The purpose of inquiry now has to be
focused on exposing this tacit network. We are
now dealing with similar cognitive processes that
we needed to explore in our own reasoning. Indeed
many of the 'techniques' of this narrative, interpretive logic parallel those we use ourselves as part of
reflective practice. Thus, our duty is to facilitate
and accompany the patient in exposing, explaining,
and challenging their deep belief structures. The clinician becomes a form of *critical companion*[3] for the
patient. The relationship is two-way, and the process of assisting the patient is of course helping
the clinician to challenge their beliefs about this alli-
ance and thus helping to find congruency between
the two sources.

The nature of inquiry and communication now
has to be more 'dialectical' (Jones & Rivett, 2005)
than confrontational. A confrontational example in
the present case has been the assertion of one
knowledge base and opinion over another. This
communication has been uni-directional (i.e. therapist to patient).

Dialectical strategies involve 'debate intended to
reconcile a contradiction without attempting to
establish either view as intrinsically truer than the
other' (Jones & Edwards, 2006, p. 290). This notion
determines a mature, discursive *conversation*
through which the problem of power inequality

---

[3]*Critical companionship* is a term usually used, in therapy
reasoning literature at least, to describe a relationship between
two clinicians (usually an expert and a less experienced clinician)
(Titchen & Higgs, 2000). However, it describes a partnership
where one person helps another on their personal, experiential
learning journey (Higgs & Titchen, 2000), and this is the nature of
partnership developed within the narrative reasoning process
between the clinician and the patient.

(authoritarianism) is addressed. A learning process is entered into and assumptions, propositions, and beliefs are adapted or replaced (Welch & Dawson, 2006; Windish et al, 2005).

The differentiator between this process and more superficial analysis is that the patient has a significant role, if the patient chooses to, in changing. In our case, in terms of attempting to change the patient's beliefs, the difference can be demonstrated as follows:

### A. SUPERFICIAL REASONING

#### Clinician's thoughts

I did a thorough assessment and reason this to be a treatable musculoskeletal condition. However, the patient thinks that it might be cancer. I therefore need to explain to the patient that because I've done a thorough assessment, and I have good experience in dealing with both musculoskeletal conditions, and cancer, that it isn't cancer. If I explain it well enough he must understand!

### B. INTERPRETIVE REASONING

#### Clinician's thoughts

Following discussion, it would appear that the patient's experience of his uncle's illness was very negative and came at a bad time for him regarding his work situation. He was close to his uncle – they were similar ages – and his illness has caused great upset. We discussed how pain experiences and beliefs can be influenced by previous events or incidents. I asked the patient to consider what his impression of his headache and neck pain might be if his uncle's situation hadn't happened. He said that he found it difficult to comprehend that, but could appreciate that it might be different. He then asked why previous treatment hadn't worked. I encouraged him to recall what his impressions of his pain were at that time. He said that actually he had always believed that this was something serious right from the onset. We then discussed the significant role that an individual's thoughts can have on the effect of treatment. He recalled that the chiropractor kept saying that his neck was quite awful – something was pressing on some nerves – he said that he used to go home and worry that it was a tumour pressing on his nerves. I think that there are quite a few negative influences dictating this patient's perception of his pain. I am now keen to propose to the patient that we work together to try and achieve a different impression of his pain. He was quite keen for me to refer him back to his GP for a scan. It may well be that this is what he still wants. At least we have had the opportunity to reconsider our beliefs.

Scenario A demonstrates a one-way process of attempting to change the patient's beliefs by externally and forcibly replacing the patient's knowledge/belief structure with that of the clinician's.

Scenario B demonstrates a deeper interpretation of the patient's thought process, and what is influencing his perception of his pain. The dialogue is two-way and any significant change opportunity is coming from within the interaction. The patient becomes empowered and encouraged to contribute towards perspectives regarding their problem, but this time in a meaningful way. At no time is the therapist trying to convince the patient that the musculoskeletal hypothesis is correct and that he therefore needs combined movement therapy. This diagnostic and treatment decision again has to be a product of the interaction and the narrative.

This final section has attempted to present a clinically meaningful overview of contemporary thought on interpretive reasoning and how the integration of this reasoning into manual therapy is essential if good clinical outcomes are to be achieved. An example of how interpretative reasoning could be demonstrated in manual therapy decision-making has been given using the ongoing case study. To reiterate, this example represents only a small component of the overall assessment and management process and it is imperative that the clinician strives to consider interpretive reasoning throughout the whole period of patient interaction. Every therapist–patient interaction should be considered a learning experience for both parties, and a time for beliefs to be challenged and new knowledge to be acquired.

# Conclusion

Clinical reasoning involves a number of complex cognitive strategies. The nature of these strategies changes as progress along the novice to expert continuum is made. However, this journey is not passive and may cease at any time. In the pursuit of expertise, and therefore best patient care, it is in the therapist's interest to understand and analyze their own practice, thoughts, and clinical behaviour. In order to do this, awareness of sound and well-documented reasoning strategies is essential. Contemporary literature on clinical reasoning in the health professions, and especially manual therapy, is excellent and is a growing source of information which clinicians can exploit to enhance their own practice. This chapter has presented an overview of a number of reasoning strategies relevant to the practice of manual therapy. A sound understanding of explicit models of reasoning (e.g. pattern recognition, hypothetico-deductive reasoning, interpretative reasoning) and the component parts of reasoning mechanisms (e.g. reflective practice, knowledge, probability theory) provides a substantial analytical platform. It is from this platform that the clinician can stop, reflect, reduce, and attempt to make sense of their practice. In doing so, practice can then be reformulated and enhanced.

Within this book are a number of case-orientated clinical reasoning exercises specific to combined movement theory. Each will present a particular problem or series of problems for the reader to solve. In doing so, the reader is encouraged to utilize clinical reasoning strategies discussed in this chapter. The reader will be able to explicitly and consciously recognize patterns (e.g. from the information regarding patient history, pain behaviour, combined movement analysis), test the patterns for validity focusing on possible illness scripts, develop hypotheses from these ideas, and test those hypotheses in a variety of ways (e.g. considering further questions, further physical examination procedures, mini-treatments). During this process, new knowledge will be developed about the patient and this knowledge will influence subsequent thought regarding the case. The reader can exploit this opportunity to challenge their own knowledge base regarding the conditions and mechanical presentations of the cases and consciously consider the sources and therefore validity of that knowledge. The application of specific diagnostic tests that may arise during these exercises provides a chance for the reader to consider the diagnostic utility of such tests and whether they are adding valuable information to the case. In order to facilitate reasoning in these exercises, a number of questions are presented which require the reader to focus their thoughts about the case and commit to what they consider to be the best judgement in that case, e.g.: regarding the next action; planning for the physical examination; severity, irritability and nature of the condition; dominant pain mechanism. It is hoped that this analytical process will be transferred into daily practice where the same tools and techniques can be used to analyze and enhance reasoning on the shop floor. It is here of course where it all matters, and it is here that the deeper process of interpretative reasoning can be utilized and analyzed.

Clinical reasoning is an ongoing learning process for the manual therapist and is integral to life-long learning, reflective practice, and continual professional development. Awareness of what is 'good' reasoning can only enhance that learning process. It is hoped that this chapter has helped in providing some of this awareness and encouraged a conscious, positive, framework by which the manual therapist can pursue a meaningful level of expertise and thus provide best patient care.

## CLINICAL REASONING CPD ACTIVITIES

After reading Chapter 3, follow these on-going CPD activities which are designed to facilitate your continual reflection of your own day-to-day clinical reasoning.

- o Ideally aim to complete these exercises once a month.
- o It is best if you pair up with a work colleague as a 'critical companion' and work through these exercises together, reciprocating each other's companionship.
- o Ideally, these tasks should be completed in 'real-time'. However, this can be inconvenient and discourteous to the patient so the exercises will often be retrospective. If you have the means, retrospective video analysis is an ideal medium to conduct these exercises as your assessment can be paused, re-played, etc to identify your thoughts and actions (remember to get the patient's consent!).
- o This document is for use in conjunction with the Clinical Reasoning in Combined Movement Therapy Reflection Sheet.
- o Your first reflection sheet should be submitted as evidence of your CMT-related CPD. This, and all subsequent sheets, should be kept as your own CPD evidence.

### EXERCISE 1 – PATTERN RECOGNITION

Identify a new patient who you have had no previous contact with. After 5 minutes of the history-taking, excuse yourself and make a list of seven plausible patterns.
Reflection pointers:

- o If you are not able to identify this number, analyze the way you are structuring your history-taking. Are you asking the right type of questions? Are you allowing the patient the right amount of freedom to tell his story? Are there gaps in your biomedical or psychosocial knowledge?
- o Qualify the plausibility of the patterns by later considering their validity based on the exact information you acquired. Were they actually plausible, or just random guesses?

o Remember, patterns could be broad diagnostic ones such as 'nerve root entrapment', 'cervical instability', 'cervical arterial dysfunction (CAD)', 'treatable NMS', or very specific ones such as 'C5 root with C5/C6 hypomobility', 'internal carotid aneurysm', 'left C3/C4 hypomobility, non-irritable, into left side-flexion/rotation/extension', etc. As you develop, try and make the patterns more and more specific.

Over time, this exercise can be progressed by either increasing the number of patterns or reducing the time. Aim for 7+/−2 (depending on the nature and complexity of the patient) in 2 minutes!

## EXERCISE 2 – ILLNESS SCRIPTS

Develop illness scripts for each of the above patterns. Ideally, this should be done in real time before you resume the history-taking. However, this may be practically difficult and unfair to the patient so will have to be done retrospectively.

Remember that an illness script consists of the:

o Enabling condition
o Fault
o Consequences of the fault

Reflection pointers:

o Were you able to provide substantial scripts to each pattern?
o If not, try and identify the gaps in your knowledge base and the reasons for those gaps.
o Record how quickly (or slowly) it took you to complete this task. Did you need substantial assistance/referral to text books etc in completing this task?

## EXERCISE 3 – VALIDATING YOUR KNOWLEDGE

Identify the sources of your knowledge used to complete the illness scripts. Where did this knowledge come from? What is the balance between sources? How valid is your knowledge?

Remember, knowledge can be broadly categorized into:

o Propositional
o Professional craft knowledge (non-propositional)
o Personal knowledge (propositional)

This exercise can be continued throughout the rest of the patient assessment and treatment.

Reflection pointers:

o What were the noticeable gaps in your knowledge base?
o Which sources were heavily relied upon, and which sources were under-used?
o Was the source appropriate for the type of knowledge? For example, if you are considering the best treatment intervention, did the knowledge to use manual therapy come from your reflective interpretation of high quality systematic reviews, or because your mate told you it worked?

## EXERCISE 4 – HYPOTHETICO-DEDUCTIVE REASONING

Continue your pattern-driven line of reasoning by listing under each pattern (which we can now call hypotheses) the best questions which could help you differentiate between the hypotheses. Use these lists to sculpt the rest of the history-taking.

Reflection pointers:

o Were the questions actually useful?
o Where did the questions come from? (Consider knowledge sources again.)
o Was there a sufficient mix of open and closed questions allowing specificity yet enough freedom for the patient to expand their story – did the history-taking 'breathe', i.e. was there a natural undulating feel to the process, or was it a bland, unilateral, monotonous procedure?
o Do you feel confident enough to continue using these questions in future assessments – do they contribute towards your 'stock' or 'library' of differentiating questions?

Remember that each patient interaction is a learning experience and you are going to learn from the patient which questions may be differentiating in the future. For example, what did that patient with the C3/C4 left side-flexion/extension hypomobility say was their worst functional activity? What was the family history of that patient with the carotid aneurysm?

## EXERCISE 5 – PROBABILITY

On reflection of the above processes, attempt to map out the key differentiating or informative details of the history and physical examination and commit yourself to quantifying your subjective opinion on the (pre-test) probability of each suspected diagnosis in line with the principles of conditional, or Bayesian, probability.

Reflection pointers:

o Compare your judgements with those of your companion.
o What accounts for the differences in your opinions?

## EXERCISE 6 – PHYSICAL TESTING UTILITY

Continue the hypothetico-deductive process throughout the physical examination once you have decided which hypotheses have 'survived' the history-taking.

Decide which physical tests you are going to perform and identify at least one to analyze from a diagnostic utility perspective.

You may choose this informally by yourself or with your critical companionship, or more formally as part of, say, an in-service training session, or even as an assignment/

project as part of a post-graduate course. Remember, not all tests used in manual therapy lend themselves to proper utility calculations as a 'gold standard' measure is required to compare clinical findings against. This does not restrict the analysis into a test utility, however. Refer to an article which has examined the utility of a manual therapy test to begin to consider how you may start to think about how good tests are.

Example of a suggested reference:

Ogince, M., Hall, T., Robinson, K., Blackmore, A.M., 2007. The diagnostic validity of the cervical flexion–rotation test in C1/2-related cervicogenic headache. Man. Ther. 12 (3), 256–262.

Reflection pointers:

- o How did you attempt to identify appropriate data?
- o What are the research gaps in this area?
- o Is there potential for more diagnostic study for this test?
- o How might you design a study which would test the utility of a study?

## EXERCISE 7 – INTERPRETATIVE REASONING

Consider what you think were key parts of the patient's story and note these down.

In order to appreciate the different levels of interpretation, discuss with your companion what you thought the patient meant at a superficial level, and then at a deeper level. Reflection pointers:

- o How did the patient's story influence your decisions?
- o How much was the patient involved in the decision-making process?
- o What was the degree of consensus?
- o How could your interaction have been changed to facilitate a greater depth of understanding of the patient's narrative?
- o What was the balance between instrumental and communicative processing within the interaction?
- o What biomedical, psychological, and sociological knowledge did you learn with the patient today?
- o How will today's experience impact on your future interactions with this, and with other patients?

Your understanding of this should be complemented with further reading, e.g.:

Jones, M.A., Edwards, I., 2006. Learning to facilitate change in cognition and behaviour. In: Gifford, L. (ed.), Topical issues in pain 5. CNS Press, Falmouth, pp. 273–310.

# References

Albert, A.D., Munson, R., Resnik, M.D., et al. (eds.), 1988. Reasoning in medicine: an introduction to clinical inference. John Hopkins University Press, Baltimore.

Altman, D.G., Bland, J.M., 1994a. Statistics Notes – Diagnostic-Tests-1 – Sensitivity and Specificity .3. Br. Med. J. 308 (6943), 1552–1557.

Altman, D.G., Bland, J.M., 1994b. Diagnostic-Tests-2 – Predictive Values .4. Br. Med. J. 309 (6947), 102–105.

Barrows, H.S., Feltovitch, P.J., 1987. The clinical reasoning process. Med. Educ. 21, 86–91.

Barrows, H.S., Tamblyn, R.M., 1980. Problem-based learning: an approach to medical education, first ed. Springer, New York.

Boshuizen, H.P.A., Schmidt, H., 2000. The development of clinical reasoning expertise. In: Higgs, J., Jones, M. (eds.), Clinical reasoning in the health professions. Butterworth Heinemann, Edinburgh.

Bouter, L.M., van Tulder, M.W., Maurits, W., et al., 1998.

Methodological issues in low back pain research in primary care. Spine 23 (18), 2014–2020.

Bradnam, L., 2002. Western acupuncture point selection: a scientific clinical reasoning model. Journal of the Acupuncture Association of Chartered Physiotherapists (March), 21–29.

Brannstrom, M., Ekman, I., Norberg, A., et al., 2006. Living with severe chronic heart failure in palliative advanced home care. Eur. J. Cardiovasc. Nurs. 5 (4), 295–302.

Butler, D.S., 2000. Clinicians and their decisions. In: The sensitive nervous system. NOI publications, Unley.

Case, K., Harrison, K., Roskell, C., 2000. Differences in the clinical reasoning process of expert and novice cardiorespiratory physiotherapists. Physiotherapy 85 (1), 14–22.

Chae, Y.M., Kim, H.S., Tark, K.C., et al., 2003. Analysis of healthcare quality indicator using data mining

and decision support system. Expert Systems Appl. 24 (2), 167–172.

Chapple, A., Ziebland, S., McPherson, A., 2006. The specialist palliative care nurse: A qualitative study of the patients' perspective. Int. J. Nurs. Stud. 43 (8), 1011–1022.

Chase, W., Simon, H.A., 1973. Perceptions in chess. Cogn. Psychol. 4, 55–81.

Craik, F.I.M., Lockart, R.S., 1972. Levels of processing: a framework for memory research. Journal of Verbal Learning and Behaviour 11, 671–681.

Crowe, M.T., O'Malley, J., 2006. Teaching critical reflection skills for advanced mental health nursing practice: a deconstructive-reconstructive approach. J. Adv. Nurs. 56 (1), 79–87.

Davidson, M., 2002. The interpretation of diagnostic tests: A primer for physiotherapists. Aust. J. Physiother. 48 (3), 227–232.

Dawkins, R., 2006. The God delusion, first ed. Bantam Press, London.

Deeks, J.J., Altman, D.G., 2004. Statistics notes – Diagnostic tests 4: likelihood ratios. Br. Med. J. 329 (7458), 168–169.

DeGroot, A.D., 1965. Thought and choice in chess, first ed. Mouton, Holland.

DeGroot, A.D., Gobet, F., 1996. Perception and memory in chess. Heuristics of the professional eye. Van Gorcum, Assen.

Doody, C., McAteer, M., 2003. Clinical reasoning of expert and novice physiotherapists in an outpatient orthopaedic setting. Physiotherapy 88 (5), 258–269.

Downing, A.M., Hunter, D.G., 2003. Validating clinical reasoning: a question of perspective, but whose perspective? Man. Ther. 8 (2), 117–119.

Edwards, I., Jones, M., Carr, J., et al., 2004. Clinical reasoning strategies in physical therapy. Phys. Ther. 84 (4), 312–330.

Edwards, I., Jones, M., Hillier, S., 2006. The interpretation of experience and its relationship to body movement: A clinical reasoning perspective. Man. Ther. 11 (1), 2–10.

Elstein, A.S., Shulman, L.S., Sprafka, S.A., et al., 1978. An analysis of clinical reasoning. Harvard University Press, Massachusetts.

Elstein, A.S., Schwarz, A., 2000. Clinical reasoning in medicine. In: Higgs, J., Jones, M. (eds.), Clinical reasoning in the health professions. Butterworth Heinemann, Edinburgh.

Elstein, A.S., Schwarz, A., 2002a. Evidence base of clinical diagnosis – Clinical problem solving and diagnostic decision making: selective review of the cognitive literature. Br. Med. J. 324 (7339), 729–732.

Elstein, A.S., Schwarz, A., 2002b. Clinical problem solving and diagnostic decision making: selective review of the cognitive literature. Br. Med. J. 324, 729–732.

Fang, L., Hipel, K.W., Kilgour, D.M., et al., 2003a. A decision support system for interactive decision making – Part I: Model formulation (Vol 33, p. 42, 2003). IEEE Transactions on Systems Man and Cybernetics Part C-Applications and Reviews 33 (2), 290–300.

Fang, L., Hipel, K.W., Kilgour, D.M., et al., 2003b. Decision support system for interactive decision making – Part II: Analysis and output interpretation (Vol 33, p. 56, 2003). IEEE Transactions on Systems Man and Cybernetics Part C-Applications and Reviews 33 (2), 290–300.

Feltovich, P.J., Barrows, H.S., 1984. Issues of generality in medical problem solving. In: Schmidt, H.G., DeVolder, M.L. (eds.), Tutorials in problem based learning: a new direction in teaching in health professionals. Van Gorcum, London.

Feynman, R.P., 1995. Six easy pieces – the fundamentals of physics explained, third ed. Penguin, London.

Fleming, M.H., Mattingly, C., 2000. Action and narrative: two dynamics of clinical reasoning. In: Higgs, J., Jones, M.A. (eds.), Clinical reasoning in the health professions. Butterworth Heinemann, Edinburgh.

Gevitz, N., 2006. Centre or periphery? The future of osteopathic principles and practices. Journal of American Osteopathy Association 106, 121–129.

Gifford, L.S., 1998. The mature organism model. In: Gifford, L.S. (ed.), Topical issues in pain 1. CNS Press, Falmouth.

Gilbert, R., Logan, S., Moyer, V.A., et al., 2001a. Assessing diagnostic and screening tests: Part 1. Concepts. West. J. Med. 174 (6), 405–409.

Gilbert, R., Logan, S., Moyer, V.A., et al., 2001b. Assessing diagnostic and screening tests: Part 2. How to use the research literature on diagnosis. West. J. Med. 175 (1), 37–41.

Gobet, F., 1998. Expert memory: a comparison of four theories. Cognition 66 (2), 115–152.

Gobet, F., Simon, H.A., 1998. Pattern recognition makes search possible: Comments on Holding (1992). Psychol. Res.-Psychol. Forsch. 61 (3), 204–208.

Gobet, F., Wood, D., 1999. Expertise, models of learning and computer-based tutoring. Comput. Educ. 33 (2–3), 189–207.

Groen, G., Patel, L., 1985. Medical problem solving: some questionable assumptions. Med. Educ. 19, 95–100.

Gross, A.R., Chesworth, B., Binkley, J., 2005. A case for evidence based practice in manual therapy. In: Boyling, J.D., Jull, G.A. (eds.), Grieve's modern manual therapy – The vertebral column. Churchill Livingstone, Edinburgh.

Guo, P.J., Zeng, D.Z., Shishido, H., 2002. Group decision with inconsistent knowledge. IEEE Transactions on Systems Man and Cybernetics Part a-Systems and Humans 32 (6), 670–679.

Harbison, J., 2006. Clinical judgment in the interpretation of evidence: a Bayesian approach. J. Clin. Nurs. 15, 1489–1497.

Heisenberg, W., 1983. The physical content of quantum kinematics and mechanics. In: Wheeler, J.A., Zuvek, W.H. (eds.), Quantum theory and mechanics. Oxford University Press, New York.

Herbert, R., Jamtvedt, G., Mead, J., et al., 2005. Can I trust this evidence? In: Practical Evidence-Based Physiotherapy (Chapter 5). Elsevier, London, pp. 106–111.

Higgs, J., Jones, M., 2000. Clinical reasoning in the health professions. In: Higgs, J., Jones, M. (eds.), Clinical reasoning in the health professions. Butterworth Heinemann, Edinburgh.

Higgs, J., Jones, M.A., 1995. Clinical Reasoning in the Health Professions, first ed. Butterworth Heinemann, Oxford.

Higgs, J., Richardson, B., Dahlgren, M.A., et al., 2004. Developing practice knowledge for health professionals. Butterworth Heinemann, Edinburgh.

Higgs, J., Titchen, A., 2000. Knowledge and reasoning. In: Higgs, J., Jones, M. (eds.), Clinical reasoning in the health professions. Butterworth Heinemann, Edinburgh.

James, G., 2001. Clinical reasoning in novices: refining a research question. British Journal of Therapy and Rehabilitation 8 (8), 286–291.

Jensen, G.M., Gwyer, J., Shepard, K.F., et al., 2000. Expert practice in physical therapy – Response. Phys. Ther. 80 (1), 49–52.

Jensen, G.M., Gwyer, J., Hack, L.M., et al., 2007. Expertise in physical therapy practice. Saunders, Missouri.

Jette, D.U., Grover, L., Keck, C.P., 2003. A qualitative study of clinical decision making in recommending discharge placement from the acute care setting. Phys. Ther. 83 (3), 224–236.

Johnson, M.R., Goode, C.D., Penny, W., et al., 2001. Lesson of the week – Playing the odds in clinical decision making: lessons from berry aneurysms undetected by magnetic resonance angiography. Br. Med. J. 322 (7298), 1347–1349.

Jones, C., Harvey, A.G., Brewin, C.R., 2006. The organisation and content of trauma memories in survivors of road traffic accidents. Behav. Res. Ther. 45 (1), 151–162.

Jones, M.A., 1994. Clinical reasoning process in manipulative therapy. In: Boyling, J.D., Palastanga, N. (eds.), Grieve's Modern Manual Therapy. Churchill Livingstone, London.

Jones, M.A., 1995. Clinical reasoning and pain. Man. Ther. 1 (1), 17–24.

Jones, M.A., 1997a. Clinical reasoning: the foundation of clinical practice. Part 1. Aust. J. Physiother. 43 (3), 167–170.

Jones, M.A., 1997b. Clinical reasoning: the foundation of clinical practice. Part 2. Aust. J. Physiother. 43 (3), 213–217.

Jones, M.A., 1997c. Clinical reasoning: the foundation of clinical practice. Part 3. Aust. J. Physiother. 43 (4), 299–303.

Jones, M.A., 1999. Orthopaedic expert practice. In: Jensen, G.M. et al., (ed.), Expertise in physical therapy practice. Butterworth Heinemann, Oxford.

Jones, M.A., Edwards, I., 2006. Learning to facilitate change in cognition and behaviour. In: Gifford, L. (ed.), Topical issues in pain 5. CNS Press, Falmouth.

Jones, M.A., Rivett, D.A., 2005. Principles of clinical reasoning in manual therapy. In: Jones, M., Rivett, D.A. (eds.), Clinical reasoning for manual therapists. Butterworth Heinemann, London.

Kaminker, M.K., Chiarello, L.A., O'Neil, M.E., et al., 2004. Decision making for physical therapy service delivery in schools: A nationwide survey of pediatric physical therapists. Phys. Ther. 84 (10), 919–933.

Kempainen, R., Migeon, M.B., Wolf, F.M., et al., 2003. Understanding our mistakes: a primer on errors in clinical reasoning. Med. Teach. 25 (2), 177–181.

King, C.M., Bithell, C., 1998. Expertise in diagnostic reasoning: a comparative study. British Journal of Therapy and Rehabilitation 5 (2), 78–87.

Knottnerus, J.A., van Weel, C., Muris, J.W., 2002. Evidence base of clinical diagnosis – Evaluation of diagnostic procedures. Br. Med. J. 324 (7335), 477–480.

Kopelman, R.I., Wong, J.B., Pauker, S.G., 1999. A little math helps the medicine go down. N. Engl. J. Med. 341 (6), 435–439.

Ladyshewsky, R., 2002. A quasi-experimental study of the differences in performance and clinical reasoning using individual learning versus reciprocal peer coaching. Physiother. Theory Pract. 18 (1), 17–31.

Marlow, T., 2006. Bayesian probabilities and the histories algebra. International Journal of Theoretical Physics 45 (7), 1289–1299.

Mattingly, C., 1998. In search of the good: narrative reasoning in clinical practice. Med. Anthropol. Q. 12 (3), 273–297.

Mezirow, J., 2000. Learning to think like an adult. Core concepts of transformation theory. In: Mezirow, J. (ed.), Learning as transformation. Critical perspectives on a theory in progress. Jossey-Bass, San Francisco.

Neisser, U., 1998. Stories, selves, and schematas: a review of ecological findings. In: Conway, M.A. et al., (eds.), Theories of memory: volume 2. Psychology Press, Hove.

Niskanen, V.A., 1999. The Fuzzy Metric-Truth reasoning approach to decision making in soft computing milieux. International Journal of General Systems 28 (2–3), 139–172.

Parry, A., 1997. New paradigms for old: musings on the shape of clouds. Physiotherapy 83 (8), 423–433.

Pewsner, D., Battaglia, D., Minder, C., et al., 2004. Ruling a diagnosis in or out with 'SpPIn' and 'SnNOut': a note of caution. Br. Med. J. 329 (7459), 209–213.

Pincus, T., 2004. The psychology of pain. In: French, S., Sim, J. (eds.), Physiotherapy: a psychosocial approach. Elsevier, Edinburgh.

Pincus, T., Morley, S., 2001. Cognitive-processing bias in chronic pain: A review and integration. Psychol. Bull. 127 (5), 599–617.

Popper, K., 1980. The logic of scientific discovery, fourth ed. Routledge, London.

Resnik, L., Hart, D.L., 2003. Using clinical outcomes to identify expert physical therapists. Phys. Ther. 83 (11), 990–1002.

Resnik, L., Jensen, G.M., 2003. Using clinical outcomes to explore the theory of expert practice in physical therapy. Phys. Ther. 83 (12), 1090–1106.

Richardson, B., 1993. Practice, research and education – what is the link? Physiotherapy 79 (5), 317–322.

Ritcher, R., Reinking, M.F., 2005. Clinical Question: How does evidence on the diagnostic accuracy of the vertebral artery test influence teaching of the test in a professional physical therapist education program? Phys. Ther. http://www.ptjournal.org/PTJournal/Jun2005/Jun05_EiP.cfm.

Rivett, D.A., Jones, M., 2004. Improving clinical reasoning in manual therapy. In: Jones, M., Rivett, D.A. (eds.), Clinical reasoning for manual therapists. Butterworth-Heinemann, London.

Robertson, L., 1996. Clinical reasoning, part 2: novice/expert differences. British Journal of Occupational Therapy 59 (5), 212–216.

Roskell, C., Cross, V., 2001. Defining expertise in cardiorespiratory physiotherapy. British Journal of Therapy and Rehabilitation 8 (8), 294–299.

Rothstein, J.M., Echternach, J.L., Riddle, D.L., 2003. The Hypothesis-Oriented Algorithm for Clinicians II (HOAC II): A guide for patient management. Phys. Ther. 83 (5), 455–470.

Round, A., 2001. Introduction to clinical reasoning. J. Eval. Clin. Pract. 7 (2), 109–117.

Sackett, D.L., Haynes, R.B., 2002. Evidence base of clinical diagnosis - The architecture of diagnostic research. Br. Med. J. 324 (7336), 539–541.

Schnelker, D.L., 2006. The student-as-bricoleur: Making sense of research paradigms. Teaching and Teacher Education 22 (1), 42–57.

Schon, D.A., 1991. The reflective practitioner: how professionals think in action. Ashgate, Aldershot.

Scott, I., 2000. Teaching clinical reasoning: a case-based approach. In: Higgs, M.A., Jones, M.A. (eds.), Clinical reasoning in the health professions. Butterworth Heinemann, Edinburgh.

Sefton, A., Gordon, J., Field, M., et al., 2000. Teaching clinical reasoning to medical students. In: Higgs, J., Jones, M.A. (eds.), Clinical reasoning in the health professions. Butterworth Heinemann, Edinburgh.

Simon, H.A., 1980. Problem solving and education. In: Tuma, D.T., Reif, F. (eds.), Problem solving and education: issues in teaching and research. Erlbaum, Hillside.

Singer, K.P., 2000. Manual therapy and science: a marriage of convenience? Man. Ther. 5 (2), 61–62.

Smart, K., Doody, C., 2006. Mechanisms-based clinical reasoning of pain by experienced musculoskeletal physiotherapists. Physiotherapy 92 (3), 171–178.

Steiner, W.A., Ryser, L., Huber, E., et al., 2002. Use of the ICF model as a clinical problem-solving tool in physical therapy and rehabilitation medicine. Phys. Ther. 82 (11), 1098–1107.

Stratford, P.W., 2001. Applying the results from diagnostic accuracy studies to enhance clinical decision-making. Physiother. Theory Pract. 17, 153–160.

Strauss, S.E., Richardson, W.S., Glasziou, P., et al., 2005. Evidence-based medicine: how to teach and practice EBM. Elsevier Churchill Livingstone, Edinburgh.

Swisher, L., 2002. A retrospective analysis of ethics knowledge in physical therapy. Phys. Ther. 82 (7), 692–706.

Tien, J.M., 2003. Toward a decision informatics paradigm: A real-time, information-based approach to decision making. IEEE Transactions on Systems Man and Cybernetics Part C-Applications and Reviews 33 (1), 102–113.

Titchen, A., Higgs, J., 2000. Facilitating the acquisition of knowledge for reasoning. In: Higg, J., Joness, M.A. (eds.), Clinical reasoning in the health professions. Butterworth Heinemann, Edinburgh.

Unwin, S., 2003. The probability of God: a simple calculation that proves the ultimate truth. Crown Forum, New York.

Weaver, N., Murtagh, M.J., Thomson, R.G., 2006. How do newly diagnosed hypertensives understand 'risk'? Narratives used in coping with risk. Family Practitioner 23 (6), 637–643.

Welch, A., Dawson, P., 2006. Closing the gap: collaborative learning as a strategy to embed evidence within occupational therapy practice. J. Eval. Clin. Pract. 12 (2), 227–238.

West, A.F., West, R.R., 2002. Clinical decision-making: coping with uncertainty. Postgrad. Med. J. 78 (920), 319–321.

Wiitavaara, B., Barnekow-Bergkvist, M., Brulin, C., 2006. Striving for balance: a grounded theory study of health experiences of nurses with musculoskeletal problems. Int. J. Nurs. Stud.

Windish, D.M., Price, E.G., Clever, S.L., et al., 2005. Teaching medical students the important connection between communication and clinical reasoning. J. Gen. Intern. Med. 20 (12), 1108–1113.

Zhou, L., Friedman, C., Parsons, S., et al., 2005. System architecture for temporal information extraction, representation and reasoning in clinical narrative reports. American Medics Informatics Association Annual Symposium Proceedings 869–873.

# Chapter Four

4

# The principles of combined movement assessment

Chris McCarthy

## CHAPTER CONTENTS

The purpose of clinical examination is not simply to gather as much information as is possible in the time available. Often the inexperienced clinician can spend an entire examination gathering data with little evaluation of its clinical relevance. As manual therapists we provide our patients with incredibly sensitive examinations. The volume and sophistication of our examination procedures is immense. However, we may occasionally fail to grasp the problem of specificity. We must find a balance between gathering enough information to prioritize the patient's most significant dysfunction whilst not being distracted by the less relevant dysfunctions we discover.

We are essentially searching for the patient's 'predominant dysfunction or fault' in order to direct our intervention towards it. The process of ranking the importance of our findings requires that we test the hypothesis of 'predominant dysfunction' throughout our interaction with our patients. In short, during the examination of patients we are considering if our hypothesis will guide treatment more effectively than the next most likely hypothesis. In addition, during treatment we should be continually considering if our chosen intervention is in fact more effective than the next most likely intervention. This process of analytical assessment is not new and was advocated by Maitland (1986) and Grieve (1988, 1991) over 30 years ago.

Simply gathering huge quantities of information that is neither discriminatory nor influential in management represents a failure in our duty of care to our patients. The purpose of clinical examination is to evaluate valid information that will facilitate the prioritization of likely diagnoses and strategies of management. In other words, our duty to our patients is to ensure we are identifying their predominant dysfunction/fault and to continually ensure that we are providing the most effective management strategy at the time. Ensuring we adhere to this principle will ensure we are facilitating recovery as quickly as possible. It could be argued that the primary objective of manual therapy is to facilitate recovery as quickly as possible. On the whole, the conservative management of most musculoskeletal dysfunctions will facilitate recovery. Manual therapy's role is in the acceleration of this process. Thus, ensuring our treatment choice is making more difference, more quickly than the next most likely choice of treatment is a crucial responsibility.

# Subjective examination

During the initial consultation the therapist will begin to form an impression of the patient based on verbal and non-verbal communication. Expert clinicians form an impression regarding diagnosis, management and expectations of the patient very quickly. Mixed methods of clinical reasoning are utilized in this process as outlined in Chapter 3.

The diverse nature of musculoskeletal dysfunction rarely allows the definitive identification of definitive patterns of presentation. The clinician is frequently required to make reasoned judgements as to the predominant dysfunction from several alternatives. Some of the typical judgements required are listed below. This is by no means an exhaustive list. The process of establishing that one treatment approach is superior to another begins during the initial consultation with the patient. Early in the initial interview with a patient, the therapist should look for answers to the following questions.

### Is this patient's presentation suitable for a manual therapy approach?

- Is this patient presentation sounding like I should explore further with an assessment of biomechanical dysfunction?
- Does this patient's presentation suggest that a more psychosocial approach may elicit effective treatment strategies?

### Which patterns of presentation does this presentation match with?

- Does the presentation fit a pattern of presentation I have encountered before?
- If so, what is it that makes this patient's presentation fit this pattern better than the next most likely pattern?
- What questions and tests do I need to use to test this hypothesis?

### Does the functional fault have a directional quality?

- In what combination of positions are symptoms reproduced?
- In what combination of positions are symptoms reduced?

### What is the likely source of the directional fault?

- Does the presentation have predominantly arthrogenic features?

- Does the presentation have predominantly myogenic features?
- Does the presentation have predominantly neurodynamic features?

### Is this predominantly a control or impairment fault?

- Does the presentation suggest a dysfunction in control of movement?
- Does the presentation suggest a dysfunction associated with limitation (or impairment) of movement?

### Is it acceptable to reproduce symptoms – are they 'severe'?

- Is the faulty position producing severe pain?
- Is positioning in the faulty position likely to cause a latent or long-term exacerbation of symptoms?
- Is there a position that will allow examination and treatment whilst avoiding unacceptable symptom reproduction?
- Is it likely that caution needs to be taken due to a patho-anatomical reason that would make the use of combined movement theory (CMT) unwise? See the contraindications to manual therapy in the box below.

### What is the predominant pain mechanism?

- Is the patient's predominant pain mechanism: nociceptive, peripheral neurogenic, central sensitivity, autonomic or affective?

A proforma planning sheet can be found on the CD. See Figure 4.1.

Prior to the conduct of a physical examination using the CMT approach the patient should be informed of your plans and the risks and benefits of the approach against other approaches.

By examining the expectations of the patient the suitability of utilizing a CMT approach can be established. If the patient's expectations of treatment are radically different to the therapist's, a discussion of future management should ensue. A detailed biomechanical assessment of spinal dysfunction may be unwarranted if the patient is expecting and consenting only to generic advice and exercise.

## Clinical point

### Contraindications to spinal passive movement that takes a joint to the end of passive range or thrust techniques

### Bone

Any pathology that has led to significant bone weakening:

- Tumour, e.g. metastatic deposits
- Infection, e.g. tuberculosis
- Metabolic, e.g. osteomalacia
- Congenital, e.g. dysplasias
- Iatrogenic, e.g. long-term corticosteroid medication
- Inflammatory, e.g. severe rheumatoid arthritis
- Traumatic, e.g. fracture

### Neurological

- Spinal cord compression
- Cauda equina compression
- Nerve root compression with increasing neurological deficit

### Vascular

- Aortic aneurysm
- Bleeding into joints, e.g. severe haemophilia
- Cervical artery dysfunction (Kerry et al, 2008a, 2008b)

### Relative contraindications

Special consideration should be given prior to the use of spinal manipulative thrust techniques in the following circumstances:

- Adverse reactions to previous manual therapy
- Disc herniation or prolapse
- Inflammatory arthritides
- Pregnancy
- Spondylolysis
- Spondylolisthesis
- Osteoporosis
- Anticoagulant or long-term corticosteroid use
- Advanced degenerative joint disease and spondylosis
- Psychological dependence upon spinal manipulative thrust techniques
- Ligamentous laxity
- Arterial calcification
- Hypertension (diastolic >95) in cervical manual therapy

(See Gibbons & Tehan, 2001a,b; Grieve, 1991.)

### Is the patient suitable for a biomechanical assessment of their movement fault?

Patient presentations suggestive of a predominant mechanical influence on symptoms are suitable for detailed biomechanical assessment and treatment.

Presentations that do not feature mechanical/movement influences on symptomology suggest that specific positions and movements may not be the predominant influences to be addressed during examination and treatment. Thus, patients who have constant symptoms, regardless of positioning, will be unlikely to benefit from management with a positional bias. Patients with central sensitization or inflammatory neurogenic pathology ('irritable' patients (Maitland, 1985) have no mechanical predominance.

### How acceptable is it to reproduce symptoms?

Patients, seeking manual therapy, present with pain and largely judge their improvement by an amelioration of their pain. In the process of assessing the effect of testing and treatment, changes in pain are assessed. However, in cases where pain is severe, it is unacceptable to reproduce pain and inappropriate to treat an underlying mechanical dysfunction whilst reproducing pain. Thus, prior to any physical testing the therapist must be clear regarding the degree to which pain is to be reproduced during their interaction with the patient. In certain presentations it may be deemed acceptable to fully reproduce the minor discomfort the patient is seeking help for, in order to fully relieve it. However, in situations where pain is severe this is unacceptable. Using positions that can reduce the likelihood of reproducing severe pain is one of the key advantages of CMT.

## Clinical relevance

If it is not acceptable to reproduce symptoms, the condition is severe. If it is acceptable it is not. Use a nominal (yes/no) approach to this decision and your clinical reasoning will be decisive and more reasonable.

### What is the functional demonstration of the positional fault?

Patient presentations, suggestive of the suitability of a CMT approach, have symptoms predominantly influenced by specific positions or movements. Patients can often demonstrate these movements or positions and reproduce them in the course of replicating a functional activity. For example, patients with anterior stretch patterns of the mid cervical spine often relate symptom reproduction with activities inducing ipsilateral lateral flexion and rotation, e.g. reversing the car. The monitoring of change in the functional demonstration, during examination and treatment is a crucial monitor of treatment effectiveness. Again, the concept of a functional demonstration is a long-established tenet of the Maitland concept (Maitland, 1986) and at the heart of CMT.

### What is the region of the spine that is likely to be faulty?

The biomechanical interpretation of patient presentation can allow the therapist to judge the location of regions of dysfunction. Careful questioning can elicit functional activities that influence specific regions of the spine. For example, the influence of breathing on thoracic movement can provide valuable inference towards spinal or rib dysfunctions.

### What is the predominant hypothesis for the source and mechanism of symptom production and the next most likely hypothesis that will be tested against it?

It is crucial to form hypotheses regarding the underlying source and mechanism of symptom production as you recognize presentation patterns. As a pattern of presentation begins to emerge the use of follow-up questions will establish a good fit with this pattern. Having identified a match with a recognizable pattern, the manual therapist should test the assumption that this hypothesis is predominant by comparing the match with the next most likely pattern. For example, having established that a patient's presentation matched an 'arthrogenic' presentation, one would expect the presentation to be less well matched with a 'myogenic' presentation. In order to facilitate this process it can be useful to develop a library of 'stock' questions and tests for common presentations.

The use of these strategies will facilitate the therapist's reasoning regarding the appropriateness of using CMT, the most likely hypotheses for aetiology of symptoms, the extent and direction of movements to be included in the examination and most importantly the starting positions in which assessment and treatment will be undertaken.

Figure 4.1 shows a suggested planning sheet for use in clinical reasoning during the CMT examination.

## Physical examination

The objective examination will follow the subjective examination and is conducted in light of the considerations and clinical reasoning process outlined in this book. The object of the physical examination is not to form a long list of impairments with little evidence of their relative contribution to the patient's dysfunction. The physical examination should allow the hypotheses, generated following the subjective examination, to be tested. Thus, the examination should be structured to allow this process to occur. In order to assess the influence of the testing procedures themselves on a patient's dysfunction the physical examination should be split into components.

The order in which components of the examination are conducted will be guided by the subjective examination. A clinician may hypothesize that the predominant mechanism of symptom production is related to a restriction in articular mobility rather than, e.g. a restriction in overlying muscle mobility. In this case, the examination would be structured to examine the articular system, assess its influence on the fault, and then assess the muscular influence and reassess that system's influence on the fault. In this way, in addition to gathering information from each component of the examination the relative influence of the components can be evaluated.

Each component begins with an assessment of movement fault (using the patient's functional demonstration), testing procedures and a subsequent reassessment of functional demonstration. See Figure 4.2.

## Observation

Observation of static posture can give valuable insight into the likely mechanical presentation of symptoms with movement. A number of static features will help in the interpretation of active movement. A deep skin crease may suggest hypermobility at the level whilst flat sections with reduced muscle bulk may suggest hypomobility. Defined muscle borders may indicate hypertonicity whilst unilateral atrophy may indicate local neuropraxia or trophic change. See Figure 4.3.

## Functional demonstration

The functional demonstration is the term given to the combination of plane movements that the patient has identified to take them into their most aggravating position. This position identifies the movement fault, whilst the quality, range and speed of movement from neutral into this position and return, should be analyzed in depth. The combination of physiological movements that constitute the functional demonstration will provide invaluable information about the starting position that should be adopted for passive movement assessment and treatment. In addition, the three-dimensional components of this position will identify the movements

| OBJECTIVE EXAMINATION PLAN |
|---|

**List your hypotheses for the nature of the condition.**

.........................................................................................................................................................................

.........................................................................................................................................................................

.........................................................................................................................................................................

**Which two hypotheses will you test against each other in the initial physical examination?**

Primary ................................................................................................................................................................

Secondary ..........................................................................................................................................................

**Is the nature of the condition severe?**

Yes ☐          No ☐

**Is the nature of the condition irritable?**

Yes ☐          No ☐

**To what point are you allowing movement to occur?**

Before pain          ☐
To pain              ☐
To end               ☐

**What is your functional demonstration/re-test marker?**

.........................................................................................................................................................................

**What is the primary pain mechanism of this patient's condition?**

Nociceptive                  ☐
Peripheral neurogenic        ☐
Central                      ☐
Autonomic                    ☐
Affective                    ☐

**To what extent will you perform a neurological exam?**

None required                                                          ☐
Local peripheral                                                       ☐
Lower motor neuron, upper motor neuron, limbs                          ☐
Lower motor neuron, upper motor neuron, limbs and cranial              ☐

**What is the weighting of the following components of the problem?**

|  | % |
|---|---|
| Arthrogenic |  |
| Myogenic |  |
| Neurogenic |  |
| Inflammagenic |  |
| Psychogenic |  |
| Sociogenic |  |
| Pathogenic |  |
| Viscerogenic |  |
| Osteogenic |  |

**Radar plot**

Arthrogenic, Myogenic, Neurogenic, Inflammagenic, Psychogenic, Sociogenic, Pathogenic, Viscerogenic, Osteogenic — 100 / 50 / 0

**Likely first treatment:**

In: ..................................................................................................................................................................

Will: ................................................................................................................................................................

**Comments/cautions:**

.........................................................................................................................................................................

.........................................................................................................................................................................

**Figure 4.1 •** Clinical reasoning form.

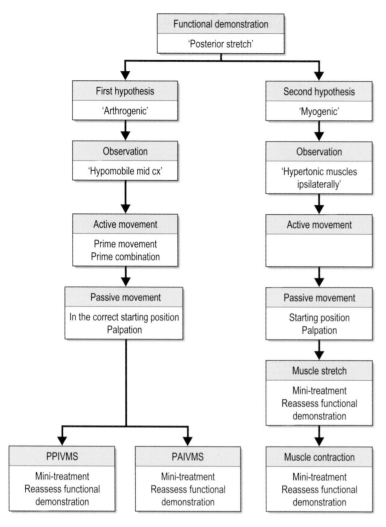

Figure 4.2 • A flow chart showing the suggested compartmentalization of the physical examination. The functional demonstration is at the head of the differentiation. Two common differentiations are displayed: primary arthrogenic versus primary myogenic.

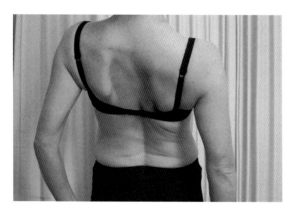

**Figure 4.3** • Active extension, right rotation, showing hypomobility of L5, L4, with movement (and skin crease) at L3. IN: standing; DID: active extension of lumbar spine. Segmental restriction of L4/L5 demonstrated.

that should be examined in isolation. Change in the range of movement and pain experienced in the functional demonstration position will most accurately reflect overall improvement in the patient's impairment.

## Active movements

Active movements should be carefully controlled by the therapist. It is important that the patient moves to a point in range that is appropriate for their severity and nature. Simply asking a patient to extend their back will not give adequate guidance about how acceptable it is to reproduce their pain. A patient with very severe pain may be eager to please the therapist and extend beyond the onset of pain causing an exacerbation, or alternatively, may be fearful of movement and not move to the point that reproduces symptoms. Variability on interpretation of incomplete commands will lead to difficulties with the reliability of testing. Thus, clear commands regarding how far to move in relation to reproduction of symptoms should be included in the commands. A decision about how acceptable it is to reproduce symptoms will need to have been made prior to undertaking this section of the examination.

## Degree of symptom reproduction deemed acceptable

Having agreed on this the therapist must use clear commands to instruct the movement conducted:

- If the agreed degree of symptom reproduction is nil, then at the completion of a combination of movements, the therapist's command should state clearly 'stop before the pain starts'.
- If the agreed degree of symptom reproduction is full, then at the completion of a combination of movements, the therapist's command should be 'move as far as you possibly can'.
- If the agreed degree of symptom reproduction is partial then at the completion of a combination of movements, the therapist's command should be 'stop when the pain starts'.

Good control of symptom reproduction will enable the combination of movements needed to fully assess the patient's movement dysfunction. Disregard of this important control will lead to situations where the patient's symptoms are exacerbated or under-evaluated.

### Clinical point

If the patient has severe pain at rest the examination will be aimed at finding the movement and position that most reduces pain and it will typically involve finding starting positions for assessment and treatment in the quadrant opposite to the dysfunctional quadrant.

## Prime movement and prime combination

Whilst observing active movements, particular attention should be paid to ensuring that the patient moves areas of the spine that are impaired. Very often a patient will have developed hypermobility above a

hypomobile section of the spine. The patient can find it difficult to move the hypomobile segments as they move at areas presenting the least resistance to movement and move only at the hyper-mobile segments. This can lead to a situation where symptoms are not reproduced as the symptomatic levels are not being tested, during the test movement. False negatives can occur unless this error in clinical reasoning is considered. Consequently, it is important to guide patients to move at regions you consider likely to be symptomatic during active movement testing. See Figures 4.4, 4.5 and 4.6.

The active movement examination is structured to examine the movements most relevant for the patient's impairment. The functional demonstration will have provided the examiner with evidence that certain movements are more important in reproducing the dysfunction than others. The functional demonstration position will justify a detailed examination of the three movements that constitute it. The next stage in examining the biomechanical features of the impairment is to examine each of the three components of the position to establish which

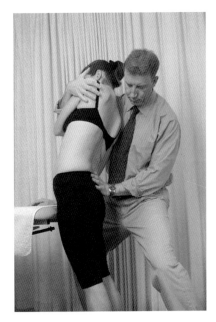

**Figure 4.4** • Active movement of the lumbar spine. Here, movement of the stiff L4/L5, L5/S1 segment is facilitated by fixing the sacrum with one hand whilst guiding movement to the low lumbar spine. IN: Standing, bed edge support, lumbar extension; DID: active right lateral flexion, range assessment. Note the wide stance required to ensure balance.

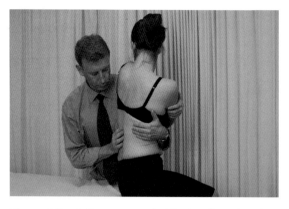

**Figure 4.5** • Active movement of the low thoracic spine. Here, movement of the stiff T10/T11 segment is facilitated by fixing the lumbar spine with one hand whilst guiding movement to the low thoracic spine. IN: sitting, lumbar neutral; DID: active left rotation, low thoracic range assessment.

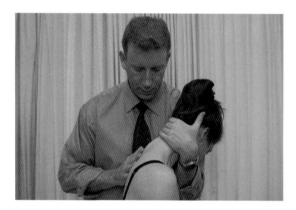

**Figure 4.6** • Active, guided low cervical flexion. IN: sitting, cervical flexion; DID: active assisted left rotation of the low cervical spine. The patient is given feedback on where to move.

two movements are the most important, and within these two movements, which is of primary importance or 'prime movement'.

The primary movement has an importance within CMT in both the classification of syndromes and in selection of starting positions for treatment. The movement itself is defined as being the movement that either reproduces the patient's signs and/or symptoms most completely (when it is appropriate to do so) or most completely relieves symptoms when the condition is too severe to reproduce symptoms.

Having established the prime movement in one plane it should be explored by repeating the movement when combined with another movement, in

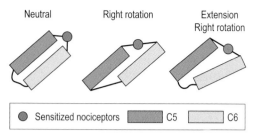

**Figure 4.7** • The illustration shows the selective tension of articular and peri-articular tissue with progressive addition of three planes of movement. A progressive increase in anterior stretch is observed with the addition of extension to right rotation (right rotation being coupled with right lateral flexion).

another plane, which will move one side of the motion segment in the same direction.

In a simplified model of spinal biomechanics extension, ipsilateral rotation and ipsilateral lateral flexion will cause the superior joint facet to move down the inferior segment's joint facet (see Fig. 4.7). Flexion, contralateral flexion and contralateral rotation will cause the superior facet to move up the inferior segment's joint facet. For example, right rotation is the patient's prime movement, reproducing right-sided neck pain. Exploring this movement by examining right rotation in extension and extension in right rotation will elicit which combination is the *primary combination*. The prime combination will closely resemble the patient's functional demonstration.

The primary combination holds a crucial place in CMT as it is the starting position where passive movement assessment is conducted. By positioning the spine in the position of dysfunction the addition of passive movements will be more influential in reproducing symptoms and more likely to alter movement dysfunction than if conducted in a neutral position. Passive movement conducted in neutral will rarely be sufficient to reproduce symptoms adequately. When performed in a position related to dysfunction, the application of passive movement or muscle contraction will provide valuable information on, not only the quality and control of movement, but also the effect of the test on the dysfunction.

Finding the primary combination is the process by which the clinician can be sure that passive movement testing will be the most informative and that treatment in this position will have the quickest effect on dysfunction. A two-dimensional equivalent would be the need to assess and treat a patient with a 10° loss of elbow extension at this position, not at 90° of elbow flexion (the equivalent of assessing in neutral).

## Muscle assessment

The assessment of muscular influences on the spinal dysfunction should involve an assessment of muscular activity (tone) in the primary combination starting position. The degree and location of hypertonicity can be readily palpated in local, deep paraspinal muscles and the overlaying, superficial, musculature (see Figs 4.8 and 4.9). At this point an assessment for trigger points (Travell & Simmons, 1998) can be

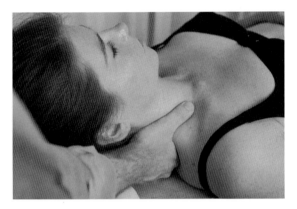

**Figure 4.8** • Palpation of anterior paraspinal muscles, fascia and neurovasular structures. IN: supine, neutral; DID: palpation of anterior low cervical musculature. Special care must be taken to ensure that the flat of the thumb is used – to avoid painful pressure.

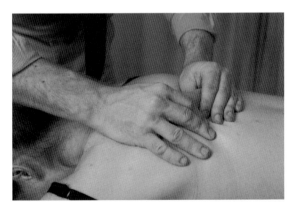

**Figure 4.9** • Palpation of upper thoracic soft tissue tone. IN: prone, neutral; DID: soft tissue tension palpation, upper thoracic spine. Firm pressure will be needed to pick and work through the superficial musculature. Bands of resistance to movement will be palpated.

**Table 4.1  Listing the musculature that becomes over or under-active in common spinal pain syndromes (Chaitow, 2006)**

| Short/facilitated/over recruited | Long/inhibited/under recruited |
|---|---|
| Occipital extensors | Upper cervical flexors (rectus capitis anterior) |
| Sternocleidomastoid | Deep cervical flexors (longus colli) |
| Scalenes | Low cervical extensors (iliocostalis) |
| Upper trapezius | Lower/middle fibres of trapezius |
| Levator scapulae | Subscapularis |
| Rhomboids | Serratus anterior |
| Pectoralis minor | |
| Pectoralis major | |
| Latissimus dorsi | |
| Iliopsoas | Gluteal muscles |
| Tensor fascia latae | Abdominal muscles |
| Quadratus lumborum | |

conducted, followed by an assessment of extensibility (Chaitow, 2006) of the superficial phasic muscles that have a tendency to become hypertonic in the presence of spinal pain. See Table 4.1.

During this process, hypertonic muscles are passively lengthened either locally, globally or both and a temporary reflexogenic reduction in muscular activity can be induced. Consequently, these tests are effectively mini-treatments of the muscular system.

The effect of this mini-treatment on the patient's functional demonstration can be immediately assessed. In this way the relative contribution of the myogenic system can be assessed against the arthrogenic system by mini-treating first one system and then another. See Figures 4.10 and 4.11.

## Passive movement and mini-treatments

Having established the optimal position to induce passive movement at the motion segments moving dysfunctionally, an assessment is made to determine which passive movement will be the most effective

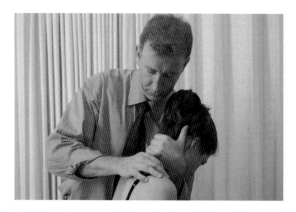

**Figure 4.10 •** Post-isometric relaxation technique for the right, posterior paraspinals. IN: sitting, thoracic flexion; DID: isometric contraction resisting left rotation of T1 on T2. The patient is told to 'Don't let me win' as the neck is moved towards more flexion and rotation. The patient will contract the extensors and right rotators. An isometric contraction can be held for 6–10 seconds.

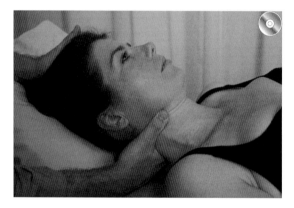

**Figure 4.11 •** Post-isometric relaxation technique for the right, anterior paraspinal muscles. IN: supine, neutral extension; DID: isometric contraction resisting extension and right rotation. The patient performs an isometric contraction in response to AP pressure. Contraction of the right anterior musculature is produced. **See video clip number 4**

at reducing the dysfunction. This will involve deciding between accessory and physiological passive movement and between particular combinations of both. One method of deciding between two likely treatment options is to compare the immediate effectiveness of using the treatments. Even a short period of treatment, if applied in the correct starting position, will have an immediate effect on movement dysfunction. The patient will be able to discriminate between the treatment effects and tell you which treatment to use!

Mini-treatment requires a degree of skill to perform. Whilst the treatment is of a short duration, in order to fit into the assessment process without becoming too time consuming, it must be enough of a 'dose' of treatment to evoke a change in muscle activity and/or joint mobility. Thus, the examiner needs the palpatory skill to be able to tell when these features have subtly changed. With practice the skilled manual therapist can be as confident in discriminating this change in mobility as they have in their ability to discriminate between a normal or hypomobile joint on initial assessment.

If we really are striving to provide treatment that is the most efficacious option we must prove that the specific treatment we are proposing is indeed more effective at reducing the dysfunction than the next most likely option. Testing one treatment against another is something we do whilst treating patients, however, the incorporation of this principle during the assessment process is of particular importance with the CMT approach.

## Assessing for the suitability of manipulative thrust techniques

Local movement impairment, specific to one or two spinal segments, can present with hypomobility in the contralateral side glide that accompanies ipsilateral lateral flexion and rotation. Acute muscle spasm or long-standing movement impairment can lead to a perceptible change in the passive range of contralateral side glide during ipsilateral lateral flexion. When visualizing the quality of resistance to passive movement the movement diagram, developed by Maitland (1986) is useful. When passively inducing lateral flexion at one spinal segment a perception of the profile of resistance to movement can be drawn. Profiles of resistance that are short in range represent a 'crisp' end feel, whilst a long range of resistance profile will feel 'bouncy'. Finally a movement that has no range of resistance and comes to a complete stop immediately resistance is felt, will feel 'solid'. See Figure 4.12. Segments that do not have this 'crisp' profile do not generally cavitate in response to a high velocity thrust.

Thus, unless the therapist assesses lateral flexion and its associated contralateral side glide the rationale for choosing a manipulation technique over a mobilization technique is less clear. The assessment of accessory glides does not afford the information to make this judgement. The assessment of

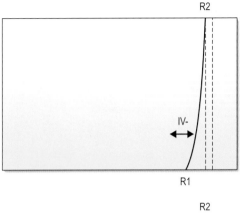

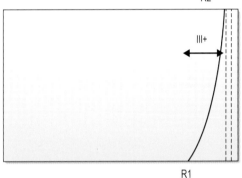

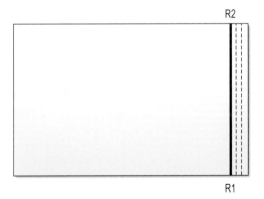

**Figure 4.12** • This illustration shows the profiles of resistance to segmental movement that can be detected with passive intervertebral movement testing. The top diagram represents a 'crisp' profile of resistance, the middle a 'bouncy' feel and the bottom figure a 'solid' feel. Only the top profile signifies that a manipulative thrust will be successful in inducing cavitation.

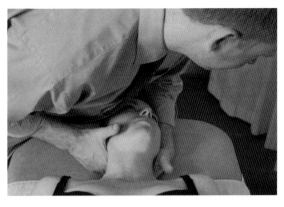

**Figure 4.13** • Assessment of the contralateral glide with right lateral flexion of the lumbar spine. IN: supine, cervical extension, left rotation, right lateral flexion; DID: passive right lateral flexion, Grade IV– thrust of the C4 segment on C5. Thrust starts before the beginning of resistance and stops just after the beginning of resistance.

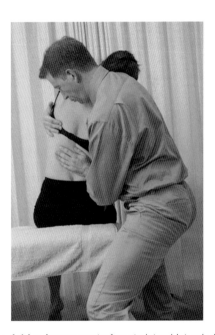

**Figure 4.14** • Assessment of contralateral lateral glide with ipsilateral lateral flexion in a combined starting position, prior to application of a IV– thrust technique. IN: sitting, thoracic extension; DID: right lateral flexion of T12 on L1. As the upper segment is ipsilaterally side-flexed the motion segment is contralaterally side glided.

segmental lateral flexion can be conducted in combined starting positions in order to fully examine for the presence of this 'crisp' profile of resistance. See Figures 4.12, 4.13, 4.14, 4.15 and 4.16.

In the following case studies there are two worked examples of the practical application of CMT approach during initial assessment, with one example from the cervical spine and one from the lumbar spine.

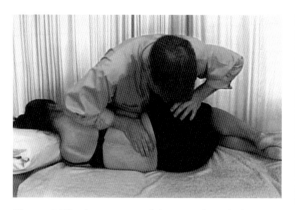

**Figure 4.15** • Assessment of the contralateral glide associated with ipsilateral flexion of the low lumbar spine. IN: left side-lying, flexion; DID: right lateral flexion with left side glide at the motion segment. As the lumbar spine is laterally flexed, firm pressure is applied towards the bed.

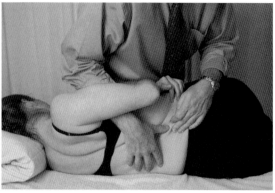

**Figure 4.16** • Assessment of resistance profile of contralateral glide in a combined position used to induce cavitation. IN: flexion, left lateral flexion, right rotation; DID: right rotation combined with contralateral glide downwards. The combined starting position for a Grade IV− rotation, thrust technique.

## CERVICAL SPINE CASE STUDY

### INITIAL INTERVIEW

### Symptomology

A 22-year-old female sought treatment for pain in the right cervical spine and right shoulder. The pain was located in the lower cervical spine and referred into the right shoulder across the right supra-scapula fossa (Fig. 4.17). The pain was not radicular in quality but severe (8/10). There was no suggestion of an upper motor neuron lesion and no indication of other red flags. There were no features suggestive of segmental cervical instability or shoulder derangement. There was no history of cervical locking, catching or weakness. There was no headache.

### Relevant history

Symptoms developed over a 6-day period following a mild, rear shunt whiplash injury, a week previously.

### Behaviour of symptoms

Pain was reproduced with low cervical flexion and left lateral flexion. Sitting with the neck in this position reproduced symptoms within 2 minutes. The symptoms were eased immediately, by positioning the lower cervical spine in extension and right lateral flexion. No latent pain was exhibited.

### Diurnal pattern

There was no stiffness in the cervical spine in the morning. Shoulder pain developed in the evening. Sleep was not disturbed.

### Special questions

The patient's general health was good. There was no weight loss, no dizziness, no dysphagia, no dysarthria,

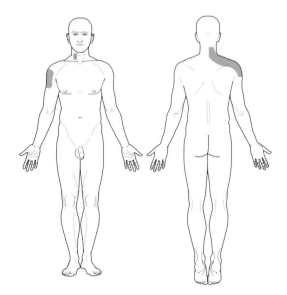

**Figure 4.17** • Cervical spine case study – pain chart.

no diplopia, no raised blood pressure, and no symptoms of cervical artery dysfunction. Radiographs of the cervical spine were normal. The patient was not currently taking any anticoagulant or steroid therapy and had received no benefit from anti-inflammatory medication. There was no history of locking, clunking or giving way of the shoulder, with no history of trauma.

See the completed planning sheet in Figure 4.18.

---

OBJECTIVE EXAMINATION PLAN

**List your hypotheses for the nature of the condition.**
1. ............................ *Posterior facet capsule sprain* ...................................................................................
2. ............................ *Posterior paraspinal strain* ...........................................................................................
3. ............................ *Posterior annular disc sprain* .......................................................................................

**Which two hypotheses will you test against each other in the initial physical examination?**
Primary ................. *Articular predominance* ......................................................................................
Secondary ........... *Myogenic predominance* .......................................................................................

**Is the nature of the condition severe?**
Yes  ☐ ✓     No  ☐

**Is the nature of the condition irritable?**
Yes  ☐     No  ☐ ✓

**To what point are you allowing movement to occur?**
Before pain        ☐
To pain             ☐ ✓
To limit             ☐

**What is the functional demonstration/primary re-test marker?**
............................ *Flexion contralateral, lateral flexion quadrant* .........................................................

**What is the primary pain mechanism of this patient's condition?**
Nociceptive                  ☐ ✓
Peripheral neurogenic   ☐
Central                          ☐
Autonomic                    ☐
Affective                       ☐

**To what extent will you perform a neurological exam?**
None required                                                               ☐
Local peripheral                                                          ☐
Lower motor neuron, upper motor neuron, limbs        ☐ ✓
Lower motor neuron, upper motor neuron, limbs and cranial   ☐

**What is the weighting of the following components of the problem?**

| | % |
|---|---|
| Arthrogenic | 50 |
| Myogenic | 40 |
| Neurogenic | 1 |
| Inflammagenic | 2 |
| Psychogenic | 1 |
| Sociogenic | 1 |
| Pathogenic | 1 |
| Viscerogenic | 1 |
| Osteogenic | 3 |

**Radar plot**

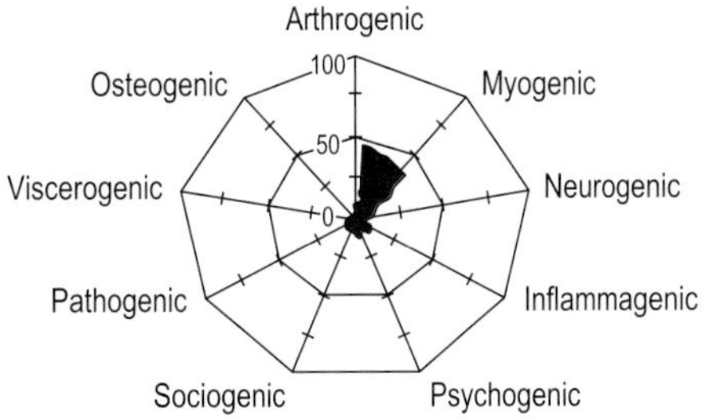

**Likely first treatment:**
In:   *Extension, right lateral flexion quadrant* .............................................................................
Will:  *Anterior capsular stretch, large amplitude movement, in resistance (Grade III)* ...........................

**Comments/cautions:**
*Pain relief approach, progressing to a stretch of the tissues driving the nociceptive pattern of presentation* ..................................
.................................................................................................................................................................

**Figure 4.18** • Objective examination plan for the cervical spine.

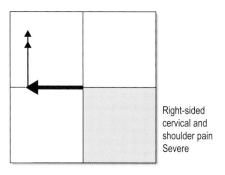

Right-sided
cervical and
shoulder pain
Severe

Prime movement = left lateral flexion
Prime combination = left lateral flexion
followed by flexion. 3/4 full range

**Figure 4.19** ● Box diagram showing the prime combination for the patient.

## PHYSICAL EXAMINATION

### Observation

There was no atrophy of the cervical musculature. There was an increase in muscle tone of the right sternocleidomastoid, upper fibres of trapezius and levator scapula and right scalenes.

### Active movement

Pain was reproduced earliest in range with left lateral flexion. Restriction to flexion was apparent at the C5/C6 level. Pain was reproduced further into range with flexion than with left lateral flexion. Restriction to movement was most obvious in the mid cervical region. See Figure 4.19.

**Figure 4.20** ● Flow chart of differential examination for the cervical spine.

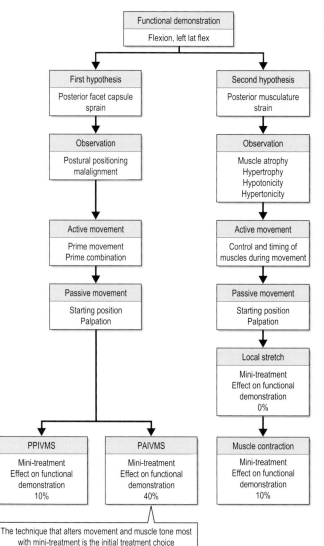

### Passive physiological intervertebral movement (PPIVMS)

Due to the severity, the examination was undertaken in right lateral flexion and extension (posterior structures off stretch) to establish the movement that most reduced pain and dysfunction. Right lateral flexion induced the greatest increase in movement and reduction in muscle tone.

*A short passive treatment, using this right lateral flexion of C5 on C6 reduced the pain produced by the functional demonstration by 10%.*

### Passive accessory intervertebral movement (PAIVMS)

Due to the severity, examination was undertaken in right lateral flexion and extension (posterior structures off stretch) to establish the movement that most reduced pain and dysfunction. Anterior pressure (AP) on C5 induced the greatest increase in movement and reduction in muscle tone (greater than induced by AP movement of C4 or C6).

*A short passive treatment, using this accessory movement reduced the pain produced by the functional demonstration by 40%.*

### Muscular assessment

In right lateral flexion and extension due to severity of pain, palpation of musculature revealed hypertonicity of deep paraspinals (C4 to C6) and hypertonicity of the region's phasic muscles. No trigger points were detected.

*Palpation and length assessment of the levator scapulae, scalenes, upper fibres of trapezius and sternocleidomastoid did not alter the functional demonstration.*

See Figure 4.20.

---

# LUMBAR SPINE CASE STUDY

### INITIAL INTERVIEW

### Symptomology

A 45-year-old male sought treatment for pain in the right back and buttock (Fig. 4.21). The pain was not radicular in quality and not severe (4/10). There was no suggestion of an upper motor neuron lesion and no indication of other red flags. There were no features suggestive of segmental lumbar instability or disc derangement. There was no history of lumbar locking, catching or weakness and there was no cauda equina syndrome.

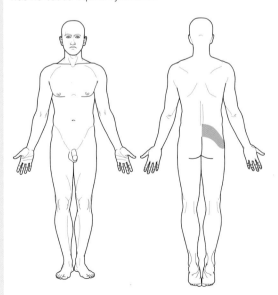

**Figure 4.21** • Lumbar spine case study – pain chart.

### Relevant history

Symptoms developed over a 6-month-period with no history of trauma.

### Behaviour of symptoms

Pain was reproduced with low lumbar extension and right lateral flexion (whilst arching his back to put on his coat). Standing reproduced symptoms within 20 minutes. Walking reproduced symptoms in 30 minutes. The symptoms were eased, immediately, by positioning the back in flexion, either by sitting or leaning over in standing. Pain was also eased by crossing the right leg over the left, in sitting. No latent pain was exhibited. Pain was also experienced whilst turning over in bed.

### Diurnal pattern

There was less than 30 minutes of stiffness in the back in the morning. Buttock pain developed in the evening. Sleep was not disturbed.

### Special questions

His general health was good. There was no weight loss, no night sweats or fever, no constant night pain (worse than during the day), no raised blood pressure, no symptoms of vascular stenosis or peripheral vascular disease. No history of cancer. The patient was not currently taking any anticoagulant or steroid therapy and had received no benefit from anti-inflammatory medication.

See the completed planning sheet in Figure 4.22.

---

### OBJECTIVE EXAMINATION PLAN

**List your hypotheses for the nature of the condition.**
1. ........................... Superior facet capsule source .............................................................
2. ........................... Sacro-iliac joint source ......................................................................
3. ........................... Anterior paraspinal muscle source ........................................................

**Which two hypotheses will you test against each other in the initial physical examination?**
Primary ................. Lumbar articular drive (75%) ........................................................................
Secondary ........... Sacro-iliac articular drive (25%) ...................................................................

**Is the nature of the condition severe?**
Yes ☐     No ☐ ✓

**Is the nature of the condition irritable?**
Yes ☐     No ☐ ✓

**To what point are you allowing movement to occur?**
Before pain     ☐
To pain     ☐
To limit     ☐ ✓

**What is the functional demonstration/primary re-test marker?**
........................... Extension, ipsilateral lateral flexion quadrant ..............................................

**What is the primary pain mechanism of this patient's condition?**
Nociceptive     ☐ ✓
Peripheral neurogenic     ☐
Central     ☐
Autonomic     ☐
Affective     ☐

**To what extent will you perform a neurological exam?**
None required     ☐
Local peripheral     ☐
Lower motor neuron, upper motor neuron, limbs     ☐ ✓
Lower motor neuron, upper motor neuron, limbs and cranial     ☐

**What is the weighting of the following components of the problem?**

| | % |
|---|---|
| Arthrogenic | 70 |
| Myogenic | 20 |
| Neurogenic | 1 |
| Inflammagenic | 4 |
| Psychogenic | 1 |
| Sociogenic | 1 |
| Pathogenic | 1 |
| Viscerogenic | 1 |
| Osteogenic | 1 |

Radar plot

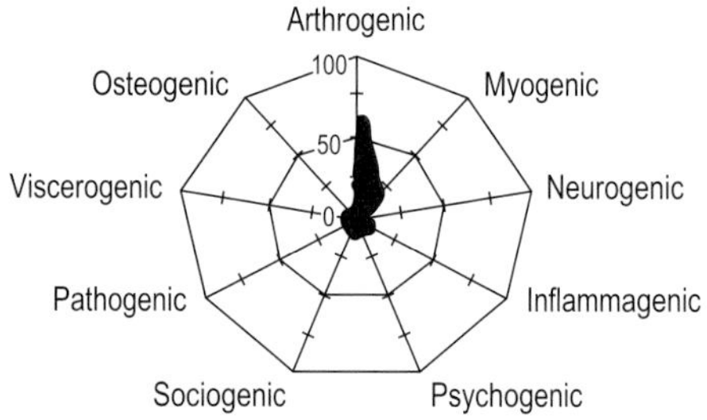

**Likely first treatment:**
In:    Extension, right lateral flexion quadrant ....................................................
Will:    Superior capsular stretch, large amplitude movement, in resistance (Grade III) .........................

**Comments/cautions:**
Pain relieving mobilization, combined with a stretch of the tissues driving the nociceptive pattern of presentation
...................................................................................................................................

**Figure 4.22** • Objective examination plan for the lumbar spine.

## PHYSICAL EXAMINATION

### Observation

There was no atrophy of the lumbar musculature. There was an increase in muscle tone of the right erectore spinae, quadratus lumborum and piriformis.

### Active movement

Pain was reproduced earliest in range with right lateral flexion. Restriction to extension was apparent at the L4/L5 level. Pain was reproduced further into range with extension than with right lateral flexion. See Figure 4.23.

### Passive physiological intervertebral movement (PPIVMS)

Right lateral flexion, in extension of L4 on L5, induced the greatest increase in movement and reduction in muscle tone, when compared with movement at L3/L4 and L5/S1.

*A short passive treatment, using this right lateral flexion of L4 on L5 reduced the pain produced by the functional demonstration by 50%.*

### Passive accessory intervertebral movement (PAIVMS)

In right lateral flexion and extension, posterior pressure (unilateral posterior-anterior angled caudad) on L4 induced the greatest increase in movement and reduction in muscle tone, when compared to the same accessory movement applied to L3 or L5.

*A short passive treatment, using this accessory movement reduced the pain produced by the functional demonstration by 20%.*

### Passive movement of the sacroiliac joint (SIJ)

In right lateral flexion and extension PA pressure on the right apex of the sacrum (encouraging nutation) reproduced symptoms and was the most restricted sacral glide, when compared to the response of moving the other three corners of the sacrum.

*A short passive treatment, using this passive movement reduced the pain produced by the functional demonstration by 10%.*

See Figure 4.24.

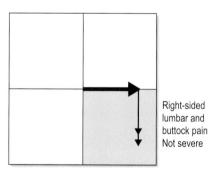

Prime movement = right lateral flexion
Prime combination = right lateral flexion
followed by extension. 3/4 full range

**Figure 4.23 •** Box diagram showing the prime combination for the patient.

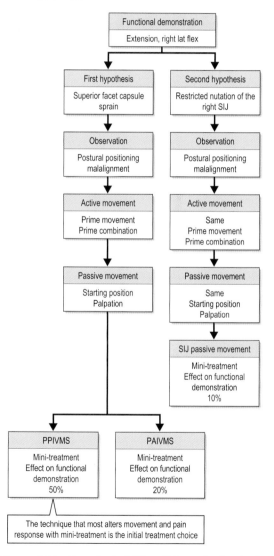

**Figure 4.24 •** Flow chart of differential examination for the lumbar spine.

# References

Chaitow, L., 2006. Muscle energy techniques. Elsevier Health Sciences, Oxford.

Gibbons, P., Tehan, P., 2001a. Patient positioning and spinal locking for lumbar spine rotation manipulation. Man. Ther. 6 (3), 130–138.

Gibbons, P., Tehan, P., 2001b. Spinal manipulation: indications, risks and benefits. Journal of Bodywork & Movement Therapies 5 (2), 110–119.

Grieve, G.P., 1988. Common vertebral joint problems. Churchill . Livingstone, New York, pp. 525–526.

Grieve, G.P., 1991. Mobilization of the spine. A Primary handbook of Clinical Method. Churchill Livingstone, Edinburgh.

Kerry, R., Taylor, A.J., Mitchell, J., et al., 2008a. Manual therapy and cervical arterial dysfunction, directions for the future: a clinical perspective. The Journal of Manual & Manipulative Therapy 16 (1), 39–48.

Kerry, R., Taylor, A.J., Mitchell, J., et al., 2008b. Cervical arterial dysfunction and manual therapy: a critical literature review to inform professional practice. Man. Ther. 13 (4), 278–288.

Maitland, G., 1986. Vertebral manipulation. Elsevier Health Sciences, Sydney.

Travell, Simmons, 1998. Travell Simons' myofascial pain and dysfunction: the trigger point manual, second ed. Lippincott Williams & Wilkins, San Francisco.

Chapter **Five**

5

# Neurological assessment

Chris McCarthy

## CHAPTER CONTENTS

## Introduction

There is no ideal neurological examination technique. There are conventional ways to perform an examination, a conventional order of examination and conventional ways to elicit particular signs (Fuller, 1993). This chapter aims to address one of the main concerns for post-graduate manipulative therapists, namely how to establish the extent of the neurological examination. The chapter is designed to supplement the more comprehensive texts on neurological examination (Donaghy, 1997; Fuller, 1993; Harrison, 1996; Perkin, 1992) and not to represent a compendium of all neurological testing procedures. The essential message of the chapter is that whilst the vast majority of patients will require a basic screening examination of both central and peripheral nervous systems the examination must be expanded if central nervous system (CNS) dysfunction is identified.

## History

An assessment of the patient's neurological function is made with every patient and during the taking of the patient's history, decisions regarding the likelihood of neurological dysfunction will be made by all but the most inexperienced therapist. During the subjective examination, hypotheses regarding the patient's primary dysfunction may be made following various models of clinical reasoning (Doody & McAteer, 2002). A process of clinical reasoning based on hypothetico-deductive reasoning and pattern recognition will enable the therapist to recognize, formulate and test likely hypotheses of dysfunction during both the subjective and the physical examinations. (See Chapter 3.)

The history has been described as the most important and most productive part of the neurological assessment, the purpose of which is to answer the questions 'where is the lesion and what is it?' and 'is it one lesion or does the condition involve a system within the nervous system?' Thus, in order to ensure high sensitivity and specificity to neurological dysfunction there are some techniques, commonly used by expert clinicians (King & Bithell, 1998), to make the subjective examination more valid. Development of an awareness of neurological time courses, patterns of presentation, and mechanisms of pain production should increase diagnostic confidence.

## Pattern recognition

Thinking of the history of a neurological dysfunction as having a shape, with an onset, a rate of evolution to maximum deficit, and a time at maximum deficit, or a rate of continuing progression or recovery to the present state, is a helpful way of visualizing a pattern of symptoms (Fuller, 1993) (Fig. 5.1).

The physical neurological examination is traditionally structured into five components: assessing alterations in tone, muscle power, coordination, reflexes, and sensory perception (Perkin, 1992). A physical examination will elicit characteristic patterns of presentation from each component which, when combined with subjective information, will enable a clinical diagnosis to be made. Developing an appreciation of subjective patterns of presentation based on these five components should increase the validity of the subjective examination. Thus, by asking about perceptions of weakness (motor power), clumsiness (coordination), limb stiffness and shaking (tone), as well as pain, there will be a greater likelihood of identifying relevant dysfunction in the physical examination. Table 5.1 shows the features typical of two spinal conditions, cervical myelopathy and cervical radiculopathy, and highlights the subjective and physical characteristics of these upper and lower motor neuron lesions as an illustration of their distinguishable features.

## Predominant symptom mechanism

The history should guide the therapist regarding the predominant mechanism of symptom production. In the case of pain, a sensitive and specific subjective examination will enable a hypothesis to be made regarding the predominant pain mechanism and thus whether a neurological examination is required. For

example, if a patient has nociceptive 'pinpoint' pain in their cervical spine and no cues from their history to suggest neurological dysfunction, a neurological examination is not necessary. However, if the pain refers to the shoulder, a neurological examination would be indicated in order that possible radicular pain production and neural conduction loss could be evaluated. Thus, if the decision to conduct an examination is based on a pain mechanism model rather than on the extent of the referred pain, a more rational approach can be adopted. Whilst there is still some debate regarding the validity of the methods of identifying predominant pain mechanisms, the definitions of pain mechanisms are well accepted (Butler, 1995) (Table 5.2).

## How much of the neurological examination should be done?

Having established that a neurological examination is required, the extent of the neurological examination needs to be clinically reasoned. It is clearly unnecessary to undertake every neurological test with all patients and thus a process of expansion or contraction of the physical examination should occur. There are a number of factors that should be considered in this process from each component of the examination. One of the primary considerations is establishing the possibility of central (CNS) or peripheral nervous system (PNS) lesions.

## Central or peripheral nervous system lesion

Following a sensitive and specific subjective examination, the therapist should have, as well as a musculoskeletal primary hypothesis, a neurological

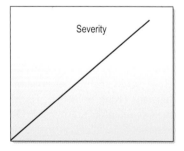 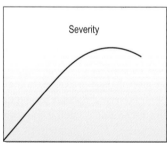 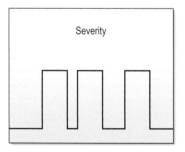

**Figure 5.1** • Typical patterns of symptom presentation. **(A)** Tumour/degenerative; **(B)** infection/inflammation; **(C)** epilepsy migraine. (Fuller, 1993)

**Table 5.1 Features of the components of the neurological examination in cervical radiculopathy and myelopathy**

| | | Tone | Motor | Coordination | Reflexes | Sensory |
|---|---|---|---|---|---|---|
| **Cervical myelopathy** | History | Arm and leg feel 'twitchy, jerky, clumsy, heavy, stiff' 'Scraping toes on floor' | Arm and leg feel 'weak, heavy, stiff, tight' | 'Dropping things, knocking over things, unable to do up fasteners' | Arm and leg feel 'twitchy, jerky, clumsy' | Arm and leg feel 'numb, dead, tingly, cold' Characteristic patterns of pain in UL and LL |
| | Physical | Reduced extensor tone in the UL Increased flexor tone in the UL Opposite pattern in the LL | Reduced in the extensors of the UL Increased in the flexors of the UL Opposite pattern in the LL | Reduced in UL and LL | Increased in the flexors of the UL Opposite pattern in the LL Plantars upgoing/Babinski +ve | Characteristic patterns of sensation loss in UL and LL |
| **Cervical radiculopathy** | History | Arm feels 'clumsy, heavy, stiff, heavy or dead' No change in legs | Arm feels 'weak, heavy' No change in legs | 'Dropping things, knocking over things, unable to do up fasteners' No change in legs | Arm feels 'slow, heavy' No change in legs | Arm feels 'numb, dead, tingly, cold' No change in legs Pain in one or two UL dermatomes but no associated pain in the LL |
| | Physical | Reduced for 1 or 2 UL myotomes No change in the LL | Reduced for 1 or 2 UL myotomes No change in the LL | Reduced in UL No change in LL | Reduced for 1 or 2 UL myotomes No change in the LL Plantars downgoing/ Babinski −ve | Loss of sensation in 1 or 2 dermatomes No change in the LL |

primary hypothesis. One of the main aims of the physical neurological examination is to try to establish the location of a potential lesion(s). In a musculoskeletal setting, one of the primary aims of the neurological examination is to establish if the patient has a lesion of the CNS or PNS. Typically, manual therapists will encounter patients with predominantly PNS dysfunction and consequently will undertake an examination weighted towards identifying the dysfunction within that system. It is imperative that therapists ensure that potential CNS dysfunction has been screened for before a clinical diagnosis is made. Some of the cardinal

features of PNS dysfunction, such as weakness, hyporeflexia and altered sensations can be elicited by CNS lesions and unless the possibility of CNS dysfunction is deliberately excluded there will be uncertainty regarding the validity of any subsequent clinical diagnosis. Within each component of the physical examination the extent of testing will be heavily influenced by the presence of CNS dysfunction.

Typically the physical examination is structured around assessment of tone, power, coordination, reflexes and finally sensation testing (Hawkes, 1996). One of the rationales for this order of testing

**Table 5.2 Describing the main mechanisms of pain**

| Pain mechanism | Description |
|---|---|
| Peripheral nociceptive | Local sources within muscles, joints and soft tissues |
| Peripheral neurogenic | Sources in peripheral nerves, nerve roots and cranial nerves |
| Central | Sources within neurons and synapses in the central nervous system |
| Efferent | Pain related to efferent mechanisms, influenced by motor neurons including those of the autonomic nervous system |
| Affective | Related to neurons and circuitry more concerned with the person's affect |

relates to the need to expand the subsequent components of the examination in the presence of potential CNS dysfunction. For example, symptoms from the history and signs of altered tone and power would indicate an expansion of coordination, reflex and sensory testing components, whilst no such signs and symptoms would suggest only a screening reflex and sensory screen was indicated. This is a principle that applies throughout all the components of the physical examination.

## Tone

The extent to which the examination of these systems is performed is governed by information obtained during the subjective examination. Assessments of tone, coordination and gait efficiency can be made as the patient enters the treatment area and during the course of the subjective examination, with more information being gained by observing the patient undressing and getting on and off the treatment couch.

Extrapyramidal disorders affecting the basal ganglia, such as Parkinson's disease, lead to a more uniform increase in tone distributed amongst flexor and extensor muscle groups with muscular rigidity in trunk and limb muscles (Perkin, 1992). Tremor and involuntary movements are common with loss of speed in intricate movement such as finger-to-thumb opposition and during gait (Harrison, 1996). The rigidity, associated with extrapyramidal lesions, and the spasticity, associated with an upper

motor neuron lesion (UMNL), can be reliably tested with two quick upper limb tests: wrist circumduction and the pronator catch test respectively (Donaghy, 1997). The wrist circumduction test involves gripping the patient's wrist with one hand and repeatedly circumducting the hand, whilst the pronator catch test involves abruptly supinating the patient's wrist and detecting a sudden jerk of resistance. If these signs are positive, an expansion of the examination of tone would be indicated, to include the lower limbs (Table 5.3).

## Motor system

The same principle applies during the motor examination. In the presence of an upper motor neuron lesion (UMNL), typical patterns of weakness and facilitation are apparent in the limbs and trunk. A UMNL lesion will typically produce a 'flexor pattern' of facilitation in the upper limbs with associated inhibition of the extensor muscle groups, with the opposite scenario being evident in the lower limbs. Thus, if the presence of a UMNL lesion has been identified through a detailed history and examination of tone, coordination and reflexes, prior to motor system testing the motor system examination would need to be expanded to evaluate all muscle groups in the limbs, neck and head (cranial nerve supply). In the absence of a CNS lesion the assessment of muscle strength can be limited to muscle groups suggested in the history, i.e. the most likely myotome and myotomes above and below it (Harrison, 1996) with a screening examination of proximal muscle power (decreased in myopathies) and distal power (decreased in peripheral neuropathy) (Table 5.4). Thus, a quick screen of power can be confined to shoulder abduction and finger abduction in the upper limb, and hip flexion with the knee straight, and ankle dorsiflexion in the lower limb. The Medical Research Council (MRC) Scale (Medical Research Council, 1990) is the conventional grading scale for muscle power when assessing the PNS and can be seen in Table 5.5.

## Coordination

Coordination is affected by proprioceptive loss (sensory ataxia) as well as cerebellar function (dysmetria, an inability to judge distance and control voluntary muscular action) and so clinical tests of coordination are not specific to cerebellar function; however, an assessment of the patient's coordination can be

**Table 5.3 The expanded and contracted tone, coordination and reflex examination**

| Examination | Test | Rationale |
| --- | --- | --- |
| *Contracted* | Observe gait, facial movement and intricate function during subjective examination<br>Wrist circumduction<br>Pronator catch<br>Plantar response<br>Comparison of deep tendon reflexes with contralateral limb | Speed and control of intricate movements of speech, gait, writing and undressing revealed prior to formal testing<br>Upper limb tests of abnormal tone quick, sensitive and reliable (Donaghy, 1997)<br>Tests for spasticity<br>Observe for isolated deep tendon reflex loss in nerve root and peripheral nerve lesions and generalized loss in peripheral neuropathy (Fuller, 1993) |
| *Expanded* | As above but expand with:<br>Lower limb tests of tone at hip, knee and ankle<br>Finger/nose and or heel/shin tests<br>Reflex testing of all four limbs and jaw jerk (cranial nerve V); also abdominal reflexes and frontal lobe release signs (Fuller, 1993). | Similar testing procedure to upper limb tests with rapid rotations of the hip and flexion/extension of the knee and ankle observing for a spastic catch or rigidity (Perkin, 1992). Cogwheel rigidity is lead-pipe rigidity that may be associated with tremor (Donaghy, 1997). Both upper and lower limb tests of coordination performed<br>Observe for patterns of increased and decreased reflexes typical of patterns in UMNL |

**Table 5.4 The expanded or contracted motor examination**

| Examination | Test | Rationale |
| --- | --- | --- |
| *Contracted* | For general screening, a proximal muscle (myopathy) should be tested with a distal muscle (peripheral neuropathy) with the specific myotomes of the peripheral nerve or root thought to be implicated (Donaghy, 1997)<br>Muscle group testing restricted to comparison with the contralateral side, not necessary to test all the limbs and neck and head muscle groups | Test mid-range isometric muscle strength to 'breaking point' which represents the muscle's maximum voluntary isometric contraction. Strong muscles like upper fibres of trapezius and quadriceps femoris should be placed in inner range to increase the mechanical advantage of the examiner. However, due to the length–tension relationship of the muscles, the starting positions for muscle testing should be standardized in order to improve the reliability of testing (Refshauge & Gass, 1995) |
| *Expanded* | Test all four limbs to examine the distribution of weakness. Patterns of weakness are particularly important in the presence of UMNL signs. In the presence of UMNL signs examine the neck and face muscles (cranial nerves) (Fuller, 1993)<br>Use repeated testing to expand strength testing into examination for fatigue of muscle (Donaghy, 1997). | There are five patterns of muscular weakness:<br>1. UMNL – increased tone, increased reflexes, pyramidal pattern of weakness (weak extensors in the UL and weak flexors in the LL)<br>2. LMNL – wasting, with or without fasciculation, decreased tone and absent or decreased reflexes<br>3. Muscle disease – wasting, decreased tone, impaired or absent reflexes<br>4. Neuromuscular junction – fatigable weakness, normal or decreased tone and normal reflexes<br>5. 'Functional weakness' normal tone, normal reflexes without wasting and with erratic performance of tests (Fuller, 1993). |

**Table 5.5 The Medical Research Council (MRC) scale for grading muscular power**

| Grade | Definition |
| --- | --- |
| 5 | Normal power |
| 4+ | Submaximal movement against resistance |
| 4 | Moderate movement against resistance |
| 4− | Slight movement against resistance |
| 3 | Moves against gravity but not resistance |
| 2 | Moves with gravity eliminated |
| 1 | Flicker |
| 0 | No movement |

quickly tested by the finger nose test and heel shin tests in the upper and lower limbs respectively (Harrison, 1996). These are conducted by asking the patient to reach out fully to touch the examiner's finger and then return their finger to their nose. The heel shin test involves the patient placing one heel accurately on their opposite knee and then running it repeatedly up and down the anterior edge of the tibia. During both tests, observations for intention tremor, overshooting and 'trick' movements to stabilize the proximal limb are made. Again, if signs of incoordination are observed with these tests, the examination would be expanded to explore the dysfunction further (see Table 5.3).

## Reflexes

An upper motor neuron lesion (UMNL) results from a disruption of the pyramidal pathway at any point between the motor cortex and the anterior horn cell, whilst a lower motor neuron lesion (LMNL) results from a disruption of the pathway from the anterior horn cell in the motor nucleus and neuromuscular junction (Perkin, 1992). The most valid single test of UMNL is the assessment of the plantar response (Donaghy, 1997). This test, also known as the Babinski test (the unfavoured term), can be present immediately a lesion has occurred, well before sufficient spasticity has developed to produce clonus or hyperreflexia (Donaghy, 1997). The plantar response is a reflex response to a noxious stimulus on the lateral margin of the sole of the foot with the normal response, after the first

year of life, being plantarflexion of the toes with dorsiflexion of the ankle (Harrison, 1996). In the presence of a UMNL the hallux dorsiflexes and the toes fan. Due to the diagnostic value of this simple test the details of conventional performance are detailed in Figure 5.2, with detail on interpretation and methods of varying the technique to account for ticklish and anxious patients. It must be remembered that, as with all examination procedures, a single test such as the plantar response, will never be perfectly accurate or adequate to form a clinical diagnosis in itself. The clinical diagnosis must be established from a synthesis of both history and physical features derived from the complete examination, and consequently, the clinician should be cautious of over interpreting this sign.

### Conventional test

The patient should be lying down and unable to see their toes. The examiner should passively examine the range of movement of the great toe to detect hallux rigidis. Draw a paperclip, thin stick or thumbnail slowly but firmly up the outer aspect of the sole and across the ball of the foot, observing for the direction of hallux movement (dorsiflexion being the abnormal and plantarflexion the normal responses; Fig. 5.2B). Observation is also made of any fanning of the little toe, which is the abnormal response (Fig. 5.2C) (Donaghy, 1997).

### Adapted methods of performing the plantar response test (Harrison, 1996)

To test for Chaddock's sign, pressure is placed very laterally on the foot and moved distally, whilst eliciting the Oppenheim sign involves running firm pressure distally along the tibia (Fig. 5.2D,E). Both can elicit an abnormal extensor response of the hallux and can be used with patients who are prohibitively anxious or ticklish (Fuller, 1993), but are not as reliable as the conventional method of testing the plantar response.

## Sensory system

The presence of a potential CNS lesion requires the expansion of the sensory examination to include the testing of light touch, pin-prick, temperature, vibration sense (pallaesthesia) and joint position sense whilst an adequate assessment of conduction with a PNS lesion can be made with just

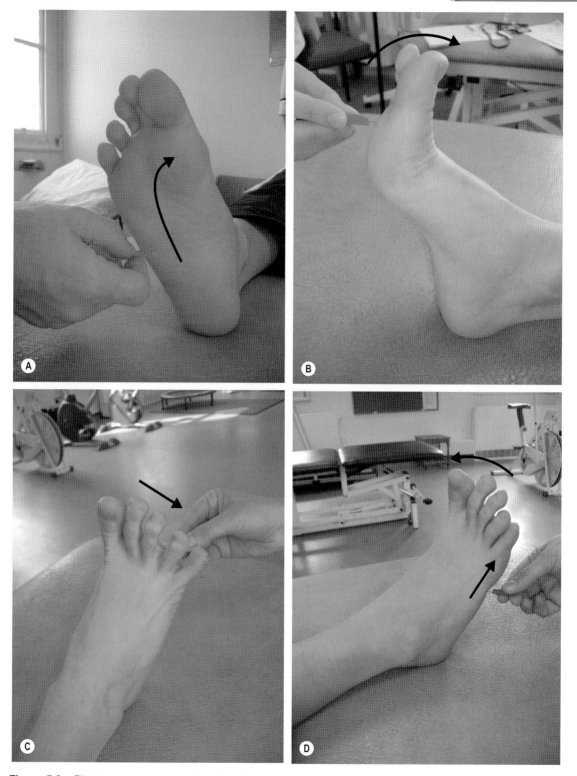

**Figure 5.2** • Plantar response: conventional and adapted methods. (A) Direction of movement; (B) hallux extension; (C) fanning of the little toe; (D) Chaddock's sign;

*continued*

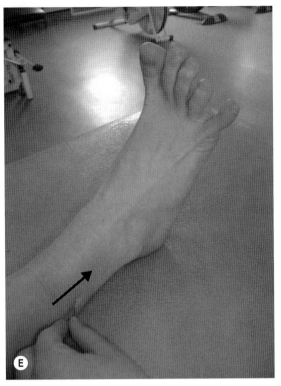

(E)

**Figure 5.2—cont'd** (E) Oppenheim's sign.

light touch and pin-prick sensations (Donaghy, 1997). Thus, having explored the presence of a CNS lesion through the assessment of tone, muscle power, coordination, and reflexes, the sensory examination can be expanded or contracted as indicated. A rationale for expansion and contraction of the sensory examination is given in Table 5.6.

## Summary

This chapter has aimed to provide guidance regarding the difficult issue of the extent of the neurological examination required for patients. A number of issues have been raised. Firstly, the physical examination is guided by the subjective examination. The subjective examination can be more sensitive and specific if patterns of presentation relating to tone, muscle power, coordination, reflexia, and of course sensation, are elucidated. Having established that there is a need to perform a neurological examination, the extent to which it is performed will be guided by interpretation of signs as the physical examination progresses. For example, assessments of tone, muscle power, coordination and reflexes will lead to justifiable expansions or contractions of the sensory system examination.

**Table 5.6 Expanding and contracting the sensory examination**

| Examination | Test | Rationale |
|---|---|---|
| *Contracted* | Light touch (large diameter afferent type II, Aβ fibres) and pin-prick (small type III, Aδ fibres), particularly at the distal area of dermatomes | Assessment of loss from fibres susceptible to ischaemic damage (large diameter fibres) and those at less risk due to a lower oxygen demand (small diameter fibres) will give an indication of the extent of the conduction impairment. Distal dermatomal loss is often observed prior to proximal loss due to greater metabolic demands of the lengthier nerve fibres |
| *Expanded* | Test light touch, joint position sense, and pallaesthesia (vibration sense) as well as temperature and pin-prick in all four limbs and head | The sensory examination is expanded in the presence of signs and symptoms indicative of a CNS lesion in order to identify characteristic patterns of loss, which enable a diagnosis of the CNS lesion to be made. The selective loss of sensations conducted in the (lateral) columns of the spinal cord (contralateral pain and temperature) with preservation of ipsilateral light touch, joint position sense and pallaesthesia would suggest normal posterior column conduction, but a lesion affecting either the (lateral) spinothalamic tracts or the decussating fibres supplying them, i.e. syringomyelia (Donaghy, 1997) |

Significantly, the absence of a potential CNS lesion, identified through the subjective examination and testing of reflexes, tone and coordination allows the physical examination to be focused on identifying the lesion(s) within the PNS, muscles and joints. Signs of CNS dysfunction require that the examination be expanded to identify the source of the lesion within both systems and is more time consuming and demanding for the patient. The subjective symptoms and physical signs, detailed in Table 5.1, should provide the therapist with clues as to how the examination for these two conditions might be conducted and is detailed below.

The cervical radiculopathy patient, with symptoms not suggestive of CNS involvement, would be screened with observation of coordination, pronator catch sign and wrist flexion/extension. In addition, the muscle power of relevant myotomes would be evaluated. Following this, the relevant upper limb deep tendon reflexes and plantar response test would be performed. Finally, after charting of light touch and pin-prick sensations, adequate information about the site and extent of a likely PNS lesion would have been gained. In contrast, symptoms and signs obtained cumulatively through the examination would lead to the cervical myelopathy patient to have tone, power, coordination, reflex and sensation components of the physical examination expanded to encompass all four limbs, trunk and head with all sensations tested.

In the clinical practice of manipulative therapists, many patients will present with neurological deficits of both the PNS and CNS. It is not clinically reasonable or necessary to conduct an over-extensive neurological examination on all patients. Through a detailed interpretation of clinical signs and symptoms the therapist can expand or contract the examination as necessary with patient examination becoming more efficient as a result.

## QUESTIONS

**1. Which sensations are conducted afferently by Aβ fibres?**

   A. Light touch and proprioceptive information

   B. Pin-prick pain

   C. Hot and cold

   D. Deep pain

**2. Cervical myelopathy typically demonstrates:**

   A. Lower limb extensor hypertonicity

   B. Lower limb extensor hypotonicity

   C. Downgoing plantar response

   D. Upgoing plantar response

**3. Cranial nerve examination is appropriate when assessing which of the following conditions?**

   A. Cervicogenic headache

   B. Facial pain

   C. Upper cervical instability

   D. Myelopathic signs and symptoms

   E. All of the above

**4. Which of the following conditions can lead to reductions in tone and coordination?**

   A. Peripheral nerve lesion

   B. Central nerve lesion affecting the extra-pyramidal system

   C. Central nerve lesion affecting the pyramidal system

   D. Muscle weakness

   E. All of the above

**Answers: 1** A; **2** A,D; **3** E; **4** E

# References

Butler, D., 1995. Moving in on pain. In: Shacklock, M.O. (Ed.), Moving in on pain. Sydney, Butterworth Heinemann.

Donaghy, M., 1997. Neurology. Oxford University Press, Oxford.

Doody, C., McAteer, M., 2002. Clinical reasoning of expert and novice physiotherapists in an outpatient setting. Physiotherapy 88 (5), 258–268.

Fuller, G., 1993. Neurological examination made easy, first ed.

Churchill Livingstone, Edinburgh.

Harrison, M.G., 1996. Clinical skills in neurology. Butterworth Heinemann, Oxford.

Hawkes, C.H., 1996. How to perform a rapid neurological examination. Medicine 24 (4), 15–17.

King, C.A., Bithell, C., 1998. Expertise in diagnostic reasoning: a comparative study. British Journal of Therapy and Rehabilitation 5 (2), 78–87.

Medical Research Council, 1990. Aids to the examination of the peripheral nervous system. Baillière, London.

Perkin, G.D., 1992. The nervous system. In: Epstein, O., Perkin, G.D., de Bono, D.P., Cookson, N. (Eds.), Gower Medical Publishing, London.

Refshauge, K., Gass, E., 1995. The neurological examination. In: Refshauge, E., Gass, E. (Eds.), Musculoskeletal physiotherapy: clinical science and practice. Butterworth Heinemann, Sydney.

# Chapter Six

6

# Haemodynamics

Roger Kerry, Alan J. Taylor

## CHAPTER CONTENTS

## Introduction

The purpose of this chapter is to provide information for the manual therapist to attempt to differentiate vascular pathology from neuromusculoskeletal (NMS) dysfunction. Furthermore, this information will help inform clinical judgement as to the likelihood of an adverse vascular event occurring following the application of combined movement techniques.

Haemodynamics is the study of the nature of blood flow in the circulatory system, the forces regulating flow, and the pathologies associated with alterations in that blood flow. This chapter reviews relevant clinical information on haemodynamics and its relationship to the application of combined movement techniques in the spine. The need for manual therapists to understand and appreciate haemodynamic principles is based on two simple premises:

1. Spinal movements can affect blood flow
2. Disease or injury to blood vessels can present with local pain patterns similar to commonly seen NMS conditions.

The first point above is not, in itself, a worrisome issue. This is quite a natural and necessary event. However, some particular manual therapy movement-based techniques performed on some people can, at times, result in unintended adverse events. The most widely known such adverse event is arguably cerebrovascular accident (stroke) occurring as a result of the application of a cervical manipulative technique. The second point concerns the recognition of those people who either are not suitable for manual therapy (because their pain is not of an NMS origin), or who may be at an increased risk of adverse vascular events if manual therapy techniques are undertaken for, say, a co-existing NMS problem. The above two points are obviously related. If a movement-based technique that alters blood flow detrimentally is applied to a patient with pain which (unknown to the clinician) is a manifestation of underlying vascular disease, the probability of an adverse event is increased. For example, pre-existing vertebrobasilar insufficiency (manifesting in pain) will increase the likelihood of that patient having a hind-brain stroke if certain movements (affecting blood flow) are performed.

This preamble therefore results in the identification of two distinct but interrelated study areas for the manual therapist:

- How does movement actually affect blood flow, and in what way (i.e. detrimentally or positively)?
- How can pain arising from a vascular source be differentiated from NMS pain?

The rest of this chapter is concerned with addressing these questions. The chapter is divided into two main sections: (1) the cervical spine, and (2) the thoraco-lumbar spine. Most reported vascular incidents related to manual therapy occur in the cervical spine, therefore the majority of this chapter is focused on this area. However, there is important clinical haemodynamic information for the manual therapist to consider when assessing and treating patients with thoracic and lumbar pain. The shorter last section is devoted to this. Each section includes clinically relevant information on vascular anatomy, associated pathologies, and methods to assess for the presence of vascular pathology.

# Haemodynamics and the cervical spine

Blood flow in the neck and head has been a contentious issue among physiotherapists for many decades. The focus of attention has primarily been on vertebrobasilar insufficiency (VBI), and complications following end-of-range cervical manipulation. Consideration of carotid (anterior) flow and the effect of treatment modalities other than end-of-range manipulation is essential for the therapist to have a complete understanding of clinical presentations of the head and neck.

This section reviews the clinical anatomy of the blood vessels in the head and neck, followed by a report of the common clinical presentations of vascular dysfunction in this region. This information will enhance clinical reasoning when assessing patients with upper cervical pain and headaches. Assessment procedures are then presented utilizing this information.

## Clinical anatomy

### The posterior vascular system of the head and neck

The hind-brain is supplied primarily by the vertebrobasilar complex. Figure 6.1 shows schematically the vertebral and basilar arteries, and how they feed into the Circle of Willis.

The verterbral artery (VA) can be divided into extra-cranial and intra-cranial sections (Fig. 6.1). Furthermore, the course of the VA is sub-divided into four anatomical divisions (Fig. 6.2): V1 (extra-cranial) – from the branch origin off the sub-clavian artery to the transverse process of C6, where the artery enters the cervical column; V2 (extra-cranial) – its course through the bony vertebral column (as it passes through the transverse foramina) from C6 to its exit at the atlantal transverse foramen; V3 (extra-cranial) – from the atlantal transverse foramen to its cranial entrance through the atlanto-occipital membrane; and V4 (intra-cranial) – from the foramen magnum to converge with the contralateral VA at the lower pontine hind-brain level to form the basilar artery. The most common sites of VA injury are V1 at its origin, and V3 as it convolutes around the posterior arch of the atlas (Savitz & Caplan, 2005).

The basilar artery (BA) runs through the cisterna pontis in a shallow median groove (known as the sulcus basilaris) from its origin to the superior pontine line (upper pontine level) where it begins to form the Circle of Willis via its bifurcation into the two posterior cerebral arteries. For a more detailed description of the vertebrobasilar arterial system, together with the many anatomical anomalies which have been noted, see Rivett (2005).

The vertebrobasilar system has branches which are responsible for both extra- and intra-cranial anatomical areas. Extra-cranially, the VA branches supply the vertebral column and spinal cord, as well as the deep upper cervical musculature. The muscular branches anastomose with the occipital artery at this region. Intra-cranially, the VA gives rise to the posterior inferior cerebellar arteries (PICA), and sometimes the anterior inferior cerebellar arteries (AICA) (although more frequently, this does not branch off until the basilar artery). The PICA and AICA (along with the tiny medullary arteries) primarily supply the superior and lateral medulla oblongata. Occlusion of flow in the PICA (or distal VA) can result in retro-olivary dorsolateral medullary, or Wallenberg, syndrome. The PICA also supplies the cerebellar hemisphere, inferior vermis, fourth ventricle, and the dentate nucleus. A branch off the AICA, or sometimes directly off the basilar artery, is the labyrinthine artery. This is responsible for supplying blood to the inner auditory and vestibular apparatus.

In addition to the AICA, the basilar artery gives rise to the pontine arteries. These are numerous

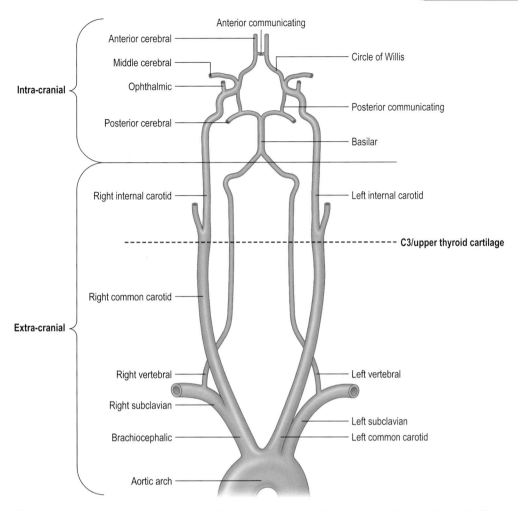

**Figure 6.1 •** Schematic representation of the vertebral and carotid arteries and their relation with Circle of Willis. (Adapted and reprinted from Drake *et al* (2005), with permission from Elsevier)

branch arteries from the basilar and supply the pons. Occlusion of the mid-basilar, and therefore the pontine arteries may result in 'locked-in syndrome', or cerebromedullospinal disconnection syndrome. Closer to the formation of the Circle of Willis are the superior cerebellar artery (SCA) and the posterior cerebral artery (PCA). The SCA supplies the pons, pineal body, mid-brain colloculi, superior medullary velum and the tela choroidea of the third ventricle. The PCA is responsible for the temporal and occipital lobe (including visual structures and pathways), and some medial and inferior cerebral structures.

Studies examining changes of blood flow in the posterior system produce variable results. Many studies have demonstrated a change in blood flow in the vertebral arteries during contralateral cervical rotation (e.g. Mitchell *et al*, 2004; Refshauge, 1994; Rivett, 1999; Rossitti & Volmann, 1995). Although there are other studies with contradictory results, contralateral rotation is the movement most consistently associated with reduction (or cessation) of VA blood flow. It is important to realize, however, that this phenomenon is likely to be a physiologically natural event and occurs in normal, asymptomatic individuals.

## The anterior vascular system of the head and neck

Figure 6.1 also shows the course of the internal carotid artery (ICA) from its origin (around the

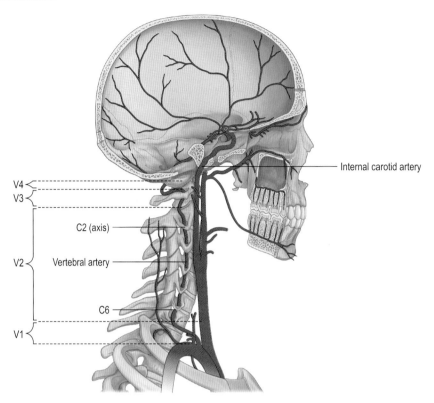

Internal carotid artery

V4
V3

C2 (axis)

V2

Vertebral artery

C6

V1

**Figure 6.2** • The course of the vertebral and internal carotid arteries through the cervical spine. The images show the classic anatomical sub-divisions of the vertebral artery: V1–V4 (see text). (Adapted and reprinted from Drake *et al* (2005), with permission from Elsevier)

C3/upper thyroid cartilage level) to its termination at the Circle of Willis. The ICA arises from the common carotid artery (CCA) which itself is a branch off the thoracic arch of the aorta (on the left), or the brachiocephalic artery (on the right). Like the VAs, the ICA can be divided into extra- and intracranial sections. Extra-cranially, the ICA begins at its bifurcation. The point of bifurcation is of great clinical importance for a number of reasons. The carotid sinus is located just superior to the bifurcation on the ICA. The carotid sinus houses nerve endings from the glossopharangeal nerve (IX) and acts as a baroreceptor controlling intra-cranial blood pressure. This is also a very common site for localized atherosclerotic lesions (Lorenz *et al*, 2006). The carotid sinus is behind the point of bifurcation and this acts as a chemoreceptor. The bifurcation area sits deep to a number of muscles which are active during cervical spine movement, jaw movement, and swallowing. This is known as the carotid triangle (a sub-division of the anterior cervical triangle) and it is where the

vessels are at their most superficial placement. The carotid triangle consists of the superior belly of omohyoid (antero-inferior border), stylohyoid and digastric (superior border), and the anterior aspect of sternocleidomastoid (posterior border). Flow changes around this section of the ICA have been demonstrated during movements that involve activity and stretching of these muscles (e.g. Foye *et al*, 2002).

As the ICA ascends towards the head, it passes anteriorly to the cervical spinal column and is adhered to the anterior body of C1. During its extra-cranial course, the vessel is adjoined posterior to longus capitis and covered throughout this section anterolaterally by the sternocleidomastoid. The vessel becomes intra-cranial as it passes through the pertrous portion of the temporal bone in the carotid canal.

Intra-cranially, the ICA is sub-divided into three parts: the pertrous part, the cavernous part, and the cerebral part. Each of these parts gives rise to a number of branches: pertous – carototympanic and pterygoid; cavernous – cavernous, hypophysial, meningeal and ophthalmic; cerebral – anterior cerebral, middle cerebral, posterior communicating and anterior choroid. The ICA joins the Circle of Willis where it is almost continuous with the middle cerebral artery (MCA) (a clinically important site as most ischaemic strokes result from occlusion of the MCA or its branches, usually as a result of embolus directly from the ICA). The ICA and its branches essentially supply the cerebral hemisphere, the eye/retina (and its accessory organs), the forehead, and the nose.

Although blood flow in the anterior vessels is commonly measured and reported upon, it is mostly in relation to the effect of disease (i.e. stenotic lesions reduce blood flow). Studies specifically examining the effect of cervical movement on carotid blood flow are less common than those examining posterior flow. However, there are several studies which demonstrate that carotid flow can be influenced (reduced) by cervical extension, and to a smaller extent, rotation (e.g. Rivett, 1999; Scheel *et al*, 2000; Schoning *et al*, 1994).

## Cranial nerves

It is important to appreciate the relationship between cervico-cranial blood flow and the cranial nerves (CN). Just as with peripheral nerves, these structures require disproportionally high amounts of blood and constant perfusion. Any interruption to this perfusion will result in symptoms of neural ischaemia. It is therefore essential that the clinician understands the roles of each cranial nerve and the manifestations of dysfunction to each nerve, as well as the specific cranial nerve tests. As the nuclei to most cranial nerves are housed in the brainstem, disruption to vertebrobasilar flow can potentially result in cranial nerve dysfunction of these nerves. ICA flow changes are unlikely to affect the nuclei of the cranial nerves, but, by virtue of the relative anatomy, can affect the nerve axons in both the extra- and intra-cranial sections of the ICA following certain vessel pathologies. The last four cranial nerves (CNIX to XII) have been reported as affected in 83% of ICA traumatic events (Chan *et al*, 2001).

## Pathophysiology

Cervical arterial dysfunction (CAD), refers to a wide variety of pathophysiological events. At one extreme are actual cerebrovascular accidents (CVA), or stroke. In the middle of this continuum are the much more subtle dysfunctions relating to transient interruption of perfusion to particular sites in the head. At the other end of the continuum is the consideration of the patient's likelihood of risk from a future cervico-cranial ischaemic event, and furthermore, calculating the chances of physiotherapy intervention contributing to such an event. It is essential that clinicians consider the full scope of this continuum.

Ischaemic strokes (as opposed to hemorrhagic strokes) account for around 80% of all young to middle-aged strokes. The majority of these strokes arise from the internal carotid artery whilst around 20% arise from the posterior system (Arnold & Bousser, 2005; Savitz & Caplan, 2005; Thanvi *et al*, 2005). These figures relate specifically to dissection events. Dissections are intimal tears that allow blood to penetrate into the vessel wall (Fig. 6.3).

These dissections may be sub-intimal, which may result in intramural haematoma formation and subsequent lumen narrowing as the intima wall is enlarged into the lumen. Others may be sub-adventitial, which may result in a gross widening of the vessel referred to as a dissecting aneurysm. There is potential for the resultant thrombus (haematoma) formation to either enlarge to the point of clinically significant stenosis or to embolize (also referred to as dissecting of the thrombus). A widened vessel, and the associated inflammation in its proximity, can also compress or stretch local

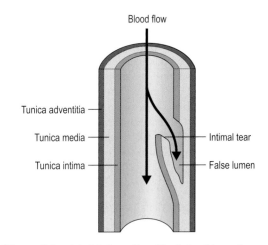

**Figure 6.3** • Arterial dissection. The intimal tear allows blood to track sub-intimally and create a false lumen. (Adapted with permission from McKeeson Health Solutions 2002)

structures resulting in a variety of symptoms, including somatic pain from non-vascular structures (Arnold & Bousser, 2005) or cranial nerve dysfunction/palsy (Leys et al, 1997). Vasculogenic pain may also arise from the deformation of nociceptive nerve endings in the adventitia of the vessel, as a result of vessel widening (Nichols et al, 1993).

Atherosclerosis is intrinsically associated with intimal dysfunction and the presence of atherosclerosis may predispose the vessel to the above pathological reactions and make dissection and thrombus formation more likely to occur (Mitchell, 2002). Furthermore, localized atherosclerotic changes may occur *as a result* of the extrinsic or intrinsic (altered haemodynamic) trauma which is responsible for the above intimal tears (Texon, 1996).

Ischaemia without embolization, or an actual embolic event, may result in retinal or brain ischaemia (anterior system), or hind-brain ischaemia (posterior system). It is the remit of the clinician to establish either if a pathological state as described above already exists *or* if there is the *potential* for such a state, and the sequelae of that state, to come about.

## Clinical presentations

Knowledge and understanding of the basic clinical anatomy, as referred to above, can significantly assist the clinician in interpreting patient presentations that display subtle signs and symptoms suggestive of either transient ischaemic event (TIE), transient ischaemic attack (TIA), ischaemic stroke, or, as stated above, the *potential* for such cervico-cranial ischaemic occurrences. This approach should be the remit of any clinician assessing and treating patients with head and/or cervical symptomology.

Examples of CAD are referred to below, and for the sake of clarity these are split into 'posterior' presentations and 'anterior' presentations. It is important to realize however that multi-vessel dysfunction exists and can present as a combination of these presentations.

### Posterior circulation presentations

These involve the posterior vertebrobasilar system as described above. Classically, the signs and symptoms related to the posterior system are considered as the '5 Ds and 3 Ns' of Coman (Coman, 1986). The signs and symptoms are presented in Table 6.1

Table 6.1 Classic signs and symptoms of vertebrobasilar insufficiency (VBI) with associated neuroanatomy. See text for the limitations of only considering these features for potential VBI

| Sign or symptom | Associated neuroanatomy |
| --- | --- |
| Dizziness (disequilibrium, giddiness, lightheadedness) | Lower vestibular nuclei (vestibular ganglion = nuclei of CN VIII vestibular branch) |
| Drop attacks (loss of consciousness) | Reticular formation of midbrain Rostral pons |
| Diplopia (amaurosis fugax; corneal reflux) | Descending spinal tract, descending sympathetic tracts (Horner's syndrome); CN V nucleus (trigeminal ganglion) |
| Dysarthria (speech difficulties) | CN XII nucleus (medulla, trigeminal ganglion) |
| Dysphagia (+ hoarseness/hiccups) | Nucleus ambiguous of CN IX and X, medulla |
| Ataxia | Inferior cerebellar peduncle |
| Nausea | Lower vestibular nuclei |
| Numbness (unilateral) | Ipsilateral face: descending spinal tract and CN V Contralateral body: ascending spinothalamic tract |
| Nystagmus | Lower vestibular nuclei + various other sites depending on type of nystagmus (at least 20 types) |

(with a ninth 'classic' sign – ataxia) together with the associated neuro-anatomical site of insult.

Unreasoned adherence to these cardinal 'classic' signs and symptoms can, however, be misleading and result in an incomplete understanding of patient presentations. A closer look at contemporary evidence and case reports shows that the typical presentation of vertebrobasilar dysfunction is not always in line with this classic picture. Clinical haemodynamic presentations can be better understood if the symptomology is broken down 'into non-ischaemic (i.e. local, somatic causes) and ischaemic (i.e. brain, or retinal) manifestations (Arnold & Bousser, 2005). The non-ischaemic presentation of vertebral dissection is typically ipsilateral posterior neck pain and/or occipital headache alone (e.g.

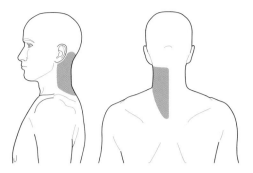

**Figure 6.4 •** Typical pain distribution relating to extra-cranial vertebral artery dissection – ipsilateral posterior upper cervical pain and occipital headache.

Arnold & Bousser, 2005; Asavasopon *et al*, 2005; Childs *et al*, 2005; Dziewas *et al*, 2006; Leys *et al*, 1997; Nichols *et al*, 1993; Savitz & Caplan, 2005; Silbert *et al*, 1995; Thanvi *et al*, 2005; Watanabe *et al*, 2001). Figure 6.4 shows a typical pain distribution for vertebral artery dissection.

This stage may then be followed by the ischaemic events associated with vertebrobasilar dysfunction. These *may* also include some of the classic 5Ds and 3Ns as stated above, but may also include any of the following (APA, 2006; Arnold & Bousser, 2005; Rivett, 2005; Savitz & Caplan, 2005):

• Vomiting
• Hoarseness
• Loss of short-term memory
• Vagueness
• Hypotonia/limb weakness (arm or leg)
• Anhidrosis (lack of facial sweating)
• Pallor, tremors, sweating
• Hearing disturbances
• Malaise
• Perioral dysthesia
• Facial dysthesia
• Photophobia
• Papillary changes
• Clumsiness and agitation, anxiety
• Disorientation.

It is rare for posterior dysfunction to manifest in only *one* sign or symptom, and isolated dizziness or transient loss of consciousness are often misattributed to posterior circulation ischaemia (Savitz & Caplan, 2005). The nature of dizziness is a differentiating factor in establishing a vascular versus non-vascular cause. Typically, posterior circulation

dizziness (as a result of the subsequent occluded flow through the AICA and labyrinthine arteries), does not present as frank vertigo (although some authors have suggested this *could* occur, e.g. Savitz and Caplan (2005). Rotation of the torso and neck as a single unit (i.e. no cervical torsion) may assist in differentiating vascular from vestibular causes of dizziness. Further detail regarding vestibular testing is beyond the scope of this chapter.

## Anterior circulation presentations

The ICA is more susceptible to atherosclerotic lesions than the VA and this is apparent in the proportion of cranial ischaemic events occurring in the carotid territory (80% anterior to 20% posterior). In addition, the anterior circulation supplies more blood to the brain than the posterior (coincidentally also around 80% anterior to 20% posterior). The vessel is larger in diameter than the VA and thus the velocity of the flow is greater, making localized intimal trauma more likely, especially around the turbulent point of the bifurcation from the common carotid to the internal and external carotid. Thus, one of the most common pathologies of the ICA is a localized atherosclerotic lesion at a point around, or proximal to, this bifurcation point, i.e. the carotid sinus and above. It is important, therefore, for manual therapists to be familiar with the clinical presentation of ICA trauma and localized lesions.

Fronto-temporal headache (cluster-like, thunderclap, migraine without aura, hemicrania continua, different from previous headaches), upper cervical or anterolateral neck pain, facial pain/facial sensitivity ('carotidynia'), Horner's syndrome, pulsatile tinnitus, and cranial nerve palsies (most commonly CN IX to XIII) are the commonest *local sign/symptoms* presentations of internal carotid dissection/thrombus formation (Arnold & Bousser, 2005; Taylor & Kerry, 2005; Zetterling *et al*, 2000). Figure 6.5 shows a typical ICA-referred pain distribution.

Less common local signs and symptoms include ipsilateral carotid bruit, scalp tenderness, neck swelling, CN VI palsy, orbital pain, and anhidrosis (Frigerio *et al*, 2003; Guillon *et al*, 1998; Lemesle *et al*, 1998; Zetterling *et al*, 2000). It is important to appreciate that most commonly, particularly in the early stages of the pathology, headache and/or cervical pain can be the sole presentations of internal carotid artery dysfunction (Biousse *et al*, 1994; Buyle *et al*, 2001; Lemesle *et al*, 1998; Mainardi *et al*, 2002; Nichols *et al*, 1993; Pezzini *et al*, 2005;

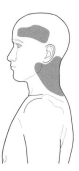

**Figure 6.5** • Typical pain distribution relating to dissection of the internal carotid artery – ipsilateral fronto-temporal headache, and upper/mid cervical pain.

Rogalewski & Evers, 2005; Silbert *et al*, 1995; Taylor & Kerry, 2005).

The local pain mechanisms involved with the internal carotid artery are again likely to be related to either deformation of nerve endings in the tunica-adventitia, or direct compression on local somatic structures (Nichols *et al*, 1993). Specifically, the terminal nerve endings in the carotid wall are supplied by the trigeminal nerve, which accounts for instances of facial pain and carotidynia. Stimulation of the trigemino-vascular system may account for this carotid-induced pain (Leira *et al*, 2001).

Cranial nerve palsies and Horner's syndrome are interesting phenomena and often pathognomonic of internal carotid artery pathology, especially if the onset is acute. The hypoglossal nerve (CN XII) is the most commonly affected, followed by the glossopharyngeal (CN IX), vagus (CN X), or accessory (CN XI) (Arnold & Bousser, 2005; Zetterling *et al*, 2000). However, all cranial nerves (except the olfactory nerve) can be affected (Zetterling *et al*, 2000). If the dissection extends into the cavernous sinus, the occulomotor (CN III), trochlear (CN IV), or abducens (CN VI) can be affected (Lemesle *et al*, 1998; Zetterling *et al*, 2000). The two most likely mechanisms for these cranial nerve palsies are (1) ischaemia to the nerve via the vasa nervorum (comparable to peripheral neurodynamic theory); and (2) direct compression of the nerve axon by the enlarged vessel (Arnold & Bousser, 2005; Lemesle *et al*, 1998; Zetterling *et al*, 2000).

Horner's syndrome has been found to be present in up to 82% of patients with known internal carotid dissection (Chan *et al*, 2001). Most commonly, this syndrome occurs *with* head, neck, or facial pain. Carotid-induced Horner's syndrome manifests as a drooping eyelid (ptosis), sunken eye

(enophthalmia), and a small, constricted pupil (miosis) and facial dryness (anhidrosis), i.e. the overbalance of parasympathetic activity in the eye. The syndrome is therefore a result of interruption to the sympathetic nerve fibres supplying the eye. In the case of carotid Horner's syndrome, the pathology is classed as post-ganglionic. The superior cervical sympathetic ganglion lies in the posterior wall of the carotid sheath, and the post-ganglionic fibres follow the course of the carotid artery before making their way deep towards the eye through the cavernous sinus. Compression or ischaemia as a result of internal carotid dysfunction will occur at the ganglion or distal to it. Some post-ganglionic sympathetic fibres that follow the course of the *external* carotid artery control facial sweating, thus accounting for the presence of anhidrosis in post-ganglionic Horner's syndrome.

The above local signs and symptoms of internal carotid pathology can precede cerebral ischaemia (TIA or stroke) or retinal ischaemia by anything from less than a week, to beyond 30 days (Biousse *et al*, 1994; Zetterling *et al*, 2000). In addition to the above early signs, it is important for the manual therapist to be aware of signs and symptoms related to cerebral and retinal ischaemia (i.e. internal carotid territory). It is unlikely that a patient with full stage cerebral ischaemic stroke will present to the manual therapist, but the more subtle presentation of retinal ischaemia might. The internal carotid artery supplies (via the ophthalmic artery) the retina, and embolus from the internal carotid can result in retinal ischaemic dysfunction: symptoms include a painless episodic loss of vision, or blackout (amaurosis fugax), and localized/patchy blurring of vision (scintillating scotoma). Orbital ischaemia syndrome, as a result of ophthalmic artery occlusion, presents as weakness of the ocular muscles (ophthalmoparesis); protrusion of the eye due to weakness of extrinsic eye muscles (proptosis); swelling of the eye or conjunctiva (chemosis) (Arnold & Bousser, 2005; Dziewas *et al*, 2006; Zetterling *et al*, 2000).

## Clinical examination of cervical arterial dysfunction

The most important part of clinical examination with regard to cervical arterial dysfunction is the history. Consideration of the information presented in this chapter is vital in facilitating pattern recognition and directing the nature of the subjective examination if serious pathology is suspected. Knowledge of anatomy, pathophysiology, and specific clinical presentations, as well as a thorough appreciation of atherosclerotic risk factors (see below), aids the clinician in developing strong decisions as to the likelihood of the presenting signs and symptoms being related to a vascular pathology. This is equally the case for the thoraco-lumbar presentations detailed in the following section of this chapter. Physical examination is used to consolidate the clinician's thoughts from the history-taking.

## Functional positioning tests

Traditionally, manual therapists' clinical examination of potential neurovascular problems associated with treatment has been confined to testing of the vertebrobasilar system for transient lack of competency. This has classically been based around the use of a functional positioning test. There are many variations of this test, but all involve a sustained re-positioning of the head and neck whilst signs and symptoms suggestive of hind-brain ischaemia are noted. Figure 6.6 shows the commonly used sustained rotation-in-lying test. Current clinical guidelines recommend the use of this testing procedure (APA, 2006).

There are two important points to be considered when performing this test, or variations of it:

**1.** The diagnostic utility of these tests has not been consistently supported by evidence. This testing procedure has been shown to have poor and variable sensitivity and specificity (Gross et al, 2005; Kerry, 2006; Kerry & Rushton, 2003; Ritcher & Reinking, 2005). Some authors have even questioned whether the test should be relied upon at all (Kerry, 2002; Thiel & Rix, 2005).

**2.** This procedure is specifically designed to test the posterior circulation, and is unlikely to stress the anterior vessels (unless combined with cervical extension). However, such a functional test for the anterior vessels has never been validated.

It is of great importance that clinicians are aware of these points when considering to what extent the result of this testing procedure should influence their clinical decisions. Chapter 3 expands on the interpretation of test results in the decision-making process. Despite these shortcomings, it is unreasonable for this testing procedure to be abandoned in clinical practice at this point in time. Functional positioning testing may have a role in informing decision-making if used in combination with other testing procedures and as part of a more holistic examination. This role is again dependent on the clinician's appreciation of the test's diagnostic utility, together with the effect of information from other sources.

## Ultrasound Doppler

As an adjunct to the functional positioning testing referred to above, the use of audible ultrasound Doppler has been suggested as a method to examine, in closer detail, the nature of blood flow in specific vessels (Haynes et al, 2005; Rivett et al, 2005). Figure 6.7 shows the use of a simple, handheld ultrasound Doppler unit in the assessment of the VA and ICA flow. Experimental work assessing the utility of ultrasound Doppler in the field of manual therapy is in its infancy, and although some reports are encouraging (e.g. Haynes et al, 2005), this testing procedure should also be used judiciously.

## Pulse palpation

Pulse palpation (Figs 6.8 and 6.9) may also be used in the assessment of suspected cervical vessel pathologies. This is a simple, quick procedure which again lacks specific support from experimental work, but could have an important diagnostic role. It is unlikely that transient changes in flow rate or velocity can be perceived in the cervical vessels by palpation. However, palpating for gross pathologies – specifically aneurysm – is feasible. An extra-cranial aneurysmal pulse will

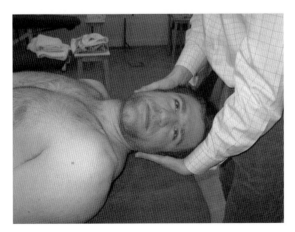

**Figure 6.6** • Functional positional testing of the vertebral artery (rotation). The patient's head is passively rotated and held for 10 seconds. Reproduction of symptoms associated with vertebrobasilar insufficiency are considered a positive test.

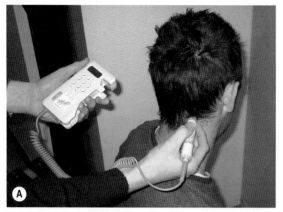

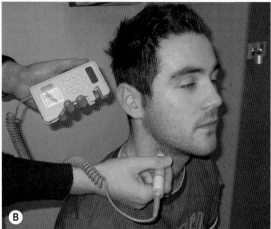

**Figure 6.7** • Use of handheld Doppler ultrasound for the examination of blood flow changes. (A) In the verterbral artery (sub-occipital site) and (B) the internal carotid artery. Interpretation of the results of Doppler examination is dependent on the skill and experience of the clinician.

classically feel like a localized mass which is more pulsatile (more noticeable) and more expandable (greater tissue excursion) than a non-pathological pulse.

## Blood pressure

Despite its limited use in the examination of manual therapy red flags, blood pressure testing has a good predictive value for arterial disease and stroke – and specifically for cervical vessel pathology (Cao *et al*, 2007; Femia *et al*, 2007; Hupp *et al*, 2007; Kurvers *et al*, 2007; Paraskevas *et al*, 2007). As with the testing procedures referred to above, a blood pressure test alone will not provide a definitive diagnostic answer. However, hypertension has a high association with both systematic and localized atherosclerotic

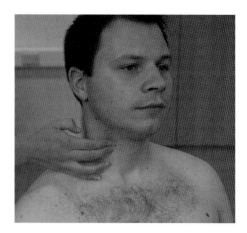

**Figure 6.8** • Palpation of the carotid artery. Pulses are found in the mid-cervical region with gentle pressure applied medial to the sternocleidomastoid muscle against the vertebral transverse process. The internal carotid pulse can be felt from the mid-cervical region upwards, whilst the more obvious carotid bifurcation is felt more distally towards the angle of the mandible. These are common sites for aneurysm formation.

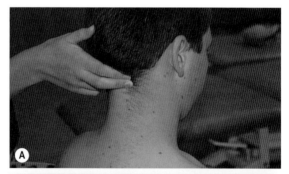

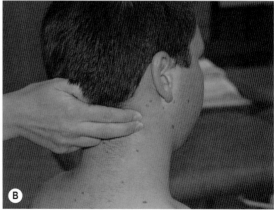

**Figure 6.9** • Vertebral artery pulse palpation sub-occipital (A) and below the mastoid process (B).

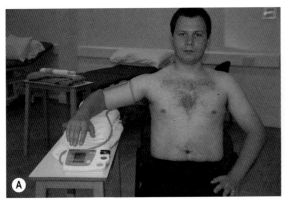 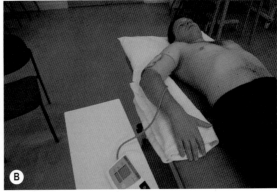

**Figure 6.10 •** (A) Blood pressure monitoring in sitting. The patient sits still for at least 5 minutes in a comfortable, stable environment. The arm is supported at a height level with the heart (mid-sternum). The cuff is applied with the correct tension (it should be possible to place two fingers in the cuff when it is deflated). At least three readings should be taken at 3-minute intervals. **(B)** Blood pressure monitoring in lying. Note that the arm is still kept level with the position of the heart. If the arm is left to drop on the plinth, an inaccurately high reading may occur.

disease, and cervical artery related stroke. An accurate blood pressure reading requires comfortable, standardized positioning and proper use of valid and reliable equipment (Fig. 6.10).

## Cranial nerve examination

The above account of pathophysiology has indicated cranial nerve dysfunction related to either posterior or anterior CAD. It therefore stands that examination of the cranial nerves serves as a useful adjunct to the physical examination of CAD. It is beyond the scope of this book to detail cranial nerve examination fully. However, Table 6.2 presents a summary of cranial nerves, their function, and relevant tests. The reader is encouraged to refer to more detailed sources of neurological examination to fully appreciate the scope and extent of cranial nerve testing.

**Table 6.2 Summary of cranial nerves, functions, and tests**

| Cranial nerve | Name | Sensory or motor | Function | Dysfuntion | Test |
|---|---|---|---|---|---|
| I | Olfactory | S | Smell | Anasomia/ parasomia | Smell test (e.g. soap) |
| II | Optic | S | Vision | Hemianopia/ quadranopia/ scotoma | Visual acuity (chart), field (finger), colour Optic disc appearance (ophthalmoscope) |
| III | Oculomotor | M > S | M – eye movements, pupil size, visual accommodation S – proprioception | Aniscoria/ diplopa Strabismus | Observe for ptosis (differentiate with sympathetic n.) Pupil reaction to light |
| IV | Trochlear | M > S | M – eye movements (superior oblique eye muscles S – proprioception | Nystagmus/ diplopia/ocular paralysis or paresis | as for CN III |

*Continued*

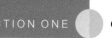

**Table 6.2 Summary of cranial nerves, functions, and tests—Cont'd**

| Cranial nerve | Name | Sensory or motor | Function | Dysfuntion | Test |
|---|---|---|---|---|---|
| V | Trigeminal | S > M | M – muscles of mastication – lower jaw (V3 – mandibular branch)<br>S – V1 – ophthalmic branch – cornea/nasal cavity<br>S – V2 – maxillary branch – nasal cavity/teeth/face | Facial paralysis/ anaesthesia/ hypoaesthesia<br>Jaw hyperreflexia/ clonus | Jaw power (bite and opening)<br>Jaw reflexes<br>Face sensation<br>Corneal reflex |
| VI | Abducens | M > S | M – lateral rectus mm of eye (abductor)<br>S – proprioception | Nystagmus/ diplopia/ocular paralysis or paresis<br>As CN III and IV | As for CN III and IV |
| VII | Facial | M > S | M – mm of facial expression<br>S – taste | Lower facial muscle paralysis/ paresis<br>Taste disturbance (also CN V) | Facial power (orbicularis oculi, blink lag, buccinator, orb oris), i.e. cheeks, eyes, smiling<br>Obvious asymmetry |
| VIII | Vestibulocochlear | S | S – vestibular – inner ear, balance – cochlear – inner ear, hearing | Hypoacusia<br>Tinnitus<br>Vertigo<br>Oscillopsia | Weber test (256 Hz fork on head)<br>Rinne's test (fork on mastoid process then by ear, i.e. bone v. air conductance)<br>Rubbing fingers by ears |
| IX | Glossopharyngeal | S = M | M – stylopharyngeus mm (swallowing and secretion)<br>S – tongue (posterior third); BP, respiration reflex control | Dysarthria/ dysphagia<br>Hoarseness | Gag reflex<br>Tongue depression<br>Swallowing |
| X | Vagus | S M | M and S – pharynx, larynx, chest and abdominal viscera, carotid body and sinus<br>S – heart, voice | Dysphonia/ dysphagia<br>Nausea/ vomiting<br>Uvula deviation | Soft palate elevation and deviation<br>Gag reflex<br>As CN IX |
| XI | Accessory | M > S | M – cranial acc. = pharynx, larynx, soft palate – spinal acc. = SCM; upper trapezius | Trapezius power/ hyperreflexia/ clonus + SCM | Shoulder elevation |
| XII | Hypoglossal | M > S | M – tongue mm<br>S – proprioception | Tongue deviation/ atrophy<br>Dysphagia | Tongue function, wasting, fasciculation, asymmetrical movement |

# Haemodynamics and the thoraco-lumbar spine

There are a small number of pathologies associated with the thoraco-lumbar arterial system which may mimic neuromusculoskeletal pain and serve as absolute contraindications to manipulative therapy. This section reviews the arterial anatomy of the trunk and considers two pathologies the manual therapist is likely to witness in practice: aortic dissection and aortic abdominal aneurysm. Although these two conditions share the same pathological basis, i.e. they are both atherosclerotic disorders, they are considered separately to facilitate the therapists' pattern recognition and management reasoning.

## Clinical anatomy

This section describes the route of the aorta from its origin at the heart to its ending at the mid-lumbar level. It is important for the therapist to appreciate this anatomy relative to surrounding structures, and in particular the aorta's relationship with the low thoracic and upper lumbar vertebrae. Functionally, the vessel can be broken down into four sections: the ascending aorta; aortic arch, the descending thoracic aorta, and the descending abdominal aorta (Fig. 6.11).

### Ascending aorta

This section begins at the base of the left ventricle of the heart and ascends behind the sternum to the level of the left second costal cartilage. The ascending aorta is enclosed within the pericardium and shares a second pericardial tube with the pulmonary trunk (short linking vessel to pulmonary arteries). It sits behind the pulmonary trunk and the right auricle and is anterior to the principal bronchus, left atrium, and right pulmonary artery. To its right lie the aortico-pulmonary bodies and the pulmonary artery. The ascending aorta has no branches.

### Arch of the aorta

This section is a continuation of the ascending aorta. Its entire pathway is within the superior mediastinum and it finishes at the left second costal cartilage, i.e. the 'arch' rises upwards and back down to the same level it started at. As it rises upwards, it travels backwards. Its descent therefore is next to the left side of the third and fourth thoracic

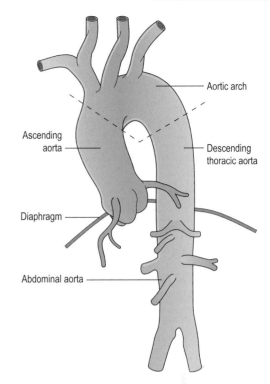

**Figure 6.11** • The aorta. Dashed lines represent anatomical landmarks between each section.

vertebra. Its highest point is at the mid-level of the manubrium. As it rises up and back, traversing to the left side of the body, it is pressed against the front of the trachea.

The arch of the aorta is defined not only by its obvious shape, but also by the important branches arising from it. From right to left these are: the brachiocephalic (or innominate) artery, which then bifurcates into the right sub-clavian and common carotid arteries; the left common carotid artery; and the left sub-clavian artery. Thus 100% of blood supplied to the brain and the upper limbs arises from the arch of the aorta.

### Descending thoracic aorta

Continuous with the aortic arch, this section begins at the fourth thoracic level. It is a descending vessel unremarkable in its pathway which finishes at the lower border of the 12th thoracic vertebra – at the aortic hiatus of the diaphragm. Its descending orientation is slightly posterior–anterior. Thus it begins lateral (left) to the vertebral column but terminates anterior to it. It approximates most consistently with the oesophagus, but shares relationships with most other posterior mediastinal structures. Visceral branches arise from this section including (in order) the pericardial, bronchial, mediastinal, phrenic, intercostals, and sub-costal arteries.

## Descending abdominal aorta

This section descends directly anterior to the lumbar vertebrae. It ends when it bifurcates into the left and right common iliac arteries at the fourth lumbar vertebra (Fig. 6.12). The angle of this bifurcation is highly variable and considered to be a factor in altering the haemodynamics at this point, in turn, contributing to aneurysm development. The average diameter of the adult descending abdominal aorta is around 2 cm. The actual diameter tapers inwards from superior to anterior. The abdominal aorta lies directly anterior to the first to fourth lumbar

vertebra and intervertebral discs, separated only by the anterior longitudinal ligament. It lies behind a number of its own branch arteries and visceral structures, including the liver, pancreas, duodenum, and peritoneum. To its right are the thoracic duct, right diaphragmatic crus, inferior vena cava, and coeliac ganglion. To its left are the left diaphragmatic crus, left coeliac ganglion, sympathetic trunk, and the fourth part of the duodenum. At its lower part, the anterior border of the left psoas major muscle may be overlapped by the vessel.

The abdominal aorta has three groups of branch arteries: anterior, lateral and dorsal. The dorsal branches are of interest to the manual therapist as this group includes the lumbar arteries which supply blood to the vertebral column and canal. Furthermore, the lumbar arteries give rise to their own dorsal branches which, in addition to supplying the cauda equina, meninges and rest of the canal,

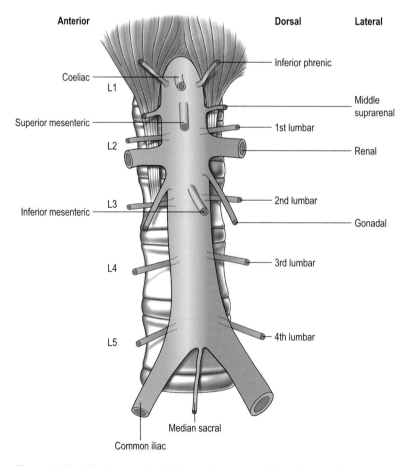

**Figure 6.12 •** The descending (abdominal) aorta and its main branch arteries. (Adapted and reprinted from Drake *et al* (2005), with permission from Elsevier)

also supply the lumbar muscles, zygoapophyseal joints, and ligaments. The anterior and lateral groups of branches supply viscera.

## Pathophysiology

### Aortic dissection

Both aortic dissection and aortic aneurysm are events related to a weakening of the vessel wall and the presence of atherosclerosis. However, they can present differently and it falls within the skill of the therapist to differentiate so the most appropriate management decision can be made, i.e. an emergency referral (dissection or aneurysmal rupture) or a routine medical referral (non-rupture aneurysm).

The dissection process in the aorta is comparable with the carotid and vertebral events referred to above. The condition is characterized by the development of a channel of blood flow developing at least a sub-intimal level. This channel is referred to as a false lumen (Coady et al, 1999; Mukherjee & Eagle, 2005) (Fig. 6.13).

The false lumen is caused by a tear in the tunica intima through which blood can run. The tear itself may be a result of weakened tissue secondary to atherosclerotic disease, hypertension, connective tissue disease (notably Marfan's syndrome, Ehlers-Danlos syndrome, and familial aortic dissection syndrome), stress on the intima from pre-existing intramural haemorrage, or trauma (Grundmann et al, 2006; Kasher et al, 2004; Lissin & Vagelos, 2002; Mukherjee & Eagle, 2005; Muluk et al, 1996). The flow within the false channel is what is referred to as the dissection. Thus, the dissection may develop (spread along the vessel), or remain localized to the site of the tear. Aortic dissections are classically categorized as either Type A or Type B depending on their anatomical site (see Fig. 6.13).

### Aortic aneurysm

Aneurysm describes an abnormal dilatation of a vessel. Vessels are defined as being aneurysmal when they increase to 50% of their normal size (Crawford et al, 2003; Hellmann et al, 2007). Although aortic aneurysm can occur anywhere along the aorta, 75% occur in the descending aorta below the line of the renal arteries (Crawford et al, 2003), otherwise known as abdominal aortic aneurysm (AAA). 90%

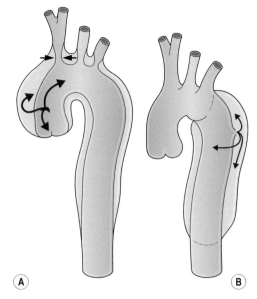

**Figure 6.13** • Aortic dissection. Blood flow through an intimal tear into a 'false lumen' (light arrows). **(A)** Type A dissection: a lesion involving the ascending aorta and aortic arch up to the left sub-clavian artery (this image shows associated stenotic lesion at the base of the brachiocephalic artery – dark arrows). **(B)** Type B dissection – involvement of the descending aorta only. (Reproduced from Coady et al (1999) with permission from Elsevier)

of AAAs are related to atherosclerosis (Johnson et al, 2005; Patel & Kettner, 2006). The remaining 10% are referred to as inflammatory AAAs (Hellmann et al, 2007). Although this distinction is pathophysiologically informative, the presentation and risk factors are similar and it should also be noted that atherosclerosis itself is an inflammatory condition (Kaperonis et al, 2006a, 2006b). The pathologies of aneurysm and dissection overlap to a significant degree, i.e. 'dissecting aneurysm' is an inter-mural haemotoma whereby the haemorrage is separating the vessel wall layers (Crawford et al, 2003). Thus, much of the histopathology is related. The aneurysmal event is associated with weakening (degradation) of the vessel wall – related either to atherosclerosis and/or inflammation as above. Although, in all but a pseudo-aneurysm, all three layers of a vessel are affected, it is the media that loses its structure most significantly, thus affecting the shape of the vessel. Elastin and collagen tissue content is reduced in the media. Thus, the vessel loses both its elasticity and its mechanical strength.

In atherosclerotic AAA, the vessel wall thins. Plasmin is associated with the production of proteolytic enzymes (elastase and collagenase) responsible for this tissue degradation. Plasmin is found in rich supply in an aneurysmal wall (Patel & Kettner 2006). A large number of proinflammatory cytokines, tissue inhibitors (most recent evidence suggests matrix metalloproteinases), vascular smooth muscle cells, leukocyte adhesion molecules, and growth factors have long been implicated in the pathogenesis of AAA. Mounting evidence also steers towards the role that infectious (bacterial and viral) agents have on atherosclerotic inflammatory mediation (Kaperonis et al, 2006a). An exaggerated immune response has also been associated with this pathology.

## Clinical presentations

### Aortic dissection

Early diagnosis of aortic dissection can be life-saving, but is often difficult (Ahmad et al, 2006; Falconi et al, 2005; Grundmann et al, 2006; Kleinfeldt et al, 2007). The most common presentation is sharp, severe chest pain. However, back pain is also commonly associated with aortic dissection (Fig. 6.14). This may be radiating but rarely to the legs or arms. In around 20% of cases, patients

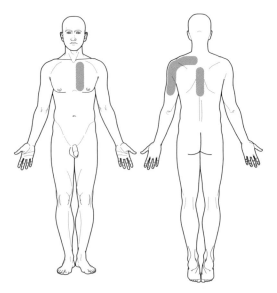

**Figure 6.14** • Potential pain sites associated with aortic dissection. Chest pain is the most common symptom, followed by back pain. If there is upper limb ischaemia as a result of the dissection event, then arm pain may occur.

have presented with syncope without a typical neurological or pain history for this (Mukherjee & Eagle, 2005). The dissection event may prevent blood from reaching its intended distal target limb. Thus, peripheral pulses may be diminished (the limb dependent of the site of the event). However, diagnosis based on peripheral pulse palpation is not definitive (Teece & Hogg, 2004). Equally, differences in upper limb blood pressure may support a diagnosis, but negative findings cannot rule the pathology out (Lissin & Vagelos, 2002). As the condition is related to atherosclerosis and hypertension, a strong history regarding these may support a diagnosis.

Suspicion of aortic dissection should alert the manual therapist to make an urgent emergency department referral where appropriate diagnostic imaging, medical (analgesia and blood pressure stabilization) and ultimately, surgical management, should be administered.

### Abdominal aortic aneurysm

As above, early detection of abdominal aortic aneurysm (AAA) is essential. AAA rupture is between the 10th and 13th most common causes of death in Western males, accounting for around 7000 UK deaths per annum with an increasing incidence (Crawford et al, 2003, Norwood et al, 2007). Prevalence is between 1.7 and 5% of the population, increasing to around 33% in first degree relatives. Back pain is common in up to 50% of pre-rupture AAA (Al-Koteesh et al, 2005; Aydogan et al, 2007; Borenstein, 1996, 1997; Brown, 2001; Crawford et al, 2003; Erdogan et al, 2005; Hellmann et al, 2007; Kaur, 2004; Kleinfeldt et al, 2007; Lissin & Vagelos, 2002) (Fig. 6.15). Because of the nature of patients seen by manual therapist (i.e. back pain), our role in this differential diagnosis cannot be understated (Borenstein, 1996, 1997; Brown, 2001; Crawford et al, 2003; Patel & Kettner, 2006; Riambau et al, 2004).

The ethical and medico-legal implications of ignoring AAA as a potential cause of back pain have been clearly expressed for the manual therapist (Crawford et al, 2003). Overriding risk factors for AAA are: being male (five times more common than in females), age (over 50 years for men, over 60 years for women), smoking, and hypertension. Additional atherosclerotic risk factors must also be considered. The clinical presentation of AAA differs depending on the stage and/or nature of the pathology.

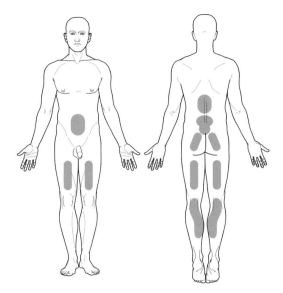

**Figure 6.15** • Potential pain sites associated with abdominal aortic aneurysm. Back pain is present in around 50% of pre-rupture aneurysms. Buttock and thigh symptoms may be referred from the vessel itself. Calf pain may be a result of distal embolization.

## Rupture

This is the most life-threatening stage of AAA and represents vessel wall failure. The diagnostic triad is classically:

- Sudden onset of abdominal and/or back pain
- Hypotension
- Pulsatile abdominal mass.

In addition, the patient may present with sudden onset of syncope or shock. Supported by a relevant history of atherosclerosis or inflammatory risk factors, the patient should receive urgent emergency medical attention.

## Stable rupture

This is when the leakage remains stabilized within the retroperitoneal space. It is less common than an unstable rupture and presents as a more chronic, gradual onset of back or abdominal pain. Additionally, there may be sciatic neuropathy due to compression by the retroperitoneal haematoma. Risk of frank haemorrhage or rupture is high in these patients, and again, immediate emergency medical attention is indicated.

## Non-rupture

The normal diameter of the abdominal aorta is around 2 cm. An aneurysm is defined at 50%

increase of normal diameter, i.e. 3 cm for the abdominal aorta. The surgical cut-off point for most AAAs (based on when risk of rupture outweighs risk of surgery) is around 5.5 cm (Golledge *et al*, 2006; Holt *et al*, 2007; Norwood *et al*, 2007; Wilson *et al*, 2006). The natural progression is for the aneurysm to expand and eventually rupture. Therefore, there is a period of time when the aneurysm is present, but not yet at the stage of rupture. This is the stage when the manual therapist is most likely to witness patients with AAA. The presentation may be either a gradual, insidious or acute (with or without trauma) onset of pain anywhere between the low thoracic and mid-lower lumbar spine. It must be remembered that the majority of AAAs are atherosclerotic. Therefore there will often be significant stenotic lesions within the lumen of the vessel as well as the distended mass. Thus, there may also be associated distal pain related either to ischaemia of the lower limb and/or buttocks (related to the degree of central stenosis), or pressure on spinal structures from the aneurysmal mass referring pain distally. Distal embolization from the central lesions may also cause leg pain. AAAs are often associated with distal aneurysms – most commonly popliteal. A classic vascular intermittent claudicant pattern may be present whereby pain is related to effort. However, the pain behavior may also be mechanical as the nociceptive mechanisms associated with the distended vessel, pressure on surrounding (anterior vertebral) structures, or vertebral erosion may influence pain perception during both flexed and extended lumbar positions and activities.

# Clinical examination of the thoraco-lumbar arterial system

In addition to a careful history regarding the onset and nature of the pain and screening for atherosclerotic risk factors (see below), a physical examination should be undertaken which may incorporate the following elements.

## Pulse palpation

Palpation of the abdominal aorta (Fig. 6.16), together with distal pulse palpation (femoral, popliteal, posterior tibial, dorsalis pedis) can provide valuable information when aortic pathology is suspected. A pulsatile, expandable mass at the site of the abdominal aortic pulse is indicative of AAA.

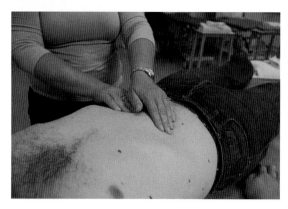

**Figure 6.16** • Palpation of the abdominal aorta. The pulse can usually be found just to the left of the mid-line next to the umbilicus. A positive finding for aneurysm is a pulsatile, expandable mass.

This positive pulse finding is occasionally witnessed in asymptomatic individuals. If this is the case, the finding should be taken seriously and medical opinion should be sought. Conversely, it is important to note that although positive findings from the above tests may support the suspicion of AAA, negative findings do not exclude the diagnosis in the presence of a strong history. As it is possible for aortic pathologies to affect the limbs, it may be warranted to assess distal peripheral pulses. Which pulses are assessed would be dependent on the distribution of symptoms and suspected pathology. It has been reported, however, that testing for deficient peripheral pulses (upper limb) does not have a high enough sensitivity to confidently rule out aortic dissection (Teece & Hogg, 2004). No studies have looked at the diagnostic utility of peripheral pulse examination for AAA.

## Blood pressure testing

As with cervical arterial system examination, because the thoraco-lumbar pathologies are atherosclerotic in nature, blood pressure testing can form an important part of the patient examination. Examination as described in Figure 6.10 will provide information regarding resting blood pressure. Additionally, an arm-to-arm difference in systolic pressure has been associated with aortic dissections (Singer & Hollander, 1996). However, the magnitude of difference is variable and a cut-off point for diagnosis has not been established. Inter-arm differences have been found in healthy subjects between 1 and 20 mmHg (Kimura *et al*, 2004; Orme *et al*, 1999).

## Atherosclerosis

A common underlying pathology to almost all of the conditions presented is atherosclerosis. This section provides a summary of the key elements of a patient's profile to attempt to identify when assessing for the likelihood of atherosclerotic-linked pathologies.

Atherosclerosis is a cascade of inflammatory events influenced by conventional inflammatory mediators and infectious microorganisms. These events are triggered by endothelial dysfunction of the tunica intima induced by chemical, mechanical, or immunological insult (Kaperonis *et al*, 2006a). Below, in list form, is a summary of evidence-based clinical atherosclerotic risk factors which need to be considered in respect of all the above conditions. Questioning during the history-taking can incorporate these evidence-based factors when there is early suspicion of a vascular pathology.

- Hypertension
- Diabetes
- Family history of atherosclerotic-related pathologies (heart disease, stroke, TIA, peripheral vascular disease)
- Smoking
- High serum low density lipoprotein (hypercholesterolemia/hyperlipidemia/high cholesterol-high fat diet)
- Hyperhomocysteinemia
- Infection by *Escherichia coli*, *Helicobacter pylori*, *Chlamydia pneumoniae*, *Streptococcus*, *Staphylococcus*, *Salmonella*, *Clostridium*, *Mycobacterium*, fungi, *Yersinia*, *Treponema*
- Mechanical trauma to vessel.

# Summary

This chapter has presented a number of vascular conditions for the manual therapist to consider in their differential diagnosis, and to identify as contraindications to manual therapy techniques. In all cases, immediate medical referral is indicated. Sound physical tests for these conditions are few and far between. The clinician must therefore rely on their clinical reasoning and the gathering of information from a number of sources. An appreciation of the anatomy, pathophysiology, and clinical presentations will go a long way to helping identify these conditions. Table 6.3 provides a summary of the vascular conditions presented including brief clinical information about the presentation and physical tests which may be used.

**Table 6.3 Summary of clinical presentations, assessment, and management for the manual therapy differentiation of vascular conditions**

|  | Vertebral artery dysfunction | Internal carotid artery dysfunction | Aortic dissection |
|---|---|---|---|
| *Clinical presentation* | Neck/occipital pain<br>Hind-brain ischaemia<br>Hypertension | Neck/temporal/parietal/frontal pain<br>Partial Horner's syndrome<br>Cranial nerve palsy (commonly CN IV–VII)<br>Hypertension | Chest pain<br>Thoracic/lumbar pain<br>Syncope<br>Arm pain/dysaesthesia<br>Hypertension |
| *Risk factors* | Local neck trauma (rotation/extension)<br>Atherosclerosis risk factors<br>Connective tissue disease<br>Upper cervical instability | Local neck trauma (extension/rotation)<br>Atherosclerosis risk factors<br>Connective tissue disease<br>Upper cervical instability | Atherosclerotic risk factors<br>Connective tissue disease<br>Familial aortic dissection syndrome<br>Chest/abdominal trauma (rare) |
| *Physical examination* | Blood pressure<br>Functional positional tests<br>Cranial nerve examination | Blood pressure<br>Carotid pulse palpation<br>Cranial nerve examination | Blood pressure (for state of hypertension)<br>Arm-to-arm blood pressure differences<br>Upper limb pulses |
| *Management* | Urgent medical referral | Urgent medical referral | Immediate urgent medical referral |

# References

Ahmad, F., Cheshire, N., Hamady, M., 2006. Acute aortic syndrome: pathology and therapeutic strategies. Postgrad. Med. J. 82 (967), 305–312.

Al-Koteesh, J., Masannat, Y., James, N.V., et al., 2005. Chronic contained rupture of abdominal aortic aneurysm presenting with longstanding back pain. Scott. Med. J. 50 (3), 122–123.

APA, 2006. Clinical guidelines for assessing vertebrobasilar insufficiency in the management of cervical spine disorders. Australian Physiotherapy Association 2006 [cited 2006] Available from http://apa.advsol.com.au/.

Arnold, M., Bousser, M.G., 2005. Carotid and vertebral dissection. Practical Neurology 5 (1), 100–109.

Asavasopon, S., Jankoski, J., Godges, J.J., 2005. Clinical diagnosis of vertebrobasilar insufficiency: resident's case problem. J. Orthop. Sports Phys. Ther. 35 (10), 645–650.

Aydogan, M., Karatoprak, O., Mirzanli, C., et al., 2007. Severe erosion of lumbar vertebral body because of a chronic ruptured abdominal aortic aneurysm. Spine J. 8 (2), 394–396.

Biousse, V., D'Anglejan-Chatillon, J., Massiou, H., et al., 1994. Head pain in nontraumatic carotid-artery dissection - a series of 65 patients. Cephalalgia 14 (1), 33–36.

Borenstein, D.G., 1996. Chronic low back pain. Rheum. Dis. Clin. North Am. 22 (3), 439–456.

Borenstein, D.G., 1997. A clinician's approach to acute low back pain. Am. J. Med. 102 (1, Suppl. 1), 16S–502.

Brown, M.J., 2001. Prevalence of pathology seen on lumbar x-rays in patients over the age of 50 years. The British Journal of Chiropractic 5 (1–2), 23–30.

Buyle, M., Engelborghs, S., Kunnen, J., et al., 2001. Headache as only symptom in multiple cervical artery dissection. Headache 41 (5), 509–511.

Cao, J.J., Arnold, A.M., Manolio, T.A., et al., 2007. Association of carotid artery intima-media thickness, plaques, and C-reactive protein with future cardiovascular disease and all-cause mortality: the Cardiovascular Health Study. Circulation 116 (1), 32–38.

Chan, C.C.K., Paine, M., O'Day, J., 2001. Carotid dissection: a common cause of Horner's syndrome. Clin. Experiment. Ophthalmol. 29 (6), 411–415.

Childs, J.D., Flynn, T.W., Fritz, J.M., et al., 2005. Screening for vertebrobasilar insufficiency in patients with neck pain: manual therapy decision-making in the presence of uncertainty. J. Orthop. Sports Phys. Ther. 35 (5), 300–306.

Coady, M.A., Rizzo, J.A., Elefteriades, J.A., 1999. Pathological variants of thoracic aortic dissections. Cardiol. Clin. 17 (4), 637–657.

Coman, W.B., 1986. Dizziness related to ENT conditions. In: Grieve, G.P. (Ed.), Grieve's modern manual therapy of the vertebral column. Churchill Livingstone, Edinburgh.

Crawford, C.M., Hurtgen-Grace, K., Talarico, E., et al., 2003. Abdominal aortic aneurysm: An illustrated narrative review. J. Manipulative Physiol. Ther. 26 (3), 184–195.

Drake, R., Vogl, W., Mitchell, A., 2005. Gray's Anatomy for students. Churchill Livingstone. Elsevier, Philadelphia.www.studentconsult.com.

Dziewas, R., Schilling, M., Konrad, C., et al., 2006. Cervical artery dissection - clinical features, risk factors, therapy, and outcome in 126 patients. J. Neurol. 250, 1179–1184.

Erdogan, A., Gilgil, E., Demircan, A., 2005. Vertebral erosion resulting from a chronic retroperitoneal rupture of an abdominal aortic aneurysm. EJVES Extra 9 (6), 113–115.

Falconi, M., Oberti, P., Krauss, J., et al., 2005. Different clinical features of aortic intramural hematoma versus dissection involving the descending thoracic aorta. Echocardiography 22 (8), 629–635.

Femia, R., Kozakova, M., Nannipieri, M., et al., 2007. Carotid intima-media thickness in confirmed prehypertensive subjects. Predictors and progression. Atherosclerosis, Thrombosis, and Vascular Pathology Jul 26 Epub.

Foye, P.M., Najar, M.P., Camme, A.J., et al., 2002. Pain, dizziness and central nervous system blood flow in cervical extension - Vascular correlations to beauty parlor stroke syndrome and salon sink radiculopathy. Am. J. Phys. Med. Rehabil. 81 (6), 395–399.

Frigerio, S., Buhler, R., Hess, C.W., et al., 2003. Symptomatic cluster headache in internal carotid artery dissection - Consider anhidrosis. Headache 43 (8), 896–900.

Golledge, J., Muller, J., Daugherty, A., et al., 2006. Abdominal aortic aneurysm - Pathogenesis and implications for management.

Arterioscler. Thromb. Vasc. Biol. 26 (12), 2605–2613.

Gross, A.R., Chesworth, B., Binkley, J., et al., 2005. A case for evidence based practice in manual therapy. In: Boyling, J.D., Jull, G.A. (Eds.), Grieve's modern manual therapy – The vertebral column. Elsevier Churchill Livingstone, Edinburgh.

Grundmann, U., Lausberg, H., Schäfers, H.J., 2006. Acute aortic dissection. Differential diagnosis of a thoracic emergency. Anaesthesist 55 (1), 53–63.

Guillon, B., Biousse, V., Massiou, H., et al., 1998. Orbital pain as an isolated sign of internal carotid artery dissection. A diagnostic pitfall. Cephalalgia 18 (4), 222–224.

Haynes, M.J., Cala, L., Melsom, A., et al., 2005. Posterior ponticles and rotational stenosis of vertebral arteries. A pilot study using Doppler ultrasound velocimetry and magnetic resonance angiography. J. Manipulative Physiol. Ther. 28 (5), 323–329.

Hellmann, D.B., Grand, D.J., Freischlag, J.A., 2007. Inflammatory abdominal aortic aneurysm. JAMA 297 (4), 395–400.

Holt, P.J.E., Poloniecki, J.D., Gerrard, D., 2007. Meta-analysis and systematic review of the relationship between volume and outcome in abdominal aortic aneurysm surgery. Br. J. Surg. 94 (4), 395–403.

Hupp, J.A., Martin, J.D., Hansen, L., 2007. Results of a single center vascular screening and education program. J. Vasc. Surg. 46 (2), 182–188.

Johnson, D., Shah, P., Collins, P., et al., 2005. Thorax. In: Standing, S. (Ed.), Gray's Anatomy: the anatomical basis of clinical practice. Elsevier Churchill Livingstone, Edinburgh.

Kaperonis, E.A., Liapis, C.D., Kakisis, J.D., et al., 2006a. Inflammation and atherosclerosis. Eur. J. Vasc. Endovasc. Surg. 31 (4), 386–393.

Kaperonis, E.A., Liapis, C.D., Kakisis, J.D., et al., 2006b. Inflammation and Chlamydia pneumoniae infection correlate with the severity of peripheral arterial disease. Eur. J. Vasc. Endovasc. Surg. 31 (5), 509–515.

Kasher, J.A., El-Bialy, A., Balingit, P., 2004. Aortic dissection: A dreaded disease with many faces.

J. Cardiovasc. Pharmacol. Ther. 9 (3), 211–218.

Kaur, R.A., 2004. Co-morbidity of low back pain and abdominal aortic aneurysm: a case report. Clinical Chiropractic 7 (2), 67–72.

Kerry, R., 2002. Pre-manipulative procedures for the cervical spine – new guidelines and a time for dialectics: knowledge, risks, evidence and consent. Physiotherapy 88 (7), 417–420.

Kerry, R., 2006. Verterbral artery testing: how certain are you that your pre-cervical manipulation and mobilisation tests are safe and specific? In: Paper read at HES 2nd International Evidence Based Practice Conference, at London.

Kerry, R., Rushton, A., 2003. Decision theory in physical therapy. Paper read at World Confederation for Physical Therapy 14th International Congress, at Barcelona.

Kimura, A., Hashimoto, J., Watabe, D., et al., 2004. Patient characteristics and factors associated with inter-arm difference of blood pressure measurements in a general population. J. Hypertens. 22 (12), 2277–2283.

Kleinfeldt, T., Ince, H., Rehders, T.C., et al., 2007. The diagnostic dilemma of acute thoracic pain. Internist 48 (1), 75–78.

Kurvers, H.A., van der Graaf, Y., Blankensteijn, F.L., et al., 2007. Screening for asymptomatic internal carotid artery stenosis and aneurysm of the abdominal aorta: comparing the yield between patients with manifest atherosclerosis and patients with risk factors for atherosclerosis only. J. Vasc. Surg. 37 (6), 1226–1233.

Leira, E.C., Cruz-Flores, S., Leacock, R.O., et al., 2001. Sumatriptan can alleviate headaches due to carotid artery dissection. Headache 41 (6), 590–591.

Lemesle, M., Beurait, P., Becker, F., et al., 1998. Head pain associated with sixth-nerve palsy: spontaneous dissection of the internal carotid artery. Cephalalgia 18 (2), 112–114.

Leys, D., Lucas, C., Gobert, M., et al., 1997. Cervical artery dissections. Eur. Neurol. 37 (1), 3–12.

Lissin, L.W., Vagelos, R., 2002. Acute aortic syndrome: a case presentation and review of the literature. Vasc. Med. 7 (4), 281–287.

Lorenz, M.W., von Kegler, S., Steinmetz, H., et al., 2006. Carotid intima-media thickening indicates a higher vascular risk across a wide age range: prospective data from the carotid atherosclerosis progression study (CAPS). Stroke 37 (1), 87–92.

Mainardi, F., Maggioni, F., Dainese, F., et al., 2002. Spontaneous carotid artery dissection with cluster-like headache. Cephalalgia 22 (7), 557–559.

Mitchell, J., 2002. Vertebral artery atherosclerosis: a risk factor for vertebrobasilar insufficiency? Phys. Res. Int. 7 (3), 122–135.

Mitchell, J., Keene, D., Dyson, C., et al., 2002. Is cervical spine rotation, as used in the standard vertebrobasilar insufficiency test, associated with a measurable change in intracranial vertebral artery blood flow? Man. Ther. 9 (3), 220–227.

Mukherjee, D., Eagle, K.A., 2005. Aortic dissection - An update. Curr. Probl. Cardiol. 30 (6), 287–325.

Muluk, S.C., Kaufman, J.A., Torchiana, D.F., et al., 1996. Diagnosis and treatment of thoracic aortic intramural hematoma. J. Vasc. Surg. 24 (6), 1022–1029.

Nichols, F.T., Mawad, M., Mohr, J.P., et al., 1993. Focal headache during balloon inflation in the vertebral and basilar arteries. Headache 33 (2), 87–89.

Norwood, M.G.A., Lloyd, G.M., Bown, M.J., et al., 2007. Endovascular abdominal aortic aneurysm repair. Postgrad. Med. J. 83 (975), 21–27.

Orme, S., Ralph, S.G., Birchall, A., et al., 1999. The normal range for inter-arm differences in blood pressure. Age Ageing 28 (6), 537–542.

Paraskevas, K.I., Stathopoulos, V., Mikhailidis, D.P., et al., 2007. Internal carotid artery occlusion: association with atherosclerotic disease in other arterial beds and vascular risk factors. Angiology 58 (3), 329–335.

Patel, S.N., Kettner, N.W., 2006. Abdominal aortic aneurysm presenting as back pain to a chiropractic clinic: a case report. J. Manipulative Physiol. Ther. 29 (5), 409.e401–409.e407.

Pezzini, A., Granella, F., Grassi, M., et al., 2005. History of migraine and the risk of spontaneous cervical artery dissection. Cephalalgia 25 (8), 575–580.

Refshauge, K.M., 1994. Rotation: a valid premanipulative dizziness test? Does it predict safe manipulation. J. Manipulative Physiol. Ther. 17 (1), 15–19.

Riambau, V., Caserta, G., Garcia-Madrid, C., 2004. Thrombosis of a bifurcated endograft following lower-back microwave therapy. J. Endovasc. Ther. 11 (3), 334–338.

Ritcher, R.R., Reinking, M.F., 2005. Clinical Question: How does evidence on the diagnostic accuracy of the vertebral artery test influence teaching of the test in a professional physical therapist education program? Phys. Ther. http://www.ptjournal.org/PTJournal/Jun2005/Jun05_EiP.cfm.

Rivett, D.A., 1999. Effect of premanipulative tests on vertebral artery and internal carotid artery blood flow: a pilot study. J. Manipulative Physiol. Ther. 22 (4), 368–375.

Rivett, D.A., 2005. The vertebral artery and vertebrobasilar insufficiency. In: Boyling, J.D., Jull, G.A. (Eds.), Grieve's Modern Manual Therapy – The vertebral column. Elsevier Churchill Livingstone, Edinburgh.

Rivett, D.A., Thomas, L.C., Bolton, P.S., 2005. Pre-manipulative testing: where do we go from here? New Zealand Journal of Physiotherapy 33 (3), 78–84.

Rogalewski, A., Evers, S., 2005. Symptomatic hemicrania continua after internal carotid artery dissection. Headache 45 (2), 167–169.

Rossitti, S., Volmann, R., 1995. Changes of blood flow velocity indicating mechanical compression of the vertebral arteries during rotation of the head in the normal human measured with transcranial Doppler sonography. Arq. Neuropsiquiatr. 53 (1), 26–33.

Savitz, S.I., Caplan, L.R., 2005. Current concepts: Vertebrobasilar disease. N. Engl. J. Med. 352 (25), 2618–2626.

Scheel, P., Ruge, C., Schöning, M., 2000. Flow velocity and flow volume measurements in the extracranial carotid and vertebral arteries in healthy adults: reference data and the effects of age. Ultrasound Med. Biol. 26, 1261–1266.

Schoning, M., Walter, J., Scheel, P., 1994. Estimation of cerebral blood flow through color duplex sonography of the carotid and vertebral arteries in healthy adults. Stroke 25 (1), 17–22.

Silbert, P.L., Mokri, B., Schievink, W.I., 1995. Headache and neck pain in spontaneous internal carotid and vertebral artery dissections. Neurology 45 (8), 1517–1522.

Singer, A.J., Hollander, J.E., 1996. Blood pressure. Assessment of interam differences. Arch. Intern. Med. 156 (17), 2005–2008.

Taylor, A.J., Kerry, R., 2005. Neck pain and headache as a result of internal carotid artery dissection: implications for manual therapists - Case report. Man. Ther. 10 (1), 73–77.

Teece, S., Hogg, K., 2004. Peripheral pulses to exclude thoracic aortic dissection. Emerg. Med. J. 21 (5), 589.

Texon, M., 1996. Haemodynamic basis of atherosclerosis: With critique of the cholesterol-heart disease hypothesis. Begell House, New York.

Thanvi, B., Munshi, S., Dawson, S.L., 2005. Carotid and vertebral artery dissection syndromes. Postgrad. Med. J. 81, 383–388.

Thiel, H., Rix, G., 2005. Is it time to stop functional pre-manipulative testing of the cervical spine? Man. Ther. 10 (2), 154–158.

Watanabe, K., Hasegawa, K., Takano, K., 2001. Anomalous vertebral artery-induced cervical cord compression causing severe nape pain - Case report. J. Neurosurg. 95 (1), 146–149.

Wilson, R.W., Choke, E.C., Dawson, J., et al., 2006. Contemporary management of the infra-renal abdominal aortic aneurysm. Surgeon 4 (6), 363–371.

Zetterling, M., Carlström, C., Konrad, P., et al., 2000. Internal carotid artery dissection. Acta Neurol. Scand. 101 (1), 1–7.

# Principles and progression of combined movements

Chris McCarthy

## Notation

Whilst the use of the IN and DID system will encourage the consideration of starting positions, the use of box diagrams is an excellent method of conveying combined movement theory (CMT) positioning. The box diagram conveys considerable amounts of information with the simple addition of two lines to a box framework (Fig. 7.1). The frame of the box diagram represents the normal range of movement in sagittal (vertical line), coronal and axial planes (horizontal line). Flexion, extension and lateral flexion movements are denoted using straight lines, and rotation by an arc. The box diagram is drawn to represent the movement pattern associated with a dysfunction. It should be accompanied by shading to identify the predominant side of pain. This process identifies the quadrant of dysfunction (the corner of possible three-dimensional movement that is painful or restricted).

In addition to the above, a judgement on severity of pain (severe or not) should be placed next to the box. The diagram signifies to another CMT therapist that a process has been undertaken in order to draw the box diagram. The significant features of the box diagram follow:

- The direction of movement that reproduces pain suggests whether the pain is an anterior or posterior stretch pattern.
- Patients finding it difficult to move towards the side of pain have anterior stretch dysfunction whilst pain produced by movement away from the side of pain is a posterior stretch dysfunction. This information ensures that the three movements that stretch either the anterior or posterior structures are examined and ranked for importance.
- The presence of two lines on the box diagram signifies that the movement not featuring was the least provocative.
- The bolder of the two arrows signifies that this is the most provocative movement, or 'prime movement'.
- A two-headed arrow simply emphasizes that this was the second movement of the primary combination, whilst a one-headed arrow shows that it was the first.
- The order of the primary combination signifies that this order has been established by comparing both combinations and ranking them.

## Treatment progression

In order to describe the reasoning process of CMT treatment we will use the cervical spine case study from Chapter 4. Take a minute to familiarize yourself again with the presentation which is detailed below.

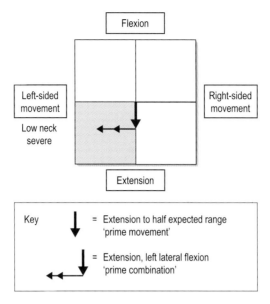

Key
↓ = Extension to half expected range 'prime movement'

= Extension, left lateral flexion 'prime combination'

**Figure 7.1** • Box diagram illustrating prime movement and prime combination.

## CERVICAL SPINE CASE STUDY

### INITIAL INTERVIEW

#### Symptomology

A 22-year-old female sought treatment for pain in the right cervical spine and right shoulder. The pain was located in the lower cervical spine and referred into the right shoulder across the right supra-scapula fossa. The pain was not radicular in quality but severe at rest and with movement (8/10). There was no suggestion of an upper motor neuron lesion and no indication of other red flags. There were no features suggestive of segmental cervical instability or shoulder derangement. There was no history of cervical locking, catching or weakness. There was no headache.

### RELEVANT HISTORY

Symptoms developed over a 6-day period following a mild, rear shunt whiplash injury, a week ago.

### BEHAVIOUR OF SYMPTOMS

Pain was reproduced with low cervical flexion and left lateral flexion. Sitting with the neck in this position reproduced symptoms within 2 minutes. The symptoms were eased, immediately, by positioning the lower cervical spine in extension and right lateral flexion. No latent pain was exhibited.

### DIURNAL PATTERN

There was no stiffness in the cervical spine in the morning. Shoulder pain developed in the evening. Sleep was not disturbed.

### SPECIAL QUESTIONS

The patient's general health was good. There was no weight loss, no dizziness, no dysphagia, no dysarthria, no diplopia, no raised blood pressure, and no symptoms of cervical artery dysfunction. Radiographs of the cervical spine were normal. The patient was not currently taking any anticoagulant or steroid therapy and had received no benefit from anti-inflammatory medication. There was no history of locking, clunking or giving way of the shoulder, and no history of trauma.

### PHYSICAL EXAMINATION

#### Observation

There was no atrophy of the cervical musculature. There was an increase in muscle tone of the right sternocleidomastoid, upper fibres of trapezuis and levator scapula and right scalenes.

Pain was reproduced earliest in range with left lateral flexion. Restriction to flexion was apparent at the C5/C6 level. Pain was reproduced further into range with flexion than with left lateral flexion. Restriction to movement is most obvious in the mid cervical region (see Fig. 7.3).

#### Passive physiological intervertebral movement (PPIVM)

Due to the severity, examination was undertaken in right lateral flexion and extension (posterior structures off stretch) to establish the movement that most reduced pain and dysfunction. Right lateral flexion induced the greatest increase in movement and reduction in muscle tone.

See the completed planning sheet in Figure 7.2.

**OBJECTIVE EXAMINATION PLAN**

**List your hypotheses for the nature of the condition.**
1. .................... *Posterior facet capsule sprain* ......................................
2. .................... *Posterior paraspinal strain* ...........................................
3. .................... *Posterior annular disc sprain* ........................................

**Which two hypotheses will you test against each other in the initial physical examination?**
Primary ............. *Articular predominance* ...............................................
Secondary ......... *Myogenic predominance* ...............................................

**Is the nature of the condition severe?**
Yes  ☐ ✓    No  ☐

**Is the nature of the condition irritable?**
Yes  ☐    No  ☐ ✓

**To what point are you allowing movement to occur?**
Before pain          ☐
To pain              ☐ ✓
To limit             ☐

**What is the functional demonstration/primary re-test marker?**
.................... *Flexion contralateral, lateral flexion quadrant* ....................

**What is the primary pain mechanism of this patient's condition?**
Nociceptive              ☐ ✓
Peripheral neurogenic    ☐
Central                  ☐
Autonomic                ☐
Affective                ☐

**To what extent will you perform a neurological exam?**
None required                                              ☐
Local peripheral                                           ☐
Lower motor neuron, upper motor neuron, limbs              ☐ ✓
Lower motor neuron, upper motor neuron, limbs and cranial  ☐

**What is the weighting of the following components of the problem?**

| | % |
|---|---|
| Arthrogenic | 50 |
| Myogenic | 40 |
| Neurogenic | 1 |
| Inflammagenic | 2 |
| Psychogenic | 1 |
| Sociogenic | 1 |
| Pathogenic | 1 |
| Viscerogenic | 1 |
| Osteogenic | 3 |

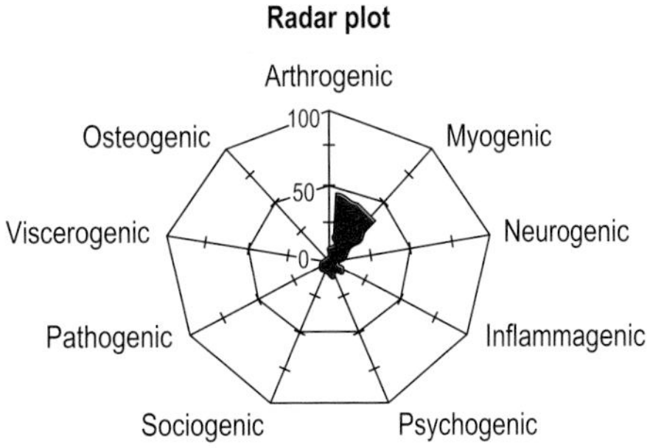

Radar plot

**Likely first treatment:**
In:   *Extension, right lateral flexion quadrant* ...........................................
Will: *Anterior capsular stretch, large amplitude movement, in resistance (Grade III)* ..............................

**Comments/cautions:**
*Pain relief approach, progressing to a stretch of the tissues driving the nociceptive pattern of presentation* ............................
........................................................................................................

**Figure 7.2 •** The objective examination plan.

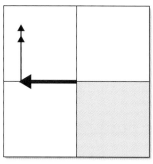

Right-sided cervical and shoulder pain Severe

Prime movement = left lateral flexion
Prime combination = left lateral flexion
followed by flexion. 3/4 full range

**Figure 7.3** • Box diagram showing the prime combination for the patient.

*A short passive treatment, using this right lateral flexion of C5 on C6 reduced the pain produced by the functional demonstration by 10%.*

The most appropriate treatment to induce greatest change in dysfunction was established to be:

Rx1    IN: right lateral flexion, extension
       DID: unilateral AP glide of C5 on C6, Grade III, 1 × 1 minute
       OUTCOME: 40% reduction in pain

### Clinical reasoning

The starting position for this technique allows the production of specific passive movement on the side and on the level of pain generation. The starting position and movement induced do not stretch the posterior aspect of the motion segment. A neurophysiologically-mediated alteration in the perception of nociceptive pain will occur (Wright, 1995). This phenomenon is rapid acting and within seconds the therapist will be able to detect a reduction in paraspinal hypertonicity and a concurrent increase in compliance to passive movement. This had occurred after 1 minute of mobilization and thus the technique was stopped, to allow reassessment of the patient's demonstration of dysfunction.

Rx2    IN: identical starting position
       DID: identical technique
       OUTCOME: no improvement

### Passive accessory intervertebral movement (PAIVM)

Due to the severity, examination was undertaken in right lateral flexion and extension (posterior structures off stretch) to establish the movement that most reduced pain and dysfunction. Anterior pressure (AP) on C5 induced the greatest increase in movement and reduction in muscle tone (greater than induced by AP movement of C4 or C6).

*A short passive treatment, using this accessory movement reduced the pain produced by the functional demonstration by 40%.*

### Muscular assessment

In right lateral flexion and extension due to severity of pain, palpation of musculature reveals hypertonicity of deep paraspinals (C4 to C6) and hypertonicity of the region's phasic muscles. No trigger points were detected.

*Palpation and length assessment of levator scapulae, scalenes, upper fibres of trapezius and sternocleidomastoid did not alter the functional demonstration.*

### Clinical reasoning

As the previous treatment technique had been so beneficial it was repeated. During the technique the therapist perceived less change in muscle tone and compliance and unfortunately it was likely that the neurophysiological pain relief induced in the previous starting position had achieved all it was going to do.

Rx3    IN: right lateral flexion, extension
       DID: unilateral PA glide of C5 on C6, Grade III, 1 × 1 minute
       OUTCOME: pain reduced by another 20%

### Clinical reasoning

As the dysfunction is much less severe, it was acceptable to begin to reproduce some of the patient's movement pain and to start to mobilize the tissues that are the nociceptive generators of pain. The change in direction of accessory glide allows the production of some anterior glide of C5 (inducing very gentle excursion into resistance and stretch of the posterior soft tissues).

Principles and progression of combined movements          CHAPTER 7

Rx4    IN: identical starting position
       DID: identical technique
       OUTCOME: no improvement

## Clinical reasoning

As the previous treatment technique had been so beneficial it was repeated. During the technique the therapist perceived less change in muscle tone and compliance to passive movement.

Rx5    IN: right side flexion, flexion
       DID: unilateral PA glide of C5 on C6,
       Grade III, 1 × 1 minute
       OUTCOME: pain reduced by
       another 40%

## Clinical reasoning

The dysfunction was now not severe and so greater afferent stimulus and mechanical stretch could be induced. This starting position induces more stretch on the posterior structures than the previous technique but is a starting position that avoided the patient's prime movement. The patient's prime movement was left lateral flexion and thus the progression of stretch was into flexion (counter-clockwise around the box) rather than into left-lateral flexion (clockwise around the box).

Rx6    IN: identical starting position
       DID: identical technique
       OUTCOME: no improvement

## Clinical reasoning

As the previous treatment technique had been so beneficial it was repeated. During the technique the therapist perceived less change in muscle tone and compliance to passive movement.

Rx7    IN: left lateral flexion, flexion
       DID: unilateral PA glide of C5 on C6,
       grade III, 1 × 1 minute
       OUTCOME: pain free when performing
       the functional demonstration

## Clinical reasoning

It was now necessary to progress the starting position for mobilization into the prime combination. The technique used maximally stretched the posterior structures and evoked maximal afferent barrage from mechanoreceptors stimulated to their maximum tension.

Rx8    Explanation and provision of a 'mimicking'
       home stretching/exercise programme

When a dysfunction has improved or resolved it is important to explain to the patient the mechanisms of this effect and to reinforce the message that the dysfunction was a simple mechanical fault. Emphasizing the benign mechanical fault aspect of their painful dysfunction will reduce anxiety and fear avoidance. It is imperative that you educate the patient about the importance of a home stretching programme that mimics what you have undertaken (see Ch. 13). This reinforces their active involvement in managing their dysfunction and ensures that they maintain the improvements in ranges and motor control they will have just gained.

## Clinical point

Expect them to return with some loss of the benefit they have just experienced if you do not undertake these vital components in their management.

This idealized progression of mobilization techniques can occur over seven visits to the clinic (if you are concerned about the need to monitor any latent effect of treatment) or over seven 1-minute treatments during one session. You will develop a feel for rate of progression once you have progressed and regressed a number of patients. Regression of patient treatment, in light of an exacerbation of pain or with excessive treatment soreness, involves reducing the afferent stimulus and stretch by changing the starting position. Reducing the pre-treatment stretch on the nociceptive generators allows continued mobilization in resistance. It is worth considering your handling technique if a patient has had excessive treatment soreness as, whilst considerable force is required to perform grade III+ mobilizations in combined positions, they should *never* be sore or tender.

Progression of mobilization involves progressive increase in stretch. If starting in the opposite quadrant to the quadrant of dysfunction, your mobilization

105

techniques are aiming to induce pain relief without stimulating nociceptive sources. As pain reduces, you progressively increase the stretch on these tissues by changing starting position. By moving your starting position around the box diagram you will increase the dose of your treatment until you are in a position where you cannot stretch the tissues any further. When moving around the box, choose the direction that adds in the prime movement last, by which time pain will have reduced with previous treatments. When regressing treatment, in light of an exacerbation, reduce the stretch on nociceptive sources by changing your starting position, but persist with mobilization into pain-free resistance to ensure rapid, neurophysiologically-mediated pain relief.

## Integration of manipulation

In relation to our case study patient, let us imagine that, during your initial lateral flexion PPIVM examination of C5/C6, you perceived the crisp resistance profile, which suggests that the segment would likely benefit from a manipulation (see Ch. 2). In addition, there is a palpable region of paraspinal muscle spasm local to C5/C6 on the right. As the patient has the passive movement indications for manipulation the therapist may wish to consider incorporating manipulative technique into a mobilization programme. Post manipulation we can be confident that the local paraspinal hypertonicity will be absent (albeit temporarily) and that the motion segment will be more mobile (Sandoz, 1976). Thus, subsequent mobilization will be more likely to induce movement of greater range and therefore greater associated afferent effect on pain perception.

Following an assessment for potential cervical artery dysfunction (see Ch. 6) and after a discussion with your patient to gain consent for a thrust technique, you would undertake a manipulative thrust technique:

IN: extension, right lateral flexion, left rotation
DID: right lateral flexion, grade IV−, thrust
OUTCOME: immediate reduction in paraspinal hypertonicity, increase in segmental range of motion and associated reduction in pain (25%)

### Clinical reasoning

As the objective of the manipulative thrust technique is not to stretch a particular component of the joint capsule or contiguous paraspinal muscle we establish the starting position, based on two features.

Firstly, the therapist may wish to avoid the quadrant of dysfunction in severely painful presentations, hence the extension emphasis of the starting position.

Secondly, the starting position and direction of thrust that offer the best chance of inducing cavitation should be chosen.

Thus, the order in which ipsilateral lateral flexion and contralateral rotation are produced is compared before the starting position is established. Finally, the direction of the thrust is established by approaching the starting position in each of three directions (lateral flexion, transverse thrust and rotation). Importantly, the thrust is initiated in the resistance-free range of the movement and flicks at the beginning of the resistance. The unnatural coupling of the segment induces gapping, not the force of the thrust. Attempting this technique at end of range will not result in cavitation as the joint capsule is too tight (Evans & Breen, 2006) to allow gapping – hence the grade IV notation. (See Ch. 9 for detail on this process.)

Having undertaken a manipulative thrust technique it is important that you assess that the physiological changes, associated with cavitation, have occurred at the level you were wishing to influence. A reassessment of the resistance profile of the starting position should reveal a change from a short, sharp, resistance profile to a longer, bouncy feel. Local, deep paraspinal muscle tone should have reduced. Provided these findings are present, you have achieved your aims and your patient should report associated reduction in pain, stiffness and spasm. You now have a temporary window of opportunity to progress to stronger (grade III+/IV+) mobilizations, following the principles of progression detailed above. Alternatively, you may wish to address other components of the patients motor control dysfunction in the period where you have inhibited painful hypertonicity and facilitated previously inhibited muscle (Herzog, 2000).

## Integration and progression of muscle tonicity techniques

Let us imagine our case study patient has firstly, a more significant change in functional demonstration following the assessment of muscle than from passive movement of the motion segment and secondly, palpable hypertonicity of posterior paraspinal muscles on the right of her neck. We may wish to evoke changes in perception in pain and reductions in hypertonicity using isometric muscle contractions:

Rx1    IN: right lateral flexion, extension – gripping C5 using the grip for an AP accessory movement

DID: gentle isometric contraction of the right, local anterior paraspinal muscles, 5–6 seconds, 3 repetitions – progressing further away from neutral

OUTCOME: 60% reduction in pain

## Clinical reasoning

Our patient has severe myogenic pain of the right posterior paraspinal muscles. It is unacceptable to place these muscles on stretch and make them contract, consequently we choose a starting position that places them off stretch and use the *reciprocal inhibition* phenomenon to evoke reduction in posterior muscle hypertonicity (Chaitow, 2006). Using the comfortable grip used for AP accessory movements (see Ch. 9) instruct the patient to 'don't let me win' and provide anterior pressure on the C5. Pressure need only be enough to evoke a contraction and the hold needs only to be a brief 5–6 seconds. When the patient relaxes, perform an AP pressure to push the upper segment back into further extension and right lateral flexion. This will evoke afferent stimulus of descending pain mechanisms and a reduction in both anterior and posterior muscle tone. Repeat this process until no further gain in range is made during relaxation (typically after 3 repetitions).

Rx2    IN: left lateral flexion, flexion

DID: gentle isometric contraction of the right, local posterior paraspinal muscles, 5–6 seconds, 3 repetitions – progressing further away from neutral

OUTCOME: no pain on performance of the functional demonstration

## Clinical reasoning

As the dysfunction is now no longer severe it is acceptable to put the right posterior paraspinal muscles on stretch and evoke *post-isometric relaxation* to reduce hypertonicity and pain. Thus, in the prime combination, using the grip used for the PA accessory glide technique (see Ch. 9) instruct the patient to 'don't

let me win' and provide posterior pressure on the C5. Pressure need only be enough to evoke a contraction and the hold needs only to be a brief 5–6 seconds). When the patient relaxes, perform a PA pressure to push the upper segment forward into further flexion and left lateral flexion. This will evoke afferent stimulus of descending pain mechanisms and a reduction in both anterior and posterior muscle tone. Repeat this process until no further gain in range is made during relaxation (typically after 3 repetitions).

Progression of treatment is similar to the approach utilized with passive movement. Starting positions are chosen that progressively increase the stretch on hypertonic muscles and directions of contractions are used that may need to avoid contraction of severely painful groups. As severity reduces it is acceptable to put hypertonic muscles on stretch and contract them against gentle resistance. In short, whether the patient's dysfunction is severe or not, you will use starting positions that require them to resist you as you attempt to move them further away from neutral to evoke appropriate isometric contractions.

Again, when a dysfunction has improved or resolved it is important to explain to the patient the mechanisms of this effect and to reinforce the message that the dysfunction was a simple muscular, mechanical fault. Emphasizing the benign mechanical fault aspect of their painful dysfunction will reduce anxiety and fear avoidance. It is imperative that you educate the patient about the importance of a home stretching programme that mimics what you have undertaken (see Ch. 13). This reinforces their active involvement in managing their dysfunction and ensures that they maintain the improvements in ranges and motor control they will have just gained.

## Clinical point

Expect them to return with some loss of the benefit they have just experienced if you do not undertake these vital components in their management.

# References

Chaitow, L., 2006.  Muscle energy
    techniques. Elsevier Health Sciences,
    Oxford.

Evans, D.W., Breen, A.C., 2006.
    A biomechanical model for
    mechanically efficient cavitation
    production during spinal
    manipulation: prethrust position
    and the neutral zone. J. Manipulative
    Physiol. Ther. 29, 72–82.

Herzog, W., 2000.  Clinical
    biomechanics of spinal manipulation.
    Churchill Livingstone, Philadelphia.

Sandoz, R., 1976. Some physical
    mechanisms and effects of spinal
    adjustments. Ann. Swiss Chiro.
    Assoc. 6, 91–141.

Wright, A., 1995. Hypoalgesia post
    manipulative therapy: a review of a
    potential neurophysiological
    mechanism. Man. Ther. 1, 11–16.

# Section 2

## Practical Combined Movement

# Chapter Eight

8

# Upper cervical spine

Gail Forrester, Chris McCarthy

## CHAPTER CONTENTS

## Introduction

Due to its unique regional anatomy and complicated biomechanics, the cranio-cervical region presents something of a challenge for manual therapists. It is the most mobile region of the spine; this allows accurate positioning of the main sensory organs but also predisposes the region to a wide range of disorders and increases its vulnerability to trauma and degenerative changes (Konig *et al*, 2005). In addition, the upper cervical spine has a unique pattern of innervation and a close relationship with the brainstem, spinal cord, cranial nerves and vertebral arteries (Standring, 2008). Consequently, dysfunction in the cranio-cervical region can manifest in a wide variety of unusual symptoms including nausea, headache, dizziness, and head, neck or facial pain (Kerry & Taylor, 2006; Maak *et al*, 2006; Nguyen *et al*, 2004; Swinkels & Oostendorp, 1996).

This combination of factors may make clinicians wary of managing conditions originating from the upper cervical spine. However, with carefully directed manual therapy it is possible to alleviate many of the distressing and often debilitating symptoms experienced by patients with neuromusculoskeletal disorders of the cranio-cervical region (Jull *et al*, 2008).

The purpose of this chapter is to assist the clinician in the safe and effective management of craniocervical disorders. The chapter will initially review relevant clinical information before outlining a systematic approach, using a combined movement theory framework, for the examination of neuromusculoskeletal dysfunction in the upper cervical spine.

## Combined movements and the upper cervical spine

Owing to the size, shape and orientation of upper cervical joint surfaces and the arrangement of the surrounding soft tissues, cranio-cervical movements occurring in one plane will result in three-dimensional movement patterns (Brolin & Haldin 2004; Catrysse *et al*, 2008; Panjabi *et al*, 1988). The combination of movements involved in this pattern is termed the 'coupling' or 'coupled movement' pattern and refers to all movements that take place alongside the primary movement (Cook *et al*, 2006; Ishii *et al*, 2006). Knowledge of the coupling patterns of the cranio-cervical junction forms the basis of examining and treating upper

cervical spinal disorders using combined movement theory (CMT).

The pattern of coupled movements in the upper cervical spine is largely opposite to the pattern observed in the lower cervical spine and it has been shown to be affected by the specific cranio-cervical anatomy, the overall upper cervical posture, the initiating movement, the pattern of neuromuscular activation, and the presence of local degenerative changes (Cook *et al*, 2006; Edmonston *et al*, 2005; Panjabi *et al*, 1993). These factors need to be taken into consideration when assessing or treating the upper cervical spine using CMT.

The following section will highlight relevant regional anatomy and biomechanics which can be integrated into the assessment process by the clinician in order to assist the identification of dysfunctional structures, movements or postures presenting in the upper cervical spine. In addition, this clinical information will help to justify the selection of appropriate rehabilitation strategies.

## Clinical anatomy and biomechanics

The cranio-cervical region is comprised of the occiput (C0) and the upper two cervical vertebrae known as the atlas (C1) and the axis (C2). Both these vertebrae are markedly atypical (Middleditch & Oliver, 2005).

### The atlas

The atlas (Fig. 8.1) is a ring-shaped vertebra without a vertebral body or spinous process. It has two superior and two inferior articulating facets which

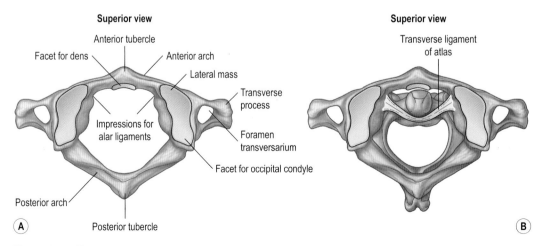

**Figure 8.1** • The atlas. (Reproduced from Drake *et al* (2005) with permission from Elsevier)

articulate with the occiput above and the axis below. In addition it has a central facet on the inside of the anterior atlas arch which articulates with the odontoid peg of C2. The atlas has an antero-posterior (A-P) diameter of approximately 3 cm which means that the spinal canal at this level is larger than anywhere else in the vertebral column (Ebraheim *et al*, 1998). The odontoid peg, transverse ligament and spinal cord occupy two thirds of the A-P diameter, leaving 1 cm of free space. This allows the large ranges of motion (ROM) to occur across the cranio-cervical junction without encroachment onto the spinal cord.

## The axis

The axis (Fig. 8.2) is the strongest and the most irregularly shaped cervical vertebra with a large vertical projection arising from the superior surface of the body of the vertebra called the dens or odontoid process. The odontoid process has an anterior and a posterior facet for articulation with the anterior arch of the atlas and the transverse ligament respectively. Laterally, the axis has two large upward and laterally-orientated articulating facets on its superior surface for articulation with the atlas above (Standring, 2008; Taylor & Twomey, 2002).

These two vertebrae, together with the occiput, form a unique triad of articulations commonly referred to as the occipital-atlanto-axial complex which consists of the atlanto-occipital joint (C0–C1) and the atlanto-axial joints (C1–C2).

## The occipito-atlanto-axial complex

The directions and amounts of movement that occur across this complex are mainly the result of the

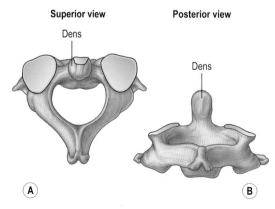

**Figure 8.2** • The axis. (Reproduced from Drake *et al* (2005) with permission from Elsevier)

orientation of the articular surfaces, the absence of intevertebral discs (IVDs) and the tension within the soft tissues.

Approximately one third of the total cervical sagittal plane movement takes place in the upper cervical spine with the movements of flexion/extension predominantly occurring at C0–C1 (Chancey *et al*, 2007; Jull *et al*, 2008). These movements are facilitated by the orientation of the joint surfaces between the occiput and the atlas, and are larger in range than at lower cervical levels.

Rotation is the dominant movement at C1–C2 and accounts for over half of the total cervical transverse plane movement. The amount of rotation at the atlanto-axial (A-A) joint is significantly larger than at any other vertebral level and again this is mainly due to the configuration of the articular surfaces (Cattrysse *et al*, 2008; Ishii *et al*, 2004; Ordway *et al*, 1999). Side-flexion occurs across both the atlanto-occipital (A-O) and A-A joints but, in contrast, it is smaller in range than at sub-axial cervical levels (Ishii *et al*, 2006; Panjabi *et al*, 2001).

The primary movements of the upper cervical spine are generally coupled with secondary movements or translations (Cattrysse *et al*, 2007; Ishii *et al*, 2006). The most significant coupled movement in the cranio-cervical complex is rotation which is coupled with lateral flexion in the opposite direction. This primarily occurs at the A-A joint but also happens to a much lesser extent at the O-A joint (Ishii *et al*, 2004). The primary movements of flexion/extension are accompanied by small, secondary plane movements of lateral flexion and rotation in a contralateral pattern (Amiri *et al*, 2003; Bogduk & Mercer, 2000). The main coupled translation which takes place across the occipito-atlanto-axial complex is lateral translation at C1–C2 during side-flexion; this occurs in the same direction as the side-flexion movement (Ishii *et al*, 2006).

## Atlanto-occipital joint

The atlanto-occipital (A-O) joint (Fig. 8.3) is essentially a uni-planar joint consisting of a pair of synovial condyloid joints between the two convex occipital condyles on the base of the skull and the two large reciprocally concave superior facets on the lateral masses of the atlas (Standring, 2008).

The joint surfaces are relatively congruous. They are long in a posterior–anterior (P–A) direction and

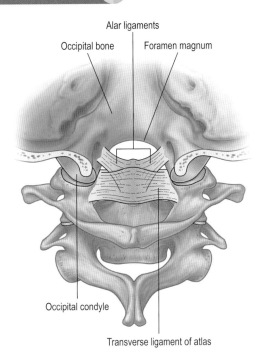

Alar ligaments

Occipital bone    Foramen magnum

Occipital condyle

Transverse ligament of atlas

**Figure 8.3 •** The atlanto-occipital joint. (Reproduced from Drake *et al* (2005) with permission from Elsevier)

narrow mediolaterally. This, together with the sagittal plane orientation of the joint and the reciprocally curved articular surfaces, primarily facilitate the movements of flexion and extension, or nodding, of the head on neck (Bogduk & Mercer, 2000). In addition, the shape of the joint surfaces is such that the anterior ends project higher than the posterior ends; this configuration permits a greater range of extension than flexion (Chancey *et al*, 2007; Panjabi *et al*, 2001).

## Kinematics of atlanto-occipital flexion and extension

Movement analysis studies of the upper cervical spine (in vitro and in vivo) report a variable range of flexion–extension at the A-O joint. Combined findings would suggest that the range of flexion is approximately 3.5°–7.0° and the range of extension is between 16.5° and 21.0°. This gives a total sagittal plane ROM at the C0–C1 segment of approximately 20°–28° (Amiri *et al*, 2003; Ordway *et al*, 1999; Panjabi *et al*, 1988, 2001). Given that the total range of flexion–extension at the C5–C6 segment is reported to be approximately 6°–10° (Goel *et al*, 1984; Goel & Clausen, 1998; Moroney *et al*, 1988; Panjabi *et al*, 2001) the C0–C1 segment demonstrates one of the largest amounts of combined flexion–extension available at any one vertebral segment.

During upper cervical flexion, the occipital condyles roll forwards and slide backwards on the atlas (Bogduk & Mercer, 2000). This movement tightens and is limited by tension developed in the posterior part of the joint capsules, the posterior neck muscles, the posterior A-O membrane, and the ligamentum nuchae. The opposite occurs during upper cervical extension. The occipital condyles roll backwards and slide forwards on the atlas (Bogduk & Mercer, 2000). This movement is mainly limited by approximation of the occiput with the sub-occipital muscles and the posterior arches of the atlas and axis but may also be restrained by tension in the anterior A-O membrane and joint capsules (Bogduk & Mercer, 2000; Palastanga *et al*, 2006) (Fig. 8.4).

Flexion–extension at the A-O joint occurs during flexion–extension of the entire cervical spine but

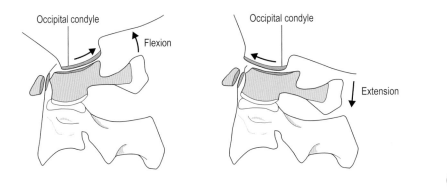

Occipital condyle

Flexion

Occipital condyle

Extension

(A)          (B)

**Figure 8.4 •** (A) Kinematics of the atlanto-occipital joint in flexion and (B) extension. (Reproduced from Palastanga *et al* (2006) with permission from Elsevier)

has been found to be at a maximum during the movements of upper cervical retraction (a posterior translation of the entire head, or 'chin in' position) and protraction (a forward translation of the entire head, or 'chin out' position) respectively (Ordway *et al*, 1999). Maximum stretch to the posterior peri-articular tissue of the A-O joint will occur in upper cervical retraction and to the anterior peri-articular structures in protraction. Clinically, it would seem appropriate to use these upper cervical movements in the assessment of the A-O joint and surrounding peri-articular structures.

### Kinematics of atlanto-occipital lateral flexion and rotation

Axial rotation and lateral flexion are not considered to be physiological movements of the A-O joint as they cannot be produced in isolation by muscle action; however, they do occur secondary to the primary movements.

Studies suggest that the available range of lateral flexion to each side is in the region of 1.9–4.5° and the amount of rotation to each side is approximately 1.7–4.9° (Bogduk & Mercer, 2000; Goel *et al*, 1988; Ishii *et al*, 2004, 2006; Panjabi *et al*, 2001). Results from in vivo studies generally produce measurements towards the lower end of the reported range whilst in vitro studies provide greater values for side-flexion and rotation; this is likely to be due to the contribution of physiological muscle tone and the effect of posture on ROM. For clinical purposes it would appear reasonable to consider that the available range of planar side-flexion and rotation at the A-O joint is approximately 2–3° to each side.

Both these movements are checked by the contralateral alar ligament and the A-O joint capsules (Bogduk & Mercer, 2000; Brolin & Halldin, 2004; Crisco *et al*, 1991b; Krakenes & Kaale, 2006).

### Coupling of movements at the atlanto-occipital joint

Planar movements of the A-O joint have been considered individually but it is perhaps of greater clinical relevance to consider these movements in combination as they would occur during normal upper cervical movement patterns. It is generally agreed that the coupling pattern of movement in the upper cervical spine is predominantly contralateral, particularly if rotation is the initiating movement (Amiri *et al*, 2003; Cook *et al*, 2006; Ishii *et al*, 2004). This is in contrast to the ipsilateral

coupling of side-flexion and rotation predictably observed in the sub-axial cervical spine (Cook *et al*, 2006).

The primary movements of the A-O joint of flexion–extension are accompanied by negligible amounts, approximately 2–3°, of rotation and side-flexion coupled in a contralateral pattern (Amiri *et al*, 2003). Clinically, these findings suggest that when the A-O joint is examined using combined movements a more consistent outcome will be achieved if the primary movements of flexion and extension are combined with rotation first and then with contralateral lateral flexion. In addition, in order to 'lock' the A-O joint the segmental position opposite to the coupled motion will be required, i.e. a combined position of flexion–extension plus rotation and ipsilateral side-flexion.

## Atlanto-axial joints

The A-A joint (Fig. 8.5) is comprised of three articulations between the atlas and the axis: two lateral and one central articulation (Palastanga *et al*, 2006; Standring, 2008).

The two lateral articulations, or facet joints, are plane synovial joints between the inferior facets of the atlas and superior facets of the axis. Their joint surfaces slope downwards and laterally from the base of the odontoid peg and are biconvex in shape. This configuration means there is little bony congruency or interlocking of the joint surfaces, a factor that contributes to the large ROM available at this level.

The central component of the A-A articulation is a synovial pivot joint where the odontoid peg of the axis articulates within an osseoligamentous ring

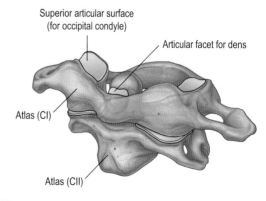

**Figure 8.5** • The atlanto-axial joint. (Reproduced from Drake *et al* (2005) with permission from Elsevier)

formed by the anterior arch of the atlas anteriorly and the strong, thick transverse ligament posteriorly. Articular cartilage covers the parts of the odontoid peg that articulate with the atlas and the transverse ligament and surrounding these areas are two separate synovial cavities (Middleditch & Oliver, 2005; Palastanga et al, 2006).

The arrangement of the three A-A joints predominantly facilitates the movement of rotation, where the head and atlas move together as a single unit rotating around the axis. In addition, due to the biconvex nature of the facet joints, small amounts of flexion–extension and lateral flexion also occur at this level (Bogduk & Mercer, 2000; Palastanga et al, 2006).

Analysis of the amount of motion and coupling patterns that occur at this joint is challenging due to the large rotational component involved. Many motion analysis studies have used two-dimensional or in-vitro study designs which, for different reasons, are not fully able to report accurate amounts of rotation or coupling patterns (Ischii et al, 2004). More recently, three-dimenisonal in-vivo studies have been carried out which provide a better picture of the range and kinematics involved during A-A rotation.

### Kinematics of atlanto-axial rotation (Fig. 8.6)

Combined findings from in vivo and in vitro movement analysis studies report a unilateral range of A-A rotation between 38° and 56° (Iai et al, 1993; Ishii et al, 2004; Panjabi et al, 2001). This large range of segmental rotation is in part made possible by the configuration of the A-A joint surfaces, the lack of an IVD and the loose joint capsules, and is in contrast to the smaller ranges of unilateral rotation of 5–7° observed sub-axially (Iai et al, 1993; Mimura et al, 1989). The total amount of unilateral cervical rotation from C0 to C7 is reported to range from 60°

to 70° (Edmonston et al, 2005). This means that approximately 60% of the total range of cervical rotation occurs at the A-A joint (Ishii et al, 2004). As a consequence, degenerative changes are seen at this joint with a much higher frequency than at the A-O joints (Konig et al, 2005).

In addition to its major contribution to cervical rotation the A-A joint has also been shown to play a key role in the initial phase of head rotation, with rotation in the sub-axial spine occurring only after the movement at C1–C2 is completed (Hino et al, 1999; Ishii et al, 2004). This may be clinically helpful in that if pain is produced on cervical rotation early in range it is likely that the dysfunction lies within the upper cervical spine; conversely, pain arising on cervical rotation later in range is likely to originate from sub-axial structures. This sequential motion pattern, however, becomes disorganized in patients with cervical segmental instability where motion in the unstable segments has been observed to precede motion in intact upper segments (Hino et al, 1999).

Rotation in the sub-axial spine is limited by the IVD disc and articular facets. The A-A joint, however, lacks an IVD and has relatively flat joint surfaces. Rotation at this level therefore is predominantly limited by ligamentous structures, in particular the contralateral alar ligament (Crisco et al, 1991a). Damage to these ligaments may permit rotational hypermobility of the A-A joint and subsequently threaten closely associated structures such as the vertebral arteries and spinal cord (Crisco et al, 1991b; Goel et al, 1990; Kerry & Taylor, 2006). Motion analysis studies suggest that 56° is the upper limit of normal unilateral rotation in the cranio-cervical region. Movement beyond this may indicate rupture of the contralateral alar ligament and thus a rotational instability of the upper cervical spine (Dvorak et al, 1987).

### Kinematics of atlanto-axial flexion–extension (Fig. 8.7)

There are few current studies reporting on the movements of flexion–extension at the A-A joint. Values for these ROMs have mainly been obtained from in vitro studies. Overall, there is consensus that the total range of sagittal plane movement is greater at the A-O segment than at the A-A segment. Analyzing the movements separately, however, shows that flexion is greatest at the A-A joint and extension is greatest at the A-O joint (Bogduk & Mercer, 2000). Approximate ranges for

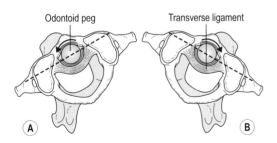

Odontoid peg    Transverse ligament

(A)    (B)

**Figure 8.6** • Kinematics of the atlanto-axial joint in rotation.

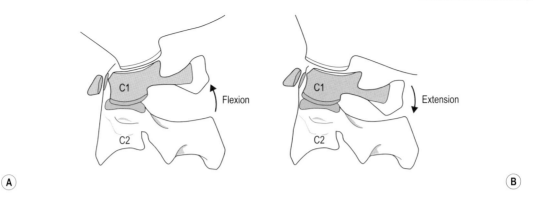

**Figure 8.7 •** (A) Kinematics of the atlanto-axial joint in flexion and (B) extension. (Reproduced from Palastanga et al (2006) with permission from Elsevier)

A-A flexion are from 6°–12° and extension from 5°–10° with in vivo studies generally recording smaller ROMs (Chancey et al, 2007; Ordway et al, 1999; Panjabi et al, 2001). A greater range of flexion–extension at the C1–C2 joint is produced through the upper cervical movements of retraction and protraction respectively (Maeda et al, 2004; Ordway et al, 1999).

### Kinematics of atlanto-axial lateral flexion

When lateral flexion is the initiating movement at the C1–C2 segment, it has a range of approximately 5°–10° and is coupled with extension and contralateral rotation, although this has not been shown to be a fully consistent pattern (Bogduk & Mercer, 2000; Cattrysse et al, 2008; Cook et al, 2006; Iai et al, 1993).

The main restraints to lateral flexion between C1–C2, and indeed across the whole complex, are the contralateral alar ligaments (Krakenes & Kaale, 2006). It has been suggested that, since axial rotation is consistently coupled with contralateral side-flexion, upper cervical rotation to one side is sufficient to tighten the alar ligaments on both sides and that the alar ligaments may be adequately tested using the movement of upper cervical rotation only (Crisco et al, 1991a). This theory has yet to be substantiated.

### Coupling of movements at the atlanto-axial joint

In basic terms, during right rotation of the A-A joint the right inferior articular surface of C1 moves backwards on the right superior facet of C2. The reverse happens on the left, the left inferior

articular surface of C1 moves forward on the left superior facet of C2. The effect of this is to increase the stretch on the anterior and posterior peri-articular structures of the left and right facet joints (Edwards, 1999).

However, due to the biconvex nature of the A-A joint surfaces, axial rotation at C1–C2 is not a pure movement, but exhibits a convex on convex behaviour. In the neutral joint position, the A-A joint surfaces contact at the height of the convexity. During right rotation, the right lateral mass of C1 will move backwards and medially as it slides down the posterior slope of its atlantial facet whilst the left lateral mass of C1 will move forward and medially as it slides down the anterior slope of its facet. This results in a double-threaded screw-like mechanism producing a vertical drop or translation at the A-A joint. This action slackens the alar ligaments and delays their limiting effect on rotation. Accompanying this vertical translation is a contralateral lateral bending of approximately 2–3° together with either flexion or extension (Cook et al, 2006; Ishii et al, 2004; Iai et al, 1993; Panjabi et al, 1993).

Whether flexion or extension occurs at C1–C2 during axial rotation depends on the position of the upper cervical spine. If the upper cervical spine is in an extended or protracted position, axial rotation will be coupled with extension; conversely if the upper cervical spine is held in a flexed or retracted position the coupled motion with axial rotation will be flexion (Edmonton et al, 2005; Panjabi et al, 1993). This key feature occurs due to the passive nature of C1 under axial loads from the head. The atlas is not bound to the axis by any ligaments and there are few muscles that act directly upon it; for this reason the atlas has frequently been likened to a passive 'washer' between the occiput and C2. As a result, the secondary movements occurring at the A-A joint are, in part, related to where the occiput sits on the atlas with reference to the line of gravity. These movements are termed 'paradoxical' movements (Bogduk, 2002a; Bogduk & Mercer, 2000; Iai *et al*, 1993). Head position therefore significantly affects movement patterns of the upper cervical spine and should be considered when testing segmental motion or treating joint limitations in this region.

### Coupling in the upper cervical spine and posture

It has been suggested by several authors that the contralateral coupling pattern seen in the upper cervical spine is, in part, a compensatory mechanism for the ipsilateral coupling pattern seen in the lower cervical spine in order to keep the head upright and facing forwards (Cook *et al*, 2006; Edmonston *et al*, 2005; Iai *et al*, 1993).

The available ROM and also the coupling pattern of movements in the occipito-atlanto-axial complex have been shown to be affected by the overall position of the head and neck (Cook *et al*, 2006; Panjabi *et al*, 1993). Available ROM in the upper cervical spine is decreased if movements are carried out in positions of protraction or retraction rather than in neutral head positions and patterns of secondary movements, particularly at the C1–C2 segment, are altered. Both these factors have a consequential effect on coupling patterns in the lower cervical spine (Edmonston *et al*, 2005). Clinicians should therefore carefully consider the position of the cranio-cervical spine during assessment and treatment of the cervical spine as this may affect the outcome.

 SUMMARY

#### Cranio-cervical anatomy and biomechanics

- Upper cervical extension occurs predominantly at C0–C1.
- Upper cervical rotation occurs predominantly at C1–C2.
- Flexion of the craniovertebral junction is almost equally distributed between C0–C1 and C1–C2.
- *When assessing flexion–extension in the upper cervical spine, manual examination should be focused on the A-O joint.*

- *When assessing rotation in the upper cervical spine, manual examination should be focused on the A-A joint.*
- Full range of upper cervical flexion occurs during retraction.
- Full range of upper cervical extension occurs during protraction.
- *Movements of retraction and protraction should be included in an upper cervical assessment in order to fully stress the surrounding soft tissues.*
- The coupling pattern in the upper cervical spine is predominantly contralateral.
- *Using the coupling pattern of flexion–extension and rotation will most effectively examine the A-O joint using CMT.*
- *Using the coupling pattern of rotation and flexion–extension will most effectively examine the A-A joint using CMT.*
- Pain on cervical rotation early in range is likely to be the result of an *upper cervical dysfunction*.
- Pain on cervical rotation beyond 45° is likely to be a *sub-axial cervical dysfunction*.
- Unilateral rotation between C1–C2 of greater than 56° suggests that the structures limiting rotation (predominantly the alar ligaments) are incompetent.
- Upper cervical posture affects cervical ROM and coupling pattern and should be considered prior to cervical spine examination.
- C1–C2 is prone to degenerative changes

# Innervation; pain generators and pain patterns of the cranio-cervical region

This section will firstly outline the different pain patterns produced by somatic craniocervical structures; upper cervical nerve roots and upper cervical peripheral nerves. It will then discuss how knowledge of these different patterns of pain referral can assist in the differential diagnosis of head, neck and facial pain.

The mechanisms of pain generation in the craniocervical region are the same as those of the lower cervical spine; however, the patterns of innervation and pain referral are different. An appreciation of the unique neuroanatomy of the upper cervical region can therefore assist the clinician in the process of differential diagnosis of head, neck and facial pain.

It is widely accepted that pain can be sub-classified based on the hypothesized mechanism of production into peripheral nociceptive, peripheral neurogenic, central sensitization or affective categories (Butler,

2000; Gifford & Butler, 1997; Loeser & Treede, 2008). This classification system can be applied to pain arising from the head, neck or face region. An understanding of the characteristic patterns of presentation for the different sub-categories of pain will allow the manual therapist to identify the dominant pain mechanism in operation and will thus help direct appropriate assessment and management strategies.

For a detailed review of the different pain mechanisms, the reader is referred to alternative texts (Butler, 2000; Gifford & Butler, 1997; Loeser & Treede, 2008). In brief, cranio-cervical or facial pain can be classified into:

- Peripheral nociceptive pain
  - Local pain due to irritation of nociceptors within local somatic tissue of the cranio-cervical region
  - Referred pain from somatic structures within the cranio-cervical spine (convergence theory)
- Peripheral neurogenic pain
  - Referred pain from irritation of cranio-cervical neural tissue (e.g. upper cervical spinal nerve roots or trunks)

(Central sensitization and affective mechanisms of pain generation will not be considered here.)

In order to be able to classify the type of pain experienced by the patient, knowledge of cranio-cervical innervation; pain referral patterns and upper cervical peripheral nerve pathways is essential.

## Cranio-cervical somatic tissue as a pain generator

Somatic structures of the cranio-cervical spine are innervated by dorsal (posterior) and ventral (anterior) branches of the first three cervical spinal nerves. Studies carried out on symptomatic and asymptomatic subjects have collectively demonstrated that irritation or dysfunction of any structure innervated by the three upper cervical nerves can potentially generate *local pain* or *referred pain* to the head, face, occipital and sub-occipital region (Bogduk, 2001; Dreyfuss et al, 1994; Dwyer et al, 1990).

On exiting, the intervertebral foramina spinal nerves divide into dorsal and ventral rami. Generally, the dorsal rami innervate structures that lie posterior to the intevertebral foramina and nerve roots (neuraxis) and the ventral rami innervate structures that lie anterior to the neuraxis (Bogduk, 2002b) (Fig. 8.8). Table 8.1 provides a summary of the structures supplied by the dorsal and ventral rami.

### Table 8.1

| Ventral rami of C1–C3 supply | Dorsal rami of C1–C3 supply |
|---|---|
| Craniocervical flexors | Suboccipital muscles |
| Scalenes | Posterior neck muscles |
| Levator scapulae | Skin over craniocervical |
| Trapezius | spine and occiput |
| Atlanto-occipital joint | Ligamentum nuchae |
| Atlanto-axial joint | |
| Transverse ligament; alar ligament; tectorial membrane | |
| Upper cervical dura mater | |
| Skin around ear and anterolateral part of neck | |

## Ventral rami innervation (Fig. 8.9)

The cervical plexus is formed by the ventral rami of the upper four cervical nerves and consists of deep muscular branches which supply the muscles and superficial branches which supply the skin (Standring, 2008). The deep branches of the cervical plexus innervate the pre-vertebral muscles (cranio-cervical flexors) as well as the scalenes; levator scapulae; trapezius and sternocleidomastoid. The A-O and A-A joints which, unlike the facet joints in the lower cervical spine, lie anterior to the intervertebral foramina, are also supplied by the cervical plexus, more specifically the ventral rami of the C1 and C2 spinal nerves respectively (Dreyfuss et al, 1994). The ligaments of the A-A region (transverse, alar and tectorial membrane) and the dura mater of the upper cervical cord are innervated by the upper three sinuvertebral nerves (SVN) (Johnson, 2004). SVNs are branches from the ventral rami which re-enter the intervertebral foramina and ascend or descend as many as four vertebral segments within the vertebral canal. As a consequence of this, they can produce varied pain patterns, making it difficult to localize the source of the pain.

The superficial cutaneous branches of the cervical plexus form the following nerves:

- **Lesser occipital nerve.** Formed from a branch of the C2 ventral ramus. It supplies the skin of the neck and scalp posterior to the ear.
- **Greater auricular nerve.** Formed from branches of the C2 and C3 ventral rami. It supplies skin around the ear and mastoid area.
- **Transverse cervical nerve.** Formed from branches of the C2 and C3 ventral rami.

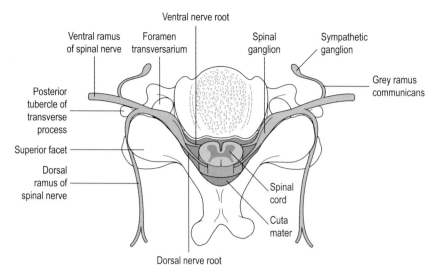

**Figure 8.8 •** A cross section through a vertebral level to show the spinal cord, spinal nerves, ventral and dorsal rami (Reproduced from Middleditch & Oliver (2005) with permission from Elsevier)

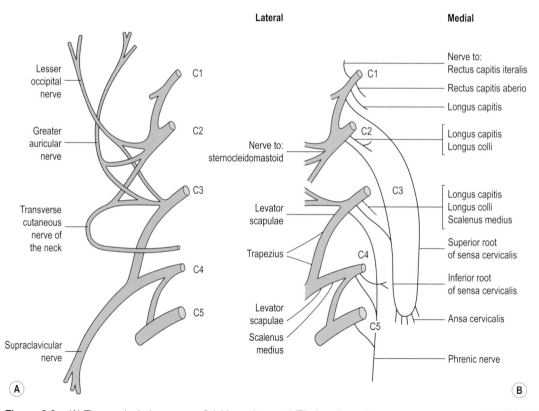

**Figure 8.9 •** (A) The cervical plexus superficial branches and (B) deep branches. (Reproduced from Palastanga et al (2006) with permission from Elsevier)

It supplies skin on the lateral and anterior part of the neck.

- **Supraclavicular nerve.** Formed from branches of the C3 and C4 ventral rami. It divides into three nerves (medial, intermedian and lateral) and supplies the skin over the sternocleidomastoid; the sternoclavicular joint, the upper chest wall, the acromion process and the upper and posterior parts of the shoulder.

## Dorsal rami innervation

The dorsal rami of the upper three cervical spinal nerves innervate the: sub-occipital muscles, the posterior neck muscles, the skin over the cranio-cervical spine and the occiput, and the ligamentum nuchae (Bogduk, 2001) (Fig. 8.10). Branches of the dorsal rami form the following nerves:

- **The sub-occipital nerve (C1).** The dorsal ramus of the first cervical nerve is called the sub-occipital nerve. It exits the spinal cord between the occiput and the posterior arch of C1. It enters the sub-occipital triangle where it supplies the sub-occipital muscles (SOMs) (Bogduk, 2001; Middleditch & Oliver, 2005; Standring, 2008). (Any changes to the SOM can potentially affect the sub-occipital nerve giving rise to a peripheral neuropathy.)

- **The greater occipital nerve (C2).** The medial branch of the C2 dorsal ramus is called the greater occipital nerve (GON). It emerges between the atlas and axis, passes through the A-A joint capsule and ascends to innervate the skin over the posterior part of the scalp as far forward as the vertex of the skull (Middleditch & Oliver, 2005; Standring, 2008). It is closely related to the posterior aspect of the A-A joint and, as a result, is susceptible to any changes occurring at this joint. Owing to its large ROM, the A-A joint is particularly prone to osteoarthritic changes, such as osteophytic growth, which may irritate the GON and result in a peripheral neuropathy frequently referred to as greater occipital neuralgia (Comley, 2003; Ehni & Benner, 1984). Additionally, the C1–C2 level is commonly affected by rheumatoid arthritis and may become unstable as a result. In this situation the GON may be the source of occipital pain due to chemical irritation from the rheumatoid disease or to mechanical impingement secondary to increased upper cervical movement.

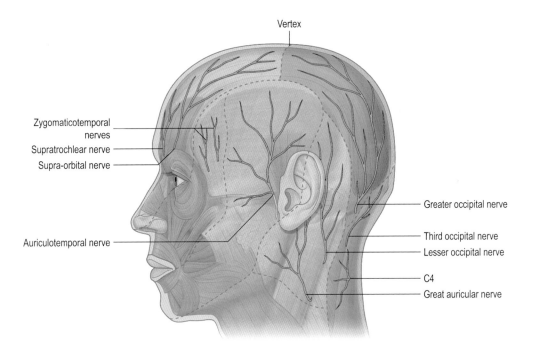

**Figure 8.10 •** Innervation of the scalp by the dorsal rami innervation of the upper three cervical spinal nerves. (Reproduced from Drake *et al* (2005) with permission from Elsevier)

- **The third occipital nerve**. The dorsal ramus of C3 divides into several branches. The superficial medial branch is called the third occipital nerve. It passes posteriorly around the articular pillar of C3, innervates the C2–C3 facet joint and supplies the skin over the sub-occipital region (Fukui *et al*, 1996; Middleditch & Oliver, 2005). Fukui *et al* (1996) demonstrated that electrical stimulation of the C3 dorsal ramus produces pain over the occiput and upper posterior cervical regions. Close association of the third occipital nerve with the C2–C3 facet joint means that any dysfunction of this joint has the potential to irritate the nerve and generate pain within its cutaneous field of distribution. The third occipital nerve has also been implicated in cervicogenic headache (Bogduk & Marsland, 1985; Lord et al, 1994).

From the preceding two sections it is clear that upper cervical somatic structures are innervated by either the ventral or dorsal rami of the first three cervical nerves. Irritation, damage or dysfunction to any of the upper cervical somatic structures will result in stimulation of the nociceptors present within that tissue and hence will produce pain in the immediate area local to or surrounding the damaged structure.

Knowledge of which structures are supplied by the ventral or dorsal rami is largely a means of being systematic and whilst it may be the case that structures innervated by the dorsal rami will refer pain differently to those structures innervated by the ventral rami, essentially what is of clinical importance is the segmental level of innervation of the structure e.g. C1/C2 or C3 and the region into which the structure can refer pain (Bogduk, 2008).

## Pain pattern from upper cervical somatic structures

Few studies, however, have been carried out to map individual referral patterns from each somatic structure. Referral patterns from facet joints have been the most commonly studied. Irritation of the A-O and A-A facet joints by injection of contrast medium has demonstrated that these joints refer pain into the upper posterolateral cervical region 100% of the time and into the occipital region 30% of the time. Irritation of the C2/C3 facet joint has been shown to produce pain more or less equally in the upper posterior cervical region, upper posterolateral cervical region and in the occipital region (Dreyfuss *et al*, 1994; Fukui *et al*, 1996) (Fig. 8.11).

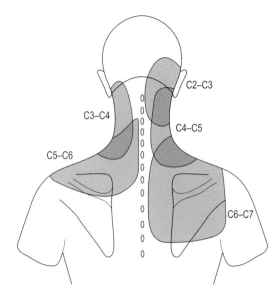

**Figure 8.11** • Pattern of referred pain from the cervical facet joints. (Reproduced from Bogduk (2002b), p. 68, Fig. 4.5, with permission from Elsevier)

Pain referral patterns of upper cervical ligaments have not been mapped out but recent MRI studies on patients following whiplash trauma have confirmed that these ligaments are an important causative factor in the neck pain associated with syndrome (Kaale *et al*, 2005).

## Referred pain from upper cervical somatic structures

In addition to producing local occipital, suboccipital and upper posterolateral neck pain, somatic structures of the craniocervical spine have been shown to refer pain to the head and face (Bogduk, 2001).

Because the boundary of innervation of the upper cervical spinal nerves does not extend much beyond the vertex of the skull (see Fig. 8.12) pain felt in the forehead and facial region as a result of upper cervical dysfunction is not transmitted via the first three cervical nerves. Consequently, fundamental to the understanding of referral of craniocervical pain to the head and face is the overlap between trigeminal nerve afferents and upper cervical afferents through the trigeminocervical nucleus (TCN). This theory of somatic pain referral is referred to as the 'convergence model' and is the most likely explanation for pain referral from the neck to the head and face (Bogduk, 1992). The trigeminal nerve (fifth cranial nerve) is the main sensory nerve of the head and face; its sensory distribution includes the scalp,

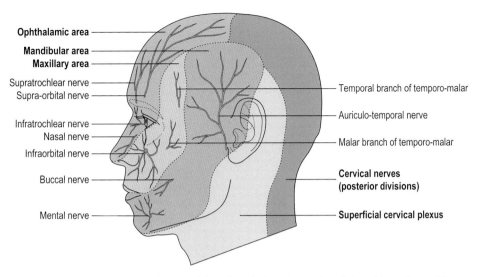

**Ophthalamic area**

**Mandibular area**

**Maxillary area**

Supratrochlear nerve

Supra-orbital nerve

Infratrochlear nerve

Nasal nerve

Infraorbital nerve

Buccal nerve

Mental nerve

Temporal branch of temporo-malar

Auriculo-temporal nerve

Malar branch of temporo-malar

**Cervical nerves
(posterior divisions)**

**Superficial cervical plexus**

**Figure 8.12** • Cutaneous distribution of the trigeminal and ventral and dorsal branches of the upper cervical nerves.

forehead, eyes, nose, cheeks, lips and teeth. It consists of three branches: the ophthalmic nerve; the maxillary nerve and the mandibular nerve which all converge on the TCN (Fig. 8.13). The TCN is a second-order neuron consisting of the spinal nucleus of the trigeminal nerve and the dorsal horns of the upper three cervical segments. It extends from the brain stem to the C3 level and receives afferent fibres from the trigeminal nerve and the upper three cervical spinal nerves. As a result of this connection, nociceptive information from the upper cervical segments may be perceived as originating from the trigeminal field of innervation, a phenomenon referred to as convergence or 'crosstalk'. Clinically this means that, via the TCN, dysfunction in the upper cervical spine may be felt as head or face pain and therefore the cranio-cervical region should be considered as a potential source of symptoms in

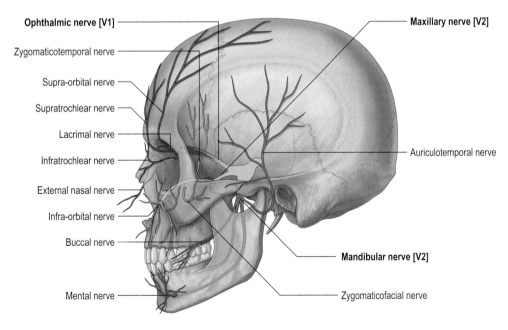

**Ophthalmic nerve [V1]**

Zygomaticotemporal nerve

Supra-orbital nerve

Supratrochlear nerve

Lacrimal nerve

Infratrochlear nerve

External nasal nerve

Infra-orbital nerve

Buccal nerve

Mental nerve

**Maxillary nerve [V2]**

Auriculotemporal nerve

**Mandibular nerve [V2]**

Zygomaticofacial nerve

**Figure 8.13** • The trigeminal nerve. (Reproduced from Drake *et al* (2005), with permission from Elsevier)

patients with these pain referral patterns (Bogduk, 2001; Busch & Wilson, 1989). The convergence model, however, may not fully explain somatic referred pain; other pain mechanisms such as central sensitization may also be involved although this has not yet been established (Jull *et al*, 2008).

## Upper cervical spinal nerve roots and peripheral nerves as pain generators

Alongside cranio-cervical somatic tissue, upper cervical spinal nerve roots and peripheral nerves can also generate pain in the head, neck and face.

Mechanical irritation (compression or traction) or chemical irritation of the *upper cervical spinal nerve roots* can cause radicular pain. Radicular pain is often described as a sharp shooting pain characteristically referred into the area innervated by the particular nerve root (dermatome) and can be associated with diminished sensation into the same area. Upper cervical nerve root irritation can therefore generate referred pain into the C1–C3 dermatomal zones (Fig. 8.14).

The first and second cervical spinal nerve roots, however, are unlikely to be affected by direct compression since they do not exit the spinal cord through intervertebral foramina and do not have any structural relations that make them susceptible to compression; nevertheless they may be vulnerable to other forms of irritation (Comley, 2003; Jull *et al*, 2008).

Pain referral patterns from the upper cervical nerve roots will be different to those from craniocervical somatic tissue. This difference can assist in the differential diagnosis of peripheral nociceptive or peripheral neurogenic mechanisms as the source of head, face and neck pain.

Irritation of *peripheral nerves* can give rise to pain and/or sensory impairment in the cutaneous distribution of the nerve (Greening & Lyn, 1998; Nee & Butler, 2006). The peripheral nerves, for example the sub-occipital nerve, lesser occipital nerve, greater occipital nerve and third occipital nerve, arise from the upper cervical nerve roots and supply the skin over the sub-occipital, occipital and posterior skull regions. As previously mentioned, it is possible that irritation of these nerves can give rise to a peripheral neuropathy and hence be a source of head and neck pain. Irritation of a peripheral nerve will give a different pain referral pattern than the dermatomal pattern associated with irritation of a nerve root. Knowledge of the cutaneous distribution of the upper cervical peripheral nerves as well as knowledge of the upper cervical dermatomes will help the manual therapist differentially diagnose the origin of cranio-cervical neurogenic pain (Figs 8.15 and 8.16).

## The vertebral artery as a pain generator

The vertebral artery is another structure that can potentially generate upper cervical pain. It is

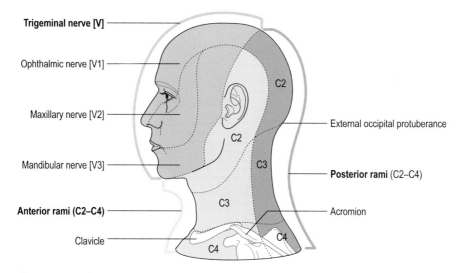

**Figure 8.14** • Dermatomes of the head and neck. (Reproduced from Drake *et al* (2005) with permission from Elsevier)

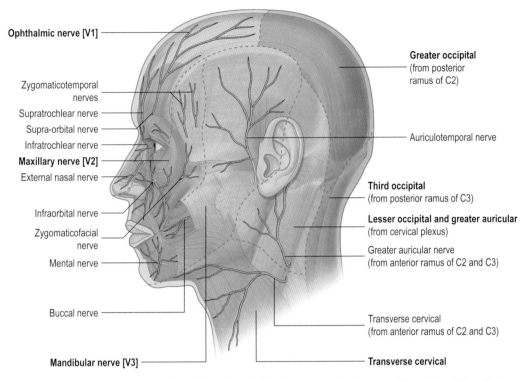

Ophthalmic nerve [V1]

Zygomaticotemporal nerves

Supratrochlear nerve

Supra-orbital nerve

Infratrochlear nerve

**Maxillary nerve [V2]**

External nasal nerve

Infraorbital nerve

Zygomaticofacial nerve

Mental nerve

Buccal nerve

**Mandibular nerve [V3]**

**Greater occipital**
(from posterior ramus of C2)

Auriculotemporal nerve

**Third occipital**
(from posterior ramus of C3)

**Lesser occipital and greater auricular**
(from cervical plexus)

Greater auricular nerve
(from anterior ramus of C2 and C3)

Transverse cervical
(from anterior ramus of C2 and C3)

**Transverse cervical**

**Figure 8.15** • Cutaneous distribution of the trigeminal and upper cervical nerves (Reproduced from Drake *et al* (2005) with permission from Elsevier)

innervated by the vertebral nerve, which is sympathetic in nature. Of particular clinical interest is the connection between the vertebral nerve in the upper cervical spine and the ventral rami of the upper cervical nerves via the grey rami communicantes (Johnson, 2004). Clinically, this means that any nociceptive information from the vertebral artery can be relayed via the vertebral nerve and ventral rami to the dorsal root ganglia of C1–C3, thus the vertebral artery can potentially refer pain into the C1–C3 field of innervation.

Arterial dissection of the vertebral artery is rare; most lesions occur at the C1–C2 level as a result of the unique vascular anatomy at this point (Johnson, 2004; Kerry & Taylor, 2006). Due to the functional neural connectivity between the artery and the upper cervical spine, arterial dissections can present similarly to occipital headache. Presenting symptoms may be described as a sudden onset of severe, sharp pain localized to the ipsilateral cranio-cervical junction and occipital region. Thus in cases of acute onset of headache 'unlike any other', especially in those that precede trauma, the clinician must be suspicious of cervical vascular pathology and thus vertebral artery dissection must be included in the differential diagnosis (Kerry & Taylor, 2006).

## SUMMARY

### Innervation; pain generators and pain patterns of the cranio-cervical region

- Pain referring to the face and anterior aspect of the head from somatic structures of the upper cervical spine will involve the trigeminal nerve. It will not directly involve the upper cervical nerves as they do not innervate this area.
- Pain felt in the posterior scalp and neck may be referred from upper cervical somatic structures; it may be radicular pain from C1–C3 spinal nerve roots or it may be a peripheral neuropathy of peripheral branches from C1–C3 spinal nerves. It will not involve the trigeminal nerve since it does not innervate this area.
- Differential diagnosis of head, neck and facial pain will be facilitated by knowledge of the following patterns of pain referral:

1. Pain referral patterns from cranio-cervical somatic tissue
2. Dermatomal zones of referral from upper cervical nerve roots
3. Cutaneous innervation fields of the upper cervical peripheral nerves

# Stability of the cranio-cervical region

This section will review the concept of spinal stability and how this can be applied to the upper cervical spine. It will then proceed to explore the structures and systems that provide the cranio-cervical region with mechanical and dynamic stability before discussing aspects of upper cervical instability.

## Spinal stability

Central to the understanding of spinal stability is the concept of the 'neutral zone' (Panjabi, 1992b). The neutral zone is a region of 'spinal laxity' around the mid position of a spinal segmental where little resistance to movement is offered by the passive spinal structures (Crawford *et al*, 1998; Panjabi *et al*, 1994). The size and control of the neutral zone has been considered an important measure of the stability of the motion segment. Studies have demonstrated that in situations of clinical instability, through injury, degeneration or segmental muscle weakness, the neutral zone enlarges and, conversely, it decreases when simulated muscle forces are applied across the segment (Kettler *et al*, 2002; Panjabi *et al*, 1989, 1994).

This change in size of the neutral zone in relation to spinal instability appears to be consistently greater than the increase in the corresponding ROM suggesting that it is likely to be a more sensitive indicator of clinical instability and ligamentous defects than ROM (Oxland & Panjabi, 1992).

Control of the neutral zone, and hence of spinal stability, requires the inter-relationship of three 'systems': the *passive system* which provides mechanical stability through the inert spinal structures such as the ligaments, capsules, joint surfaces and passive properties of the spinal muscles; the *active system* which provides dynamic stability through the muscles acting on the spine and the *neural system* which provides neurological control and coordination of spinal muscle activity to maintain normal joint ROM (Panjabi *et al*, 1992a). The combined action of the active and the neural systems of control is currently referred to as *sensorimotor control*.

Within the neutral zone, the control of spinal segmental motion is largely provided by coordination of the surrounding muscles (active and neural systems), whilst at the end of spinal segmental ROM, it is the spine's passive structures that

control the movement (Bogduk, 1997; Panjabi, 1992b).

If the passive stability of the spine is compromised through injury, disease or degeneration, spinal stability can be maintained to a certain extent by the activation of the active and neural systems, that is to say that dynamic stability or sensorimotor control can compensate in part for a lack of mechanical stability (Panjabi, 1992a,b).

## Cranio-cervical stability

A particular characteristic of the cranio-cervical joints is their large neutral zones; a good example of this is at C1–C2 where 75% of the total axial rotation occurs within the neutral zone (Goel *et al*, 1990; Panjabi *et al*, 1988). Consequently, a large proportion of upper cervical movement occurs before the onset of ligamentous resistance and therefore the cranio-cervical ligaments are lax during much of the functional movement in this region (Zhang *et al*, 2006). As a result, the cranio-cervical spine is highly dependent on the surrounding muscles for stability during movements around the mid position and on the upper cervical ligaments for stability at the extremes of motion (Edmonston *et al*, 2005; Goel *et al*, 1990; Panjabi *et al*, 1988). Indeed it has been estimated that the osseoligamentous system of the cervical spine provides approximately 20% of the spinal stability, whilst the cervical musculature contributes approximately 80% (Panjabi *et al*, 1998). Although the upper cervical ligaments do not provide mechanical stability during normal ROM, they will provide a certain amount of proprioceptive information which will assist in the sensorimotor control of cranio-cervical joint stability.

Clinically, more effective cranio-cervical ligamentous testing, therefore, can be achieved by applying the instability tests outside of the neutral zone towards the end of ROM in positions where ligamentous resistance should be expected. Additionally, stability testing of the upper cervical spine should include examination of the active and neural systems or sensorimotor control.

 SUMMARY

**Stability of the cranio-cervical region**

- The cranio-cervical joints have large neutral zones.
- The upper cervical spine is heavily reliant on coordination of the cranio-cervical muscles to provide stability during normal ROM.

- The cranio-cervical ligamentous complex provides stability at the end of ROM.
- Effective cranio-cervical ligamentous testing should be carried out towards end of ROM in positions where ligamentous resistance should be expected.
- Assessment of upper cervical sensorimotor control should form part of an examination of upper cervical stability.

## Mechanical stability of the cranio-cervical region

As previously acknowledged, the craniovertebral ligament system plays an essential role in stabilizing the upper cervical spine at extremes of ROM (Brolin & Halldin, 2004; Krakenes et al, 2003b). Injury to any component of the ligamentous complex will affect the kinematics of the cranio-cervical junction and may lead to instability, pain and disability (Krakenes & Kaale, 2006; Krakenes et al, 2003a,b; Maak et al, 2006). Careful assessment of the mechanical stability of the cranio-cervical spine is usually indicated in situations where instability is suspected. Signs and symptoms of upper cervical instability and indications for testing will be discussed later on.

Chief mechanical restraints of the cranio-cervical region are the transverse and alar ligaments with other ligaments such as the tectorial membrane, capsular ligaments, ligamentum flavum, A-A ligaments, apical ligament, ligamentum nuchea, posterior A-O membranes and A-A membranes acting as secondary stabilizers (Crisco et al, 1991a,b; Dvorak & Panjabi, 1987; Goel et al, 1990; Krakenes et al, 2003a,b; Tubbs et al, 2007). An appreciation of the functional anatomy of these ligaments can assist in the effective assessment of upper cervical stability.

### Transverse ligament

Biomechanically, the transverse ligament (Fig. 8.16) is the strongest ligament in the cranio-cervical region (Dvorak et al, 1988; Krakenes et al, 2003a). It is a tight, broad collagenous band, which extends across the ring of the atlas, arching behind the odontoid process and attaching to the medial aspect of each lateral mass of C1 (Dvorak et al, 1998; Meadows, 1998; Krakenes et al, 2003a). The ligament divides the atlas ring into two parts and importantly, separates the odontoid peg from the spinal cord. The smaller anterior part of the atlantal ring contains the dens, and the

larger posterior part contains the spinal cord and meninges; the anterior and posterior spinal arteries; the spinal root of the accessory nerve (cranial nerve XI) and approximately 1 cm of free space (Ebraheim et al, 1998). The transverse ligament provides the major mechanical stability for the A-A joint in the anterior–posterior plane; it acts like a sling holding the odontoid peg against the anterior arch of C1 and prevents anterior subluxation of C1 on C2 (Dickman et al, 1991; Krakenes et al, 2003a). In addition, it serves as an articular surface for the odontoid peg.

The transverse ligament also has vertical fibres running superiorly to the occiput and inferiorly to the posterior part of the axis, which blend in with the tectorial membrane. These vertical bands contribute to the stability of the region by limiting flexion, and in conjunction with the transverse ligament, are often referred to as the atlantal cruciform ligament (Dvorak et al, 1988; Krakenes et al, 2001).

Inflammatory disease and high speed trauma can both affect the competence of the transverse ligament and thus threaten the sagittal plane stability of the cranio-cervical junction (Dickman et al, 1991; Krakenes et al, 2003a). The synovial articulations between the odontoid peg, transverse ligament and anterior atlantal arch make the ligament more susceptible to degenerative changes from inflammatory disease such as rheumatoid arthritis (RA) which can considerably weaken the ligament and render it insufficient. Consequently, cervical subluxations such as A-A subluxation are common in patients with RA and are reported to occur in 43–86% of all patients with the disease (Roche et al, 2002; Swinkels et al, 1996).

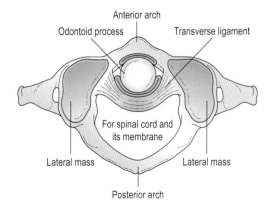

**Figure 8.16** • The transverse ligament.

Hyperflexion injuries of the upper cervical spine can strain or rupture the transverse ligament. The ligament is therefore more likely to be damaged by severe, head-on road traffic accidents (RTAs) than by small impact, rear-end collisions (Krakenes *et al*, 2003a; Maak *et al*, 2006). As many as 30% of whiplash patients with upper cervical injuries have been shown to have anterior A-A instability due to transverse ligament rupture following an RTA, with up to 26% of these injuries remaining radiographically undetected in one group of patients (Dickman *et al*, 1991,1996).

Clinically, the relationship between transverse ligament injuries and neck pain has been investigated. A study correlating abnormal transverse ligament findings on MRI scan with Neck Disability Index (NDI) scores has demonstrated that lesions to the transverse ligament can be a source of neck pain and disability but that they tend to be less disabling to patients than injuries to the alar ligaments (Krakenes & Kaale, 2006).

## Alar ligaments

Anatomically, the alar ligaments (Fig. 8.17) consist of two well-defined cords of collagenous fibre, approximately 1 cm in length, which originate from the posterior lateral aspect of the odontoid peg of C2 and extend superiorly and laterally to attach onto the medial surfaces of the occipital condyles (Crisco *et al*, 1991a; Krakenes *et al*, 2001). Previous cadaveric studies have observed an additional band of the alar ligament running from the odontoid process to the atlas; however, more recent MRI studies have failed to identify this (Dvorak & Panjabi, 1987; Panjabi *et al*, 1991; Krakenes *et al*, 2001).

The chief function of these ligaments is to limit rotation and side-bending across the cranio-cervical junction to the contralateral side. Hence, the right alar ligament limits left rotation and left side-bending whilst the left alar ligament limits rotation and side-bending to the right (Dvorak *et al*, 1988; Goel *et al*, 1990; Krakenes & Kaale, 2006). Biomechanical studies have shown the alar ligaments to be lax in the mid-position and maximally tightened in 90° cervical rotation as they twist around the odontoid peg. A further stretch can be added to the alar ligaments with the addition of flexion to upper cervical rotation (Dvorak & Panjabi; 1987; Dvorak *et al*, 1988; Krakenes & Kaale, 2006; Panjabi *et al*, 1991). Consequently, the alar ligaments are particularly vulnerable to hyperflexion trauma when the head is in a rotated position (Krakenes & Kaale, 2006).

Damage to the alar ligaments can result in increased axial rotation in the occipito-atlanto-axial complex. Alar ligament resection has been shown to cause upper cervical instability by increasing A-A rotation by approximately 30% of intact values (Panjabi *et al*, 1991). Axial rotation between C1–C2 beyond 55° will damage the ligaments and beyond 65° will cause A-A dislocation (Crisco *et al*, 1991a; Dvorak *et al*, 1987; Goel *et al*, 1990).

Abnormally large A-A rotation is known to reduce blood flow in the contralateral vertebral artery (Kerry & Taylor, 2006). Thus a rotatory instability in the upper cervical spine can cause signs and symptoms of cervical artery dysfunction (CAD) suggesting that the assessment of upper cervical stability should be included in the examination of a patient presenting with signs and symptoms of CAD. The most common symptom of alar ligament damage, however, is pain. Indeed, injury to the alar

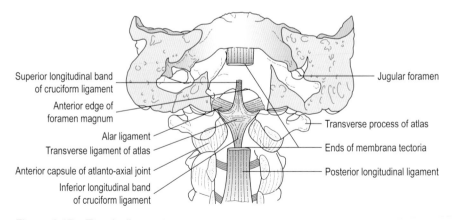

Superior longitudinal band of cruciform ligament

Anterior edge of foramen magnum

Alar ligament

Transverse ligament of atlas

Anterior capsule of atlanto-axial joint

Inferior longitudinal band of cruciform ligament

Jugular foramen

Transverse process of atlas

Ends of membrana tectoria

Posterior longitudinal ligament

**Figure 8.17** • The alar ligaments.

ligaments has been shown to be an important cause of pain and disability in patients following severe whiplash trauma and appears to cause greater pain and disability in patients, measured by the NDI, compared to the same grade of injury occurring in the transverse ligament (Krakenes *et al*, 2006).

## Tectorial membrane

The tectorial membrane (Fig. 8.18) is the cranial continuation of the posterior longitudinal ligament. It is a strong, broad band, approximately 1 mm in thickness and is composed of collagen and elastic fibres. Previously, it has been described as originating from the posterior aspect of the odontoid peg but more recent anatomical and radiological studies have suggested that this is not the case. Instead it has been reported to attach to the posterior surface of the body of C2 and to run vertically upwards to insert onto the basilar groove of the occipital bone. The membrane covers the posterior aspect of the dens, the atlantal cruciform ligament and the alar ligaments and gives off two lateral bands which blend with the A-O joint capsules on reaching the foramen magnum (Krakenes & Kaale, 2006; Krakenes *et al*, 2003b; Tubbs *et al*, 2007).

Owing to its high proportion of elastic fibres the tectorial membrane has been likened to the ligamentum flavum (Tubbs *et al*, 2007). Its exact role in craniovertebral stability has been debated but due to its position and its high elastic content it is proposed to act as a second line of defence in limiting hyperflexion in the craniovertebral joints (Dvorak & Panjabi, 1987; Tubbs *et al*, 2007). Indeed, incision of the tectorial membrane has been shown to increase translation into flexion (Harris *et al*, 1993). The method by which the ligament limits flexion has been suggested as an indirect 'hammock style' mechanism whereby on flexion of the head, the middle portion of the tectorial membrane is stretched over the odontoid peg like a 'hammock', thus preventing the dens from moving posteriorly towards the spinal canal and encroaching on the spinal cord or dura mater (Tubbs *et al*, 2007). The ligament has been found to be fully taut at 15° of upper cervical flexion and 20° of upper cervical extension, and in addition to its contribution to stability in the sagittal plane, it is also proposed to support the alar ligaments in limiting axial rotation and side-bending (Brolin & Halldin, 2004; Dvorak & Panjabi, 1987).

Hyperflexion injuries sustained during whiplash trauma by patients with whiplash associated disorder (WAD) of grade 2 and above were shown on MRI scan to have damaged the tectorial membrane indicating that this ligament may be a source of upper cervical pain and instability. The extent of pain and disability experienced by patients following injury to the tectorial membrane as indicated by NDI scores, however, has been shown to be less than for the alar and transverse ligaments (Krakenes *et al*, 2003b).

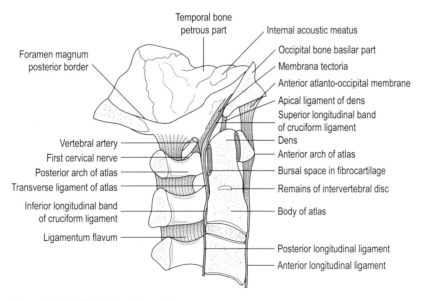

**Figure 8.18** • The tectorial membrane.

From a clinical perspective, specific testing of the tectorial membrane should be carried out in positions of both upper cervical flexion and extension. Also some 'give' should be expected on testing on end-feel owing to the high elastic content and moreover, the effect on testing of increased tone in the SOM should also be considered.

## Capsular ligaments

The capsular ligaments attach to the margins of the C0–C1–C2 facet joints and are thin and loose. Their principal role is to contain the synovial fluid but they also have a mechanical role in stabilizing the occipito-atlanto-axial joint complex (Crisco et al, 1991b). In vitro and finite element model (FEM) studies have demonstrated that the C1–C2 capsular ligaments are important mechanical restraints for rotation at this joint (Brolin & Halldin, 2004; Crisco et al, 1991b; Goel et al, 1990). Transection of C1–C2 capsular ligaments, even when the alar ligaments and transverse ligament remain intact, has been shown to increase the range of C1–C2 axial rotation but interestingly, it does not affect the neutral zone and the joint does not become unstable. Additional cranio-cervical ligamentous damage must occur to bring about A-A subluxation or dislocation (Crisco et al, 1991b). Thus, it is hypothesized that damage to the capsular ligaments brings about hypermobility, not instability, and that the capsular ligaments play a secondary role to the alar ligaments in limiting rotation in the cranio-cervical region. Alongside their primary role in limiting rotation, the capsular ligaments have also been shown to influence flexion, extension and lateral-bending and thus have the largest effect of the entire ligament complex on general upper cervical kinematics (Brolin & Halldin, 2004).

## Apical ligament

The apical ligament (Fig. 8.19) is a thin fibrous cord passing from the tip of the dens to the anterior inferior margin of the foramen magnum. It is reported to be absent in 20% of cases and is thought to be a vestigial structural (Standring, 2008; Tubbs et al, 2000). Finite element models of the upper cervical spine suggest that the apical ligament may influence upper cervical extension although its contribution to the stability of the cranio-cervical region, in general, is thought to be minimal (Tubbs et al, 2000; Brolin & Halldin, 2004). Clinically, the apical ligament is

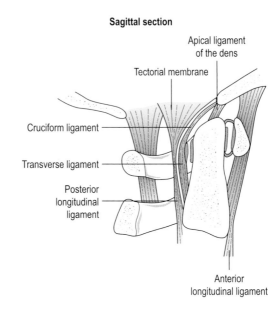

**Sagittal section**

Apical ligament of the dens

Tectorial membrane

Cruciform ligament

Transverse ligament

Posterior longitudinal ligament

Anterior longitudinal ligament

**Figure 8.19** • The apical ligament. (Reproduced from Palastanga et al (2006) with permission from Elsevier)

unlikely to be the source of pain or instability in the cranio-cervical region and therefore direct testing would not appear to be necessary.

## Ligamentum nuchae

The ligamentum nuchae (Fig. 8.20) in the cervical spine is a continuation of the supraspinous ligament from lower spinal levels. It is a dense, triangular fibroelastic ligament which runs from the external occipital protuberance to the posterior tubercle on the posterior arch of C1 and then to the spinous process of C2 before extending down to the spinous process of C7 (Middleditch & Oliver, 2005; Standring, 2008). Based on its position it is proposed to limit upper cervical flexion but its high elastic content may mean that it does not play a major role in upper cervical stability.

## Anterior atlanto-occipital membrane

The anterior A-O membrane (Fig. 8.21) is a continuation of the anterior longitudinal ligament (ALL). It is a broad, thick, elastic membrane which connects the anterior arch of C1 (atlas) with the anterior margin of the foramen magnum. It overlies and blends with the capsule of the A-O joint (Krakenes et al, 2001). Anatomical and FEM studies have shown that it limits extension of the upper cervical spine as would be expected. Transection of this membrane alone does not result in cranio-cervical instability; however, major instability does result when it is transected in conjunction with the tectorial membrane and the posterior A-O membrane (Brolin & Halldin, 2004; Harris *et al*, 1993; Krakenes et al, 2003b). Together with its high elastic content, this would suggest that it is unlikely to be a primary stabilizer of the cranio-cervical region.

## Posterior atlanto-occipital membrane

The posterior A-O membrane (Fig. 8.21) is an extension of the highly elastic ligamentum flavum. It is a broad, relatively thin, elastic membrane which runs from the posterior arch of C1 to the posterior margin of the foramen magnum (Krakenes *et al*, 2001, 2003b). It blends with the postero-medial capsule of the A-O joints and laterally it arches over the vertebral artery and C1 nerve as they cross the posterior arch of C1. Cadaveric and FEM studies have demonstrated that the posterior A-O membrane helps to limit upper cervical flexion and this has been confirmed by MRI studies which have identified lesions in the membrane following hyperflexion trauma after frontal collisions (Brolin & Halldin, 2004; Krakens & Kaale, 2006; Krakenes *et al*, 2001, 2003b). Its role in cranio-cervical stability is not fully established although, owing to its high elastic content, it is more likely to act as a reinforcement than a primary restraint for flexion.

Other cranio-cervical ligaments, for example the atlanto-axial ligaments, are small and lax and contribute little to overall cranio-cervical stability (Nightingale *et al*, 2002).

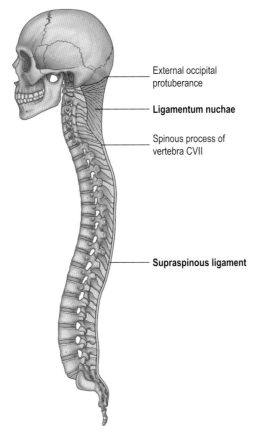

**Figure 8.20** • Ligamentum nuchae. (Reproduced from Drake *et al* (2005) with permission from Elsevier)

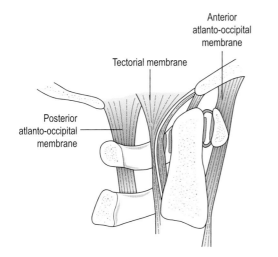

**Figure 8.21** • The anterior and posterior atlanto-occipital membranes. (Reproduced from Palastanga *et al* (2006) with permission from Elsevier)

Labels for Figure 8.20:
- External occipital protuberance
- **Ligamentum nuchae**
- Spinous process of vertebra CVII
- **Supraspinous ligament**

Labels for Figure 8.21:
- Anterior atlanto-occipital membrane
- Tectorial membrane
- Posterior atlanto-occipital membrane

### SUMMARY

#### Mechanical stability of the cranio-cervical region

- The craniovertebral ligaments play an important role in the stability of the upper cervical spine at the end of ROM.
- The primary restraint to:
  - *Anterior translation* of the atlas on the axis: transverse ligament
  - *Lateral translation* of the atlas on the axis: odontoid peg, transverse ligament and bony ring of the atlas
  - *Cranio-cervical rotation*: alar ligaments reinforced by the A-A joint capsules and the tectorial membrane

○ *Cranio-cervical flexion*: transverse ligament and the alar ligaments reinforced by the tectorial membrane, P-O membrane and ligamentum nuchae

○ *Cranio-cervical lateral flexion*: alar ligaments reinforced by the A-A joint capsule and the tectorial membrane.

- Trauma, degenerative disease and inflammation of the cranio-cervical spine can affect the ligamentous structures.
- The cranio-cervical ligaments have been shown to be an important source of pain and disability in patients with neck pain following high-speed whiplash trauma.
- The alar ligaments are the most frequently injured ligaments in whiplash trauma and cause greater pain and disability to patients than injury to the other upper cervical ligaments or membranes.
- Excessive rotational mobility of the cranio-cervical spine may reduce blood flow in the vertebral arteries and cause signs and symptoms associated with cervical artery dysfunction (CAD).
- Manual assessment of the mechanical stability of the cranio-cervical spine is normally indicated when instability is suspected and when signs and symptoms of CAD are present.

# Dynamic stability/sensorimotor control

Sensorimotor control is the term applied to the coordination and integration of sensory, motor and central processing systems involved in regulating joint stability. It is achieved through the complex interplay of several different neural processes including proprioception and neuromuscular control. Proprioception forms part of the sensory information arising from peripheral areas of the body Myers *et al*, 2006). It involves information detected by mechanoreceptors regarding joint position sense, orientation and movement. Mechanoreceptors are the primary sensory receptors involved in proprioception and are found in ligaments, muscle, fascia, joint capsules and skin around joints.

Afferent input from visual and vestibular systems in the periphery is integrated with *proprioceptive* information from the mechanoreceptors. This combined information is processed in the central nervous system (CNS) and used to elicit appropriate efferent or motor responses from the postural muscles around a joint. This efferent response is referred to as *motor control* and involves the subconscious activation of the dynamic joint restraints

(muscles) in preparation for and in response to joint movement with the aim of maintaining joint stability (Riemann & Lephart, 2002a,b; Van Vliet & Heneghan, 2006; Treleaven, 2008).

# Sensorimotor control of the cranio-cervical region

There is an abundance of mechanoreceptors found in the cervical spine, however, their distribution is not uniform. A higher density of mechanoreceptors is found in the upper cervical spine suggesting that this region has an important role in providing proprioceptive information during postural and dynamic functions of the head and neck. Interestingly, the distribution of cranio-cervical mechanoreceptors is greater in muscle tissue than in joints, indicating that the muscle receptors of the upper cervical spine are likely to be the most important sensory receptors with additional afferent information provided by the joint receptors (Boyd-Clarke *et al*, 2001, 2002; Jull *et al*, 2008; McPartland & Brodeur, 1999). Afferent input to the CNS from the receptors in cranio-cervical muscle tissue provides the primary information about static cranio-cervical joint position and about direction, amplitude and velocity of cranio-cervical joint movements. Specific connections exist between the cervical mechanoreceptors, particularly the muscle spindles in the SOM, and the vestibular and visual apparatus via the vestibular nuclei, and hence information from all three sources is integrated and involved in various postural reflexes (Armstrong *et al*, 2008; Kristjansson, 2004; Treleaven, 2008). Consequently, the mechanoreceptors found in upper cervical muscle tissue, and to a lesser extent in upper cervical joints, have a major proprioceptive role in maintaining dynamic stability of the cranio-cervical spine and in control of balance. Any dysfunction therefore of these cervical receptors will alter their afferent input to the CNS and this will subsequently have an effect on sensorimotor control of the cervical spine and on postural stability.

The cranio-cervical flexor (CCF) muscle group which includes rectus capitus anterior and lateralis, longus capitus and longus colli (Fig. 8.22), and the sub-occipital muscle (SOM) group which includes rectus capitus posterior major and minor and obliqus capitus superior and inferior (Fig. 8.23), are all short, deep, segmental muscles.

They are reported to provide segmental control and support for the cervical joints, with longus colli

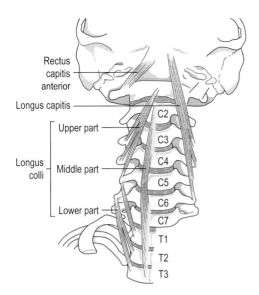

**Figure 8.22** • The cranio-cervical flexor muscle group. (Reproduced from Palastanga *et al* (2006) with permission from Elsevier)

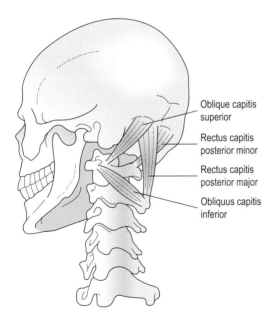

**Figure 8.23** • The sub-occipital muscle group. (Reproduced from Middleditch & Oliver (2005) with permission from Elsevier)

having an additional role in supporting the cervical lordosis (Falla, 2004; Jull *et al*, 2004a,b). Indeed, the highest density of muscle receptors, in particular muscle spindles, is found in the SOM, with large spindle densities also recorded in the CCF muscle

group. In comparison to this, the larger cervical muscles used for gross movement, such as the sternocleidomastoid and trapezius, are comparatively devoid of muscle spindles. These findings would indicate that the shorter and deeper muscles with large spindle densities are predominantly designed and ideally located to control and monitor head and neck movements and positions but that they have only a minimal role to play in phasic movements (Boyd-Clark *et al*, 2001, 2002; Kettler *et al*, 2002; McPartland & Brodeur, 1999). Strengthening this argument further, is the observation that the CCF and SOM are involved in a feedforward mechanism whereby they contract within 50 ms of the onset of head and neck movement in order to stabilize the cranio-cervical joints and prepare them for action (Falla, 2004; Van Vliet & Heneghan, 2006).

In summary, the cranio-cervical spine has a rich supply of mechanoreceptors, particularly in the CCF and SOM. In addition, these muscles are in close proximity to the cranio-cervical joints and therefore play a key role as proprioceptive monitors and dynamic stabilizers of the upper cervical spine. Moreover, information primarily from the CCF and SOM is involved in postural reflexes and hence in the control of balance. Any deficits in CCF or SOM function will therefore affect dynamic stability of the cervical spine and postural control and may lead to symptoms of neck pain and dizziness.

## Sensorimotor control and neck pain

It has been acknowledged that sensorimotor control has a major role to play in controlling and maintaining spinal stability by preserving the neutral zone within normal physiological limits. Alteration to any part of this proprioceptive–neuromuscular control system through dysfunction or injury, may compromise the region's stability, potentially leading to further tissue damage and pain (Treleaven, 2008; Van Vliet & Heneghan, 2006).

In support of this is a growing body of evidence indicating that deficits in sensorimotor control are apparent in patients with acute and chronic neck pain; cervical vertigo; cervical injury and disease (Falla, 2004; Falla *et al*, 2004; Jull *et al*, 2004a, 2004b; Loudon *et al*, 1997; Sterling *et al*, 2004; Treleaven *et al*, 2003;). In this group of patients the *proprioceptive changes* that are seen are jerky, inconsistent neck movements, poor preparation for movement and poor position sense awareness

(Sjolander *et al*, 2008). Disturbances in other sub-modalities of sensorimotor control, such as postural stability and eye movement control, have also been noted but are beyond the scope of this text; for a comprehensive review of these sensorimotor functions the reader is referred to Jull *et al* (2008). The observed proprioceptive changes in neck pain patients may be due to a combination of factors. Injury or degenerative changes in the cervical spine may disrupt the region's mechanical stabilizers, which will affect the amount and accuracy of afferent information transmitted from their mechanoreceptors and hence, affect proprioceptive functioning and motor control. In addition to this, information relayed from nociceptors in response to tissue damage may override proprioceptive information from the cervical mechanoreceptors (Hallgren *et al*, 1994; Treleaven, 2008). Furthermore, studies on symptomatic patients have shown that there is atrophy of the deep cervical stabilizing muscles and that some of the damaged muscle tissue is replaced by fatty tissue. It has been suggested that this loss of muscle tissue may cause a decrease in the density of the muscle spindles resulting in a further deficit in proprioceptive abilities of the affected region (Hallgren *et al*, 1994).

*Impaired motor control* of the cervical spine in patients with neck pain has been demonstrated, particularly in the CCF. Deficits found in the CCF of symptomatic patients include decreased muscle strength and decreased endurance capacity (O'Leary *et al*, 2007). In addition, a delayed onset in CCF activation has been observed, suggesting a dysfunction in the normal feedforward mechanism which initiates early contraction of the CCF in order to stabilize the cervical joints prior to movement (Falla, 2004). Furthermore, normal patterns of coordination present between deep and superficial flexor muscles appear to be altered in patients with neck pain, with increased activity noted in the superficial cervical muscles such as sternocleidomastoid and the scalenes, and decreased activity in the deep cervical muscles (Falla et al, 2004; Jull 2000; Jull et al, 2004a,b). These motor control impairments will undoubtedly have an effect on the dynamic control of the neutral zones and hence on cranio-cervical joint stability, with the potential of producing upper cervical pain and dysfunction.

Importantly, both the proprioceptive and motor control deficits identified seem to be present in all patient groups with head or neck pain of neuromusculoskeletal origin. Moreover, these changes in

sensorimotor control appear to occur soon after the onset of pain and do not necessarily resolve spontaneously on the resolution of the pain (Sterling *et al*, 2003). This would suggest that early on in the episode of neck pain, patients may have a decreased ability to control and monitor head and neck movements and positions, which may result in further tissue damage and ongoing or repeated episodes of neck pain or headaches.

Although deficits in sensorimotor control have generally been observed to arise as a consequence of neck pain, there is evidence to suggest that asymptomatic changes in proprioception and neuromuscular control are linked to the development of upper cervical disorders, such as cervicogenic headache, and therefore asymptomatic altered sensorimotor control may be a precursor to the development and maintenance of postural neck pain (Edmonston et al, 2005).

Clinically, the evidence presented suggests that the specific assessment and subsequent rehabilitation of sensorimotor control should be included in the management of all patients with neck pain. Indeed, proprioceptive exercises have been found to be effective in reducing pain and disability in the cervical spine, and together with the retraining of motor control deficits, may help to restore sensorimotor control and hence cervical joint stability (Jull *et al*, 2004b; Kettler *et al*, 2002; Revel *et al*, 1994; Taimela *et al*, 2000).

 ## SUMMARY

### Sensorimotor control in the cervical spine

- Sensorimotor control is the integration of coordinated muscle activity in response to proprioceptive information used to regulate joint stability.
- The SOM and CCF are short, deep, segmental muscles, ideally placed to control joint movement.
- The SOM and CCF have high densities of mechanoreceptors.
- The SOM and CCF have connections with vestibular and visual systems and the CNS.
- The SOM and CCF are important proprioceptive monitors and dynamic stabilizers of the cranio-cervical spine around neutral and mid-range positions and have a role in postural stability.
- Dysfunctions of the CCF or SOM can lead to deficits in sensorimotor control of the cranio-cervical spine and balance, potentially resulting in neck pain and dizziness.

- Deficits in proprioception and motor control are apparent in all neck pain patients from early on in the onset of the condition and do not always resolve spontaneously.
- Specific assessment of proprioception and motor control and the subsequent treatment of any observed deficit should be integrated into the clinical management of neck pain.

# Spinal instability

Following on from the concept of spinal stability related to the size and control of the neutral zone, Panjabi *et al* (1992b) redefined spinal instability as:

> ... a significant decrease in the capacity of the spine to maintain the intervertebral *neutral zones* within the physiological limits so that there is no neurological dysfunction, no major deformity and no incapacitating pain. (Panjabi *et al*, 1992b, p. 395)

Clinical instability is therefore regarded as an increased size and a loss of control of the neutral zone by the active, passive or neural spinal systems due to trauma, degenerative changes or disease processes. It is the combination of the enlarged neutral zone with the inadequate control that is proposed to cause pathology in the surrounding neural and soft tissues thus producing the signs and symptoms associated with spinal instability.

Importantly, Panjabi *et al*'s (1992b) definition of spinal instability provides a clear distinction between clinical instability and hypermobility. The former relates to a painful pathological situation where the overall physiological ROM may be normal or even decreased but the amount of joint 'play' around the neutral zone is increased. Pain with instability is generally felt within the ROM rather than at the end of range. Hypermobility on the other hand does not relate to a pathological situation and does not necessarily produce pain. The overall physiological ROM of a hypermobile joint is increased but the size of the neutral zone is within normal ranges and the neutral zone motion is adequately controlled, so the joint is stable. If pain is present it will normally be felt at the end of range, possibly due to overstretch of the periarticular tissues.

## Cranio-cervical instability

Cranio-cervical instability is characterized by excessive movement across the occipito-atlanto-axial complex. The most commonly affected level is C1–C2 owing to the oblique facet joint orientation and the lack of bony interlocking to prevent subluxation in the presence of ligamentous or capsular destruction. Instability of the cranio-cervical spine can occur as a result of trauma, degenerative changes, disease processes or congenital abnormalities.

## Trauma

Upper cervical fractures and ligament damage through trauma are well recognized, with ligamentous incompetence following whiplash trauma being far more prevalent than bone fractures (Dickman *et al*, 1996; Krakenes *et al*, 2003a,b; Krakenes & Kaale, 2006; Maak *et al*, 2006). Earlier cadaveric studies explored craniovertebral ligament failure rates and investigated the effect of transection of the craniovertebral ligaments on overall upper cervical spinal motion (Dvorak and Panjabi, 1987; Dvorak *et al*, 1987; Dvorak *et al*, 1988; Crisco *et al*, 1991). Combined findings from these studies confirm that the craniovertebral ligaments are vulnerable to loading with the alar ligaments failing at lower loads than the transverse ligament and that sequential sectioning of the ligaments and membranes results in upper cervical instability. The degree and direction of instability depends on which ligament is transected. Instability in the sagittal plane has been shown to occur following transection of the transverse ligament or a combination of the transverse ligament and tectorial membrane (Dickman *et al*, 1991; Dvorak *et al*, 1988; Krakenes *et al*, 2003a,b; Tubbs *et al*, 2007). Rotatory instability and instability in the coronal plane have been shown to occur following sectioning of the alar ligaments or a combination of the alar ligaments, capsular ligaments, tectorial membrane and A-O membranes (Goel *et al*, 1990; Crisco *et al*, 1991b).

More recent in vivo studies using MRI scans have directly explored the effect of whiplash injuries on the upper cervical ligaments (Krakenes *et al*, 2003a,b; Krakenes & Kaale, 2006). Findings from these studies have identified structural changes in the craniovertebral ligaments of whiplash patients compared to non-injured individuals. When the structural changes were correlated to clinical findings these studies suggest that there is an association between the lesions observed and symptoms reported. These studies therefore provide strong evidence that whiplash trauma can damage the craniovertebral ligaments and that these lesions may be responsible for some of the symptoms experienced by whiplash patients.

Based on the presented findings from the in vivo and in vitro studies, it is reasonable to assume that the ligament lesions identified on MRI following whiplash trauma could destabilize the upper cervical spine and therefore clinicians should be alert to the possible presence of upper cervical instability in patients following severe whiplash trauma.

The alar ligaments appear to be more frequently affected by whiplash injuries than the transverse ligament, with incidences of alar ligament injury observed in whiplash patients ranging from 50–75% (Krakenes et al, 2002; Volle & Montazem, 2001). Importantly, if one alar ligament is injured the normal mechanism of limitation of axial rotation to either side becomes non-functional (Crisco et al, 1991a). The chief mechanism of injury of the alar ligaments is stated to be a flexion–extension mechanism whilst the head is in slight rotation. Higher grade lesions in the alar ligaments have been observed following rear-end collisions rather than frontal collisions (Krakenes & Kaale, 2006; Kaale et al, 2005). Lesions in the alar ligaments have been associated with higher NDI scores than lesions in other craniovertebral ligaments suggesting that injury to these ligaments may be an important causative factor of pain and disability in whiplash (Kaale et al, 2005).

Structural abnormalities have been identified in the transverse ligament, tectorial and posterior A-O membranes several years after whiplash injury indicating that these upper cervical structures may also be affected by the forces generated in high speed trauma. The principal mechanism of injury for damage to these structures is hyperflexion (Krakenes et al, 2003a,b). Indeed, high-grade lesions of the transverse ligament and posterior A-O membrane appear to be more common following frontal collisions than rear-end collisions and may occur in as many as 30% of patients who have sustained a severe impact trauma (Dickman et al, 1991). Transverse ligament lesions are associated with higher NDI scores than lesions of the craniovertebral membranes. Cadaver studies have shown that sectioning the tectorial and A-O membranes together results in gross instability (Harris et al, 1993); however, lesions in these structures do not appear to produce the same degree of pain and disability as lesions within the principal craniovertebral ligaments (Kaale et al, 2005).

## Inflammatory causes

The cranio-cervical region has a large number of synovial joints and consequently is frequently targeted by rheumatoid arthritis (RA). Upper cervical involvement usually begins early in the disease process and the severity of involvement is linked to the extent of peripheral disease activity (Nguyen et al, 2004). The erosive synovitis associated with RA destroys cartilage, ligament, tendon and bone which can lead to instability. Atlanto-axial instability (AAI) is the most common instability affecting the upper cervical spine of rheumatoid patients and is responsible for approximately 65% of all cervical subluxation in this patient group (Nguyen et al, 2004; Roche et al, 2002). The rheumatoid inflammation and pannus can invade the medial and lateral A-A joints causing erosion and weakening of the transverse ligament and the odontoid peg. Incompetence of either of these two passive restraints will disrupt the mechanism limiting anterior subluxation of the atlas and will result in AAI. Instability at the C1–C2 level can also occur in a lateral or posterior direction but rotatory instabilities in the rheumatoid population are less common. Deformities involving the O-A joint do not normally lead to instability but instead produce cranial settling or occipito-atlanto-axial impaction due to bony erosion of the occiput, C1 and C1–C2 joint surfaces.

Other systemic inflammatory disorders that may predispose the upper cervical spine to instability include ankylosing spondylitis, scarlet fever and rheumatic fever. More rarely, upper cervical instability may be caused by infections of the upper respiratory tract, middle ear, teeth and nose due to lymphatic connections with the upper cervical region (Swinkels et al, 1996).

## Degeneration

Degenerative changes in the cranio-cervical junction can also lead to instability. Owing to its large ROM the A-A joint has a greater mechanical exposure than the A-O joint and is therefore more vulnerable to degenerative changes. As a result, upper cervical instability secondary to degenerative changes is most prevalent at C1–C2 (Konig et al, 2005).

## Congenital

Various congenital craniovertebral skeletal anomalies have been observed which can lead to upper cervical instability. The most common is fusion of two or more upper cervical vertebrae, for example occipitalization of the atlas. Fusion of two vertebral levels places greater stress on adjacent levels, predisposing them to ligament laxity through overstretch or degenerative changes, both of which may lead to instability. Presence of odontoid anomalies including complete absence, hypoplasia and os odontoideum will affect the stabilizing mechanism between the odontoid peg, transverse ligament and anterior atlantal arch (Swinkels & Oostendorp, 1996).

Down's syndrome is the commonest source of congenital cranio-cervical instability; it is associated with congenital laxity of the transverse ligament, leading most commonly to anterior AAI. The reported incidence of upper cervical instability in Down's syndrome is approximately 7–30% (Cattrysse et al, 1997).

## Signs and symptoms of cranio-cervical instability

Proximity to vital structures such as the spinal cord, brain stem and vertebral arteries, plus the unique pattern of innervation and referral of the upper cervical spine means that cranio-cervical instability can manifest in a variety of symptoms. Classically, neck pain is found at the cranio-cervical junction and is associated with other cranial pain such as occipital headache due to compression of upper cervical nerve roots or facial, mastoid or ear pain due to pain referral mechanisms involving the trigeminocervical nucleus. Cord compression may produce myelopathic symptoms such as upper limb weakness, loss of dexterity, gait disturbances, paraesthesias of the hands or L'Hermitte's sign (electric shock type symptoms). Vascular compromise due to compression of the vertebral arteries or localized cervical artery atherosclerotic changes secondary to increased upper cervical movement may produce a range of symptoms including tinnitus, dizziness, nausea, facial numbness, visual disturbances, diplopia, dysphagia, drop attacks and cognitive impairment (Kerry & Taylor, 2006; Maak et al, 2006; Nguyen et al, 2004).

## Examination of cranio-cervical instability

It has been established that the upper cervical spine is highly dependent on the cranio-cervical ligamentous system and on sensorimotor control to maintain the neutral zones of the cranio-cervical joints within normal limits. Anything that threatens either of these systems will threaten the stability of the

region. Correct identification of upper cervical instability may not always be straightforward. Gross disruption of the passive restraints to cranio-cervical motion usually results in major instability with associated severe pain, neurological signs and symptoms or vascular compromise and therefore should be relatively easy to detect. However, more minor instabilities which may simply be due to a lack of dynamic control of neutral zone motion without any major ligamentous disruption are generally harder to diagnose clinically. They may present with more subtle signs and symptoms such as headache, neck pain, weakness and poor muscle control. Additionally, physical examination may not identify any particular changes in active or passive upper cervical ROM. Thus, in order to comprehensively assess the stability of the cranio-cervical region, tests aimed at exploring the control of the neutral zone should be performed. These include tests examining upper cervical proprioception; upper cervical motor control and upper cervical ligamentous control (Kaale et al, 2008). In addition, tests assessing upper cervical and cranial nerve function and cervical artery function should also be included. The outcomes of testing should then be put into context with history findings and results from any radiographic investigations.

 SUMMARY

### Spinal instability and cranio-cervical instability

- Spinal instability is an increased size and loss of control of the neutral zone.
- Clinical instability is a different condition to hypermobility.
- Trauma, degenerative changes, inflammatory and congenital causes can threaten the mechanical and dynamic stability of the cranio-cervical spine and result in instability.
- Cranio-cervical instability can produce a range of symptoms ranging from pain to neurological and vascular signs and symptoms depending on the extent of the disorder.
- Manual examination should include:
  - Tests of upper cervical mobility in positions that stress ligamentous structures
  - Tests of cervical proprioception and motor control
  - A neurological examination of cervical and cranial nerve conductivity
  - Screening tests for cervical artery function.

# Assessment of the upper cervical spine

## Active movements

The active movements to be examined will be derived from the patient's functional demonstration. Patterns of movement that will stretch anterior or posterior articular and peri-articular structures are listed in Table 8.2.

Due to the differing biomechanics at the atlanto-occipital and atlanto-axial joints the therapist should examine both directions of rotation in either flexion or extension, guided by the direction of the functional demonstration (Figs 8.24, 8.25, 8.26, 8.27). Active movement can be encouraged in the upper cervical spine by limiting mid cervical range of movement during assessment.

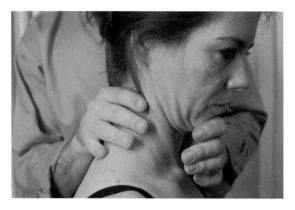

**Figure 8.25** • IN: sitting, upper cervical flexion. DID: right rotation of C0/C2.

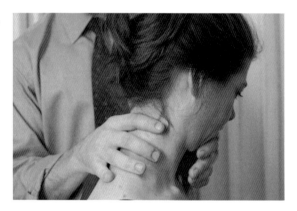

**Figure 8.26** • IN: sitting, upper cervical flexion. DID: left rotation of C0/C1.

**Table 8.2** The atlanto-occipital joint is a convex on concave joint, thus maximum capsular stretch requires opposite rotation to the atlanto-axial and upper cervical spine articulations

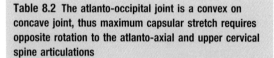

| Anterior stretch C0/C1 | Posterior stretch C0/C1 |
|---|---|
| Extension | Flexion |
| Contralateral rotation | Ipsilateral rotation |
| **Anterior stretch C1–C3** | **Posterior stretch C1–C3** |
| Extension | Flexion |
| Ipsilateral rotation | Contralateral rotation |

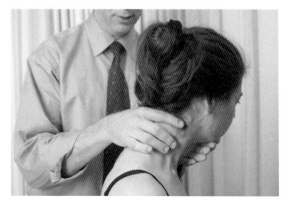

**Figure 8.24** • IN: sitting, upper cervical extension. DID: left rotation of C0 to C2.

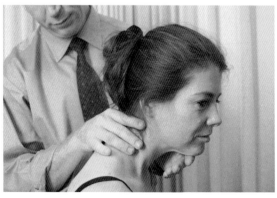

**Figure 8.27** • IN: sitting, upper cervical extension. DID: right rotation of C0/C2.

# Passive movements

Having established the prime movement and primary combination, if it is acceptable to reproduce symptoms, the passive movement examination will be conducted in this position.

## Passive accessory movements

Figure 8.28 shows induction of maximum posterior capsular stretch for the left C0/C1.

## Passive physiological intervertebral movement

Having established the effects of accessory movements on the functional demonstration, the effect of physiological assessment on the functional

demonstration should be assessed. Again, the physiological movements that should be assessed will be governed by the functional demonstration (Figs 8.29, 8.30, 8.31, 8.32).

# Testing mechanical stability of the cranio-cervical spine

Owing to their orientation, many of the craniovertebral ligaments are multifunctional in that they limit craniovertebral movements in more than one direction. The transverse and alar ligaments are the primary restraints in the sagittal, coronal and axial planes. The other craniovertebral ligaments and membranes act as secondary restraints reinforcing limitation of these movements. Consequently mechanical stability of this region is the result of a complex interplay between all of the upper cervical

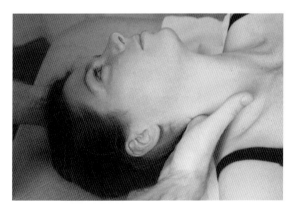

**Figure 8.28** • IN: prone, upper cervical flexion, left rotation. DID: unilateral left, posterior accessory glide on C1.

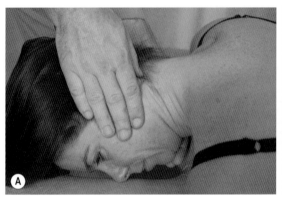

**Figure 8.29** • IN: supine, upper cervical extension. DID: left rotation of C1/C2.

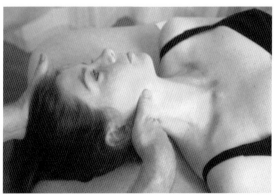

**Figure 8.30** • IN: supine, upper cervical extension, left rotation. DID: right anterior pressure on C1.

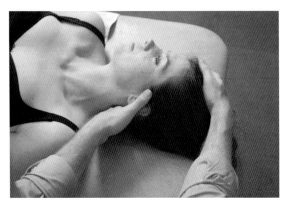

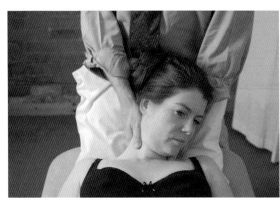

**Figure 8.31** • IN: supine, upper cervical extension. DID: right rotation of C0 on C1. (Pressure angled cephalad towards the eye.)

**Figure 8.32** • IN: supine, upper cervical flexion. DID: left rotation of C1 on C2.

ligaments (Brolin & Halldin, 2004; Crisco *et al*, 1992b; Kaale *et al*, 2008; Yoganandan *et al*, 2001). It is perhaps unrealistic, therefore, to expect to be able to stress specific ligamentous structures in isolation on manual testing. It is, however, reasonable to expect to be able to detect increased cranio-cervical mobility in a specific direction or directions and from this infer the structure or structures which may be incompetent. Adopting an approach to testing cranio-cervical stability in planes of movement instead of testing specific ligaments individually may provide manual therapists with a better understanding of the clinical consequences of any ligamentous insufficiency. In this way, structures limiting a specific movement can be grouped together and tested simultaneously. Appropriate rehabilitation and stabilization strategies related to the direction of increased movement can then be identified (Fig. 8.33).

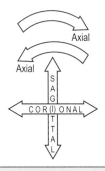

**Anterior**
- Transverse ligament
- Alar ligaments
- Tectorial membrane
- Posterior A-O membrane
- Ligamentum nuchae
- Posterior aspect C0–C2 joint capsules

**Side flexion and rotation**
- Alar ligaments
- A-A joint capsules
- Tectorial membrane
- A-O membranes

**Side flexion and rotation**
- Alar ligaments
- A-A joint capsule
- Tectorial membrane
- A-O membranes

**Posterior**
- Anterior A-O membrane
- Anterior aspect C0–C2 joint capsules
- Apical ligament

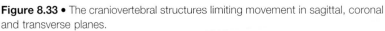

**Figure 8.33** • The craniovertebral structures limiting movement in sagittal, coronal and transverse planes.

## Diagnostic validity of craniovertebral stress testing

There are a number of manual tests commonly used in clinical practice to specifically assess the individual cranio-cervical ligaments. Pettman (1994), Aspinall (1996) and Kaale *et al* (2008) have comprehensively described these tests, however, little is actually known about their diagnostic validity. Only three published studies have been carried out in the last 20 years investigating the reliability and validity of the various cranio-cervical stress tests (Cattrysse *et al*, 1997; Kaale *et al*, 2008; Uitvlugt & Indenbaum, 1988). Cattrysse *et al* (1997) investigated the reliability of the Sharp-Purser test (SPT) on nine children with Down's syndrome, Uitvlught and Indenbaum (1988) explored the validity of the SPT on 123 patients with RA and Kaale *et al* (2008) investigated the diagnostic validity of a range of four craniovertebral stress tests on 92 patients with and 30 without WAD.

Given that reliability is considered a pre-requisite for validity, the findings of the two studies investigating the SPT are contradictory (Sim & Wright, 2000) The study by Cattrysse et al (1997) demonstrated poor inter-therapist reliability whilst the study by Uitvlugt and Indenbaum (1988) concluded that the SPT showed an acceptable level of diagnostic validity compared to X-ray. Differences exist between these two studies, for example in terms of population group studied, sample size, study objectives, criteria and outcome measures used to diagnose instability, which make it difficult to compare the studies or synthesize their findings.

The more recent study carried out by Kaale et al (2008) as part of a series of studies investigating cranio-cervical instability in patients with WAD (Krakenes & Kaale, 2006; Krakenes *et al*, 2002, 2003a,b; Kaale *et al*, 2005) found that when the proposed manual tests were graded, based on a set of criteria, as normal or abnormal there was good agreement between clinical examination and MRI findings in the assessment of upper cervical instability.

The Kaale *et al* (2008) study provides perhaps the best evidence to date to suggest that it is possible to detect lesions of the craniovertebral ligamentous structures by clinical examination and more specifically to determine which directions of craniovertebral mobility are affected.

There is, however, very little available evidence relating to cranio-cervical stability testing to guide clinical practice. Consequently additional reliability and validity studies are required to further develop clinical test procedures.

## Clinical assessment techniques for assessing cranio-cervical stability/mobility

The cranio-cervical complex allows and limits the range of flexion and extension in combinations of rotation and lateral flexion. Equivocally, the region limits rotation and lateral flexion in combinations of rotation. As previously mentioned, it is unreasonable to expect specific combined movements to stress specific anatomic structures. It is, however, realistic to expect manual therapists to be able to perceive differences in resistance free range and the profile of resistance to movement in the combined positions limited by these structures (Fig. 8.34).

In order to assess the passive mobility of the upper cervical spine the spinal segments should be assessed in the following positions and in the following directions. In order to assess AP glide of the atlas on the axis, the SPT should be undertaken. Antero-posterior glide of the atlas on the axis should be accompanied by an assessment of the lateral glide of the atlas between the occiput and the axis. These sagittal and coronal movements are performed in neutral, sagittal and coronal range to assess the maximal neutral zone. Assessments of functional range of movement can be made by examining the range and resistance to movement occurring in positions that will maximally stress ligamentous and muscular resistance. The corners of combined flexion and rotation with combined extension and rotation will provide biomechanical cues to

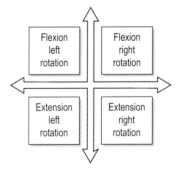

**Figure 8.34 •** A schematic diagram of the combinations of movement and accessory glides to be considered in the assessment of the available passive movement in the upper cervical spine.

treatment and alert the therapist to excessive range of movement or lack of control. Figure 8.34 depicts the planes and combined positions in which upper cervical mobility should be assessed, particularly in the presence of concerns regarding hypermobility.

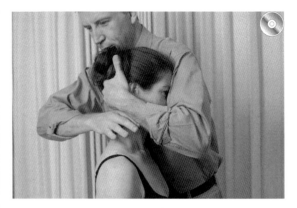

**Figure 8.35** • IN: sitting, neutral flexion/extension; DID: PA glide of the head and C1 on a fixed C2. The Sharp-Purser test. See video clip number 1

## Safety note

The majority of tests aimed at assessing the mechanical stability of the cranio-cervical region are potentially harmful and thus should be performed with care.

Patients presenting with signs and symptoms consistent with major upper cervical instability, such as severe pain in the cranio-cervical region, gross neurological deficits and/or vascular compromise **should not** be exposed to mechanical testing. In addition, these tests, with the exception of the Sharp Purser Test, are not suitable to be carried out on patients suffering from rheumatoid arthritis, particularly those patients in the more advanced stages of the disease.

Diagnosis of cranio-cervical instability in these patient groups is more appropriately and safely achieved through history findings and results from diagnostic imagery.

The tests outlined below are, however, indicated for patients with suspected minor instabilities although it is assumed that the clinician will exercise sound clinical judgement in the appropriate selection and application of these tests.

## Sagittal plane stability

### 1. Antero-posterior translation test (SPT) (adapted from Aspinall, 1996; Pettman, 1994; Sharp & Purser, 1961)

*Aim of test*

This test is a relocation test and assesses the amount of anterior-posterior translation between the atlas and the axis. The test is based on the stabilizing mechanism between the odontoid peg and the transverse ligament. If both these structures are competent, they will prevent the atlas translating anteriorly on the axis during cervical flexion. However, if these structures are insufficient, the atlas will be allowed to slide in an anterior direction in relation to the axis on cervical flexion.

*Test procedure (Fig. 8.35)*

C2 is stabilized by placing the first interosseous web space of the right hand over the spinous process of C2 with the thumb and fingers gripping the articular pillars of C2 bilaterally using a lumbrical grip. The

patient's forehead rests against the examiner's shoulder and the left hand holds the patient's occiput. The test movement is performed by applying a posterior glide of the head/C1 on a fixed C2. The test is repeated in upper cervical flexion–extension and neutral.

*Test interpretation*

If the structures that limit anterior translation of C1 on C2 are intact, there should be no appreciable posterior gliding motion of the head/C1 on C2 beyond the normal uptake of the soft tissues and there should be a hard end-feel. This should be the case in all three positions tested: flexion–extension and neutral.

If the structures that limit anterior translation of C1 on C2 are insufficient, an excessive posterior gliding motion of the head/C1 on C2 beyond the normal uptake of the soft tissues will be detected when the test is carried out in flexion. When the test is carried out in neutral and extension there should be no posterior gliding motion detected. The different test outcome appreciated in flexion compared to extension is related to the stabilizing mechanism between the odontoid peg and the transverse ligament and is important in order to classify the test as abnormal. Any significant posterior gliding motion detected when the test is carried out in flexion represents relaxation of the subluxed atlas.

### 2. Tectorial membrane test (Kaale *et al*, 2008)

*Aim of test*

This test assesses the amount of flexion and distraction between the occiput, atlas and axis. It is based on biomechanical studies which have shown the

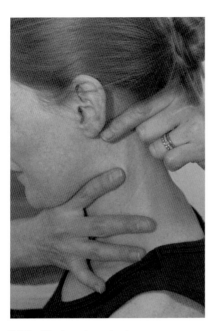

**Figure 8.36** • Flexion stress test.

tectorial membrane to limit hyperflexion. The alar ligaments, posterior A-O membrane and ligamentum nuchae will also act as restraints to this movement.

### Test procedure (Fig. 8.36)

C2 is stabilized with the left hand using a frontal grip. This is performed by fixing the antero-lateral aspects of the C2 articular pillars using the thumb on one side and fingers two and three on the other. The right hand grips around the base of the occiput. The test movement is performed by the right hand applying traction and a flexion motion to the occiput. The test is repeated in different angles of flexion.

### Test interpretation

Excessive motion in the test direction is indicative of a positive test.

## Coronal plane stability

### 1. Lateral stability stress test (Pettman, 1994)

#### Aim of test

This test assesses the amount of physiological lateral flexion across the occipito-atlanto-axial complex. The structures limiting lateral flexion are primarily the alar ligaments reinforced by the tectorial membrane and A-A joint capsules.

### Test procedure

In supine, C2 is stabilized by placing the first interosseous web space of the left hand over the spinous process of C2 with the thumb and fingers gripping the articular pillars of C2 bilaterally using a lumbrical grip (Figs 8.37 and 8.38).

The right hand grips the crown of the patient's head (Fig. 8.39) and applies the test movement of upper cervical side-flexion to the right. This movement is performed by adding slight vertical compression through the crown of the head followed by a side-bending motion where the right ear is pushed towards the left side of the neck. The test is repeated in upper cervical flexion, extension and neutral (Figs 8.40, 8.41 and 8.42).

Hand holds are then reversed and the test is performed into left side-flexion in the same three starting positions.

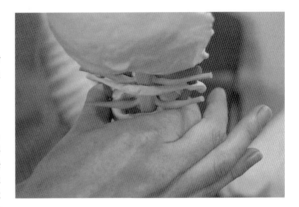

**Figure 8.37** • Fixation of C2 using lumbrical grip – posterior view.

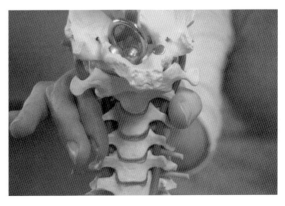

**Figure 8.38** • Fixation of C2 using lumbrical grip – anterior view.

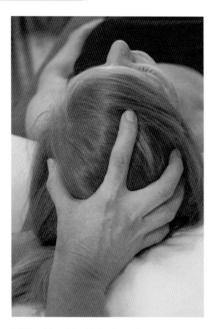

**Figure 8.39** • Hand hold for lateral and rotational stress tests.

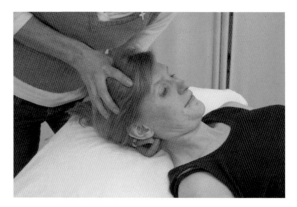

**Figure 8.41** • Lateral stability stress test in flexion.

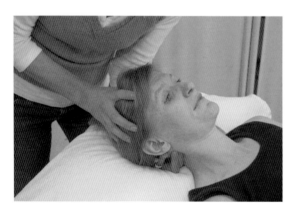

**Figure 8.40** • Lateral stability stress test in neutral.

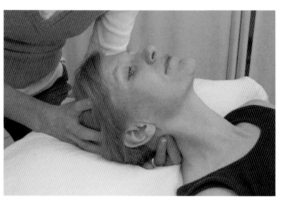

**Figure 8.42** • Lateral stability stress test in extension.

### Test interpretation

If the structures limiting lateral flexion are intact, and C2 is adequately stabilized, no movement of the head will occur.

## 2. Lateral translation stress test

### Aim of test

This test assesses the amount of accessory lateral translation of the atlas on the axis. The key structure that limits this movement is the odontoid peg. If the odontoid peg is intact, no discernible movement should be detected on application of the test.

### Test procedure

In the supine position, the right lateral aspect of C2 is stabilized using the index finger of the right hand. Contact is made with the left lateral aspect of C1 using the index finger of the left hand. The occiput is cradled by fingers three to five of the left hand. The test movement is performed by applying a contralateral side glide (from left to right) of C1 on C2 (Figs 8.43 and 8.44).

### Test interpretation

If the structures limiting this movement are intact, no movement should be detected.

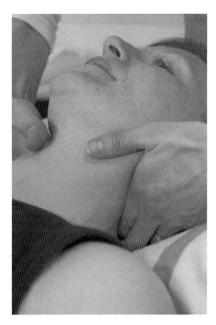

**Figure 8.43** • Lateral translation stress test.

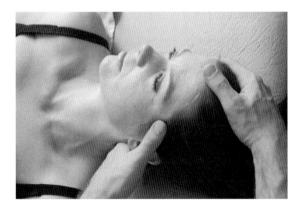

**Figure 8.44** • IN: supine, upper cervical neutral. DID: contralateral side glide in neutral flexion, left lateral flexion C0/C1.

## Transverse plane stability

### Rotational stress test

#### Aim of test

This test assesses the amount of rotation across the occipito-atlanto-axial complex. Based on biomechanical studies, cranio-cervical axial rotation in excess of 55° indicates insufficiency in the structures that limit rotation, principally the alar ligaments reinforced by

the A-A joint capsules and the tectorial membrane (Crisco *et al*, 1992b; Goel *et al*, 1990; Krakenes & Kaale, 2006).

#### Test procedure

In supine. C2 is strongly stabilized by placing the first interosseous web space of the left hand over the spinous process of C2 with the thumb and fingers gripping the articular pillars of C2 bilaterally, using a lumbrical grip (see Figs 8.37 and 8.38). The right hand grips the crown of the patient's head (see Fig. 8.39) and the test movement of rotation to the right is applied. The test is repeated in flexion, extension and neutral. Hand holds are then reversed and the test is performed into left rotation in the same three starting positions (Fig. 8.45).

#### Interpretation of test

If the structures limiting cranio-cervical rotation are intact, and C2 is adequately stabilized, rotation of the head will stop between 25° and 45°. Axial rotation of greater than 55° indicates insufficiency of the passive restraints suggestive of a rotational instability. Excessive rotation may be more obvious when the test is performed in flexion since the alar ligaments are maximally stressed in this position (Dvorak & Panjabi, 1987; Krakenes & Kaale, 2006).

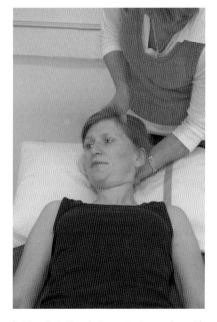

**Figure 8.45** • Rotational stress test – end position.

# Assessment of increased tone of cervical muscle tissue

## Muscle assessment

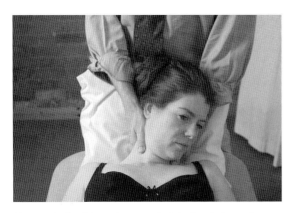

**Figure 8.46** • IN: supine, cervical flexion, left rotation. DID: post-isometric relaxation technique of the right posterior para-spinal musculature. See Chapter 7

# Assessment for Grade IV−: manipulation of the upper cervical spine

## Flexion

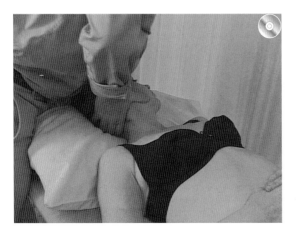

**Figure 8.47** • IN: supine, upper cervical flexion, left rotation. DID: right lateral flexion C0/C1. See video clip number 56

# Extension

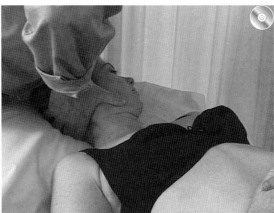

**Figure 8.48** • IN: supine, upper cervical extension, left rotation. DID: right lateral flexion C0/C1. See video clip number 57

## SUMMARY

### Assessment of the upper cervical spine

- The patient's functional demonstration will direct the examination of active movements used in combination to stretch anterior and posterior articular and peri-articular structures.
- Once the prime movement and primary combination have been identified, passive movement examination will be carried out in this position (dependent on severity/irritability of symptoms). The effects of both passive accessory and passive physiological movements on the functional demonstration should be assessed.
- The mobility and stability of the cranio-cervical spine should be assessed in the sagittal, coronal and transverse planes.
- Cervical muscle tone using post-isometric relaxation should be assessed.
- Assessment for manipulation of the cranio-cervical spine can be carried out.

## QUESTIONS

### 1. Cranio-cervical biomechanics

A. Where does extension mainly occur in the cranio-cervical spine?
   i. Atlanto-occipital joint
   ii. Atlanto-axial joint
   iii. Across both levels

B. Where does flexion mainly occur in the cranio-cervical spine?
   i. Atlanto-occipital joint
   ii. Atlanto-axial joint
   iii. Across both levels

C. Where does rotation mainly occur in the cranio-cervical spine?
   i. Atlanto-occipital joint
   ii. Atlanto-axial joint
   iii. Across both levels

D. How are movements coupled in the craniocervical spine?
   i. Ipsilaterally
   ii. Contralaterally

### 2. Cranio-cervical innervation

A. What are the mechanisms of pain referral from somatic upper cervical tissue to the head and face?
   i. Irritation of the cervical plexus
   ii. Convergence with the Vth cranial nerve at the trigeminal cervical nucleus
   iii. Compression of the brachial plexus

B. Can upper cervical nerve roots refer pain to the face?
   i. Yes
   ii. No

C. Where can the vertebral artery refer pain to?
   i. The shoulder
   ii. The sub-occipital region
   iii. The forehead

### 3. Cranio-cervical stability

A. Which structures provide most stability for the cranio-cervical spine in neutral and mid-range positions?
   i. Cranio-cervical muscles
   ii. Cranio-cervical ligaments
   iii. Intervertebral discs

B. Should the assessment of motor control form part of the assessment of cranio-cervical stability?
   i. No
   ii. Yes

C. What would you suspect if a patient had more than 55° rotation between C1–C2?
   i. The patient has full ROM at C1–C2
   ii. The patient has a congential abnormality of the odontoid peg
   iii. The patient has alar ligament insufficiency

D. What structure/s limit flexion?
   i. Alar ligaments
   ii. Transverse ligament, alar ligament and tectorial membrane
   iii. Anterior A-O membrane

E. Is there evidence to demonstrate that the craniovertebral ligaments can be a source of pain and disability following whiplash?
   i. Yes
   ii. No

### 4. Cranio-cervical assessment

A. If you want to apply a stretch to the posterior part of the C0–C1 capsule, which upper cervical movements would you combine?
   i. Extension and ipsilateral rotation
   ii. Flexion and ipsilateral rotation
   iii. Extension and ipsilateral lateral flexion

B. Which assessment techniques would you include in the assessment of a mechanical upper cervical disorder?
   i. Neurological examination and neurodynamic testing
   ii. Functional demonstration, active movements, passive accessory and passive physiological movements
   iii. Glenohumeral instability tests

C. If you performed rotation in upper cervical flexion, which ligaments would you expect to limit the movement?
   i. Transverse ligament
   ii. Anterior A-O membrane
   iii. Alar ligaments

**Answers: 1A** i; **1B** iii; **1C** ii; **1D** ii; **2A** ii; **2B** i; **2C** ii; **3A** i; **3B** ii; **3C** iii; **3D** ii; **3E** i; **4A** iii; **4B** ii; **4C** iii

# References

Amiri, M., Jull, G., Bullock-Saxton, J., 2003. Measurement of upper cervical flexion and extension with the 3-space fastrak measurement system: a repeatability study. The Journal of Manual and Manipulative Therapy 11 (4), 198–203.

Armstrong, B., McNair, P., Taylor, D., 2008. Head and neck position sense. Sports Med 38 (2), 101–117.

Aspinall, W., 1996. Clinical testing for the craniovertebral hypermobility syndrome. J. Orthop. Sports Phys. Ther. 12 (2), 47–54.

Bogduk, N., 1992. The anatomical basis for cervicogenic headache. J. Manipulative Physiol. Ther. 15, 67–70.

Bogduk, N., 1997. Clinical anatomy of the lumbar spine and sacrum, third ed. Churchill Livingstone, New York.

Bogduk, N., 2001. Mechanisms and pain patterns of the upper cervical spine. In: Vernon, H. The cranio-cervical syndrome. Butterworth Heinemann, Oxford.

Bogduk, N., 2002a. Biomechanics of the cervical spine. In: Grant, R. (Ed.), Physical therapy of the cervical and thoracic spine, third ed. Churchill Livingstone, New York.

Bogduk, N., 2002b. Innervation and pain patterns of the cervical spine. In: Grant, R. (Ed.), Physical therapy of the cervical and thoracic spine, third ed. Churchill Livingstone, New York.

Bogduk, N., 2008. Email correspondence with Gail Forrester.

Bogduk, N., Marsland, A., 1985. Third occipital headache. Cephalalagia 5 (Suppl. 3), 310.

Bogduk, N., Mercer, S., 2000. Biomechanics of the cervical spine. I: normal kinematics. Clin. Biomech. 15, 633–648.

Boyd Clark, L., Briggs, C., Galea, M., 2001. Comparative histochemical composition of muscle fibres in a pre and post-vertebral muscle of the cervical spine. J. Anat. 199, 709–716.

Boyd Clark, L., Briggs, C., Galea, M., 2002. Muscle spindle distribution, morphology and density in longus colli and multifidus muscles of the cervical spine. Spine 27 (7), 694–701.

Brolin, K., Halldin, P., 2004. Development of a finite model of the upper cervical spine in a parameter study of ligament characteristics. Spine 29 (4), 376–385.

Busch, E., Wilson, P., 1989. Atlanto-occipital and atlanto-axial injections in the treatment of headache and neck pain. Regional Anaesthesia Journal 14 (Suppl. 2), 45.

Butler, D., 2000. The sensitive nervous system. NOI Group Publications, Adelaide, Australia (Chapter 3, 4 and 6).

Catrysse, E., Swinkels, R., Oostendorp, W., 1997. Upper cervical instability: are clinical tests reliable. Man. Ther. 2 (2), 91–97.

Catrysse, E., Baeyens, J., Clarys, J., et al., 2007. Manual fixation versus locking during upper cervical segmental mobilisation. Part 1: An in vitro three-dimensional arthrokinematic analysis of manual flexion-extension mobilisation of the atlanto-occipital joint. Man. Ther. 12 (4), 353–362.

Catrysse, E., Baeyens, J.P., Kool, K., et al., 2008. Does manual mobilisation influence motion coupling patterns in the atlanto-axial joint? J. Electromyogr. Kinesiol. 18 (5), 838–848.

Chancey, V., Ottaviano, D., Myers, B., et al., 2007. A kinematic and anthropometric study of the upper cervical spine and the occipital condyles. J. Biomech. 40, 1953–1959.

Comley, L., 2003. Chiropractic management of greater occipital neuralgia. Clinical Chiropractic 6, 120–128.

Cook, C., Hegedus, E., Showalter, C., et al., 2006. Coupling behaviour of the cervical spine: a systematic review of the literature. J. Manipulative Physiol. Ther. 29 (7), 570–575.

Crawford, N., Peles, J., Dickman, C., 1998. The spinal lax zone and neutral zone. Measurement techniques and parameter comparisons. J. Spinal Disord. 11 (5), 416–429.

Crisco, J., Panjabi, M., Dvorak, J., 1991a. A model of the alar ligaments of the upper cervical spine in axial rotation. J. Biomech. 24 (7), 607–614.

Crisco, J., Oda, T., Panjabi, M., et al., 1991b. Transections of the C1-C2 joint capsular ligaments in the cadaveric spine. Spine 16 (10), S474–S479.

Dreyfuss, P., Michaelsen, M., Fletcher, D., 1994. Atlanto-occipital and lateral atlanto-axial joint pain patterns. Spine 19 (10), 1125–1131.

Dickman, C., Mamourian, A., Sonntag, B., et al., 1991. Magnetic resonance imaging of the transverse atlantal ligament for the evaluation of atlantoaxial instability. J. Neurosurg. 75, 221–227.

Dickman, C., Greene, K., Sonntag, V., 1996. Injuries involving the transverse atlantal ligament; classification and treatment guidelines based upon experience with 39 injuries. Neurosurgery 38, 44–50.

Drake, R., Vogl, W., Mitchell, A., 2005. Gray's Anatomy for students. Churchill Livingstone, Elsevier, Philadelphia.

Dvorak, J., Panjabi, M., 1987. Functional anatomy of the alar ligaments. Spine 12 (2), 183–189.

Dvorak, J., Hayek, J., Zehnder, R., 1987. CT-functional diagnostics of the rotatory instability of the upper cervical spine: 2. An evaluation on healthy adults and patients with suspected instability. Spine 12, 726–731.

Dvorak, J., Schneider, E., Saldinger, P., et al., 1988. Biomechanics of the cranio-cervical region; the alar and transverse ligaments. J. Orthop. Res. 6, 452–461.

Dwyer, A., Aprill, C., Bogduk, N., 1990. Cervical zygopophyseal joint pain patterns I: a study in normal volunteers. Spine 15, 453–457.

Ebraheim, N., Lu, J., Yang, H., 1998. The effect of translation of the C1/2 on the spinal canal. Clin. Orthop. Relat. Res. 351, 222–229.

Edmonston, S., Henne, S., Loh, W., et al., 2005. Influence of cranio-cervical posture on three-dimensional motion of the cervical spine. Man. Ther. 10, 44–51.

Edwards, B., 1999. Manual of combined movements. Butterworth Heinemann.

Ehni, G., Benner, B., 1984. Occipital neuralgia and C1-C2 arthrosis. N. Engl. J. Med. 310, 127.

Falla, D., 2004. Unravelling the complexity of muscle impairment in chronic neck pain. Man. Ther. 9 (3), 125–133.

Falla, D., Jull, G., Hodges, P., 2004. Feedforward activity of the cervical flexor muscles during voluntary arm movements is delayed in chronic neck pain. Exp. Brain Res. 157, 43–48.

Fukui, S., Ohseto, K., Shiotani, M., et al., 1996. Referred pain distribution of the cervical zygopophyseal joints and cervical dorsal rami. Pain 68, 79–83.

Gifford, L., Butler, D., 1997. The integration of pain sciences in to clinical practice. J. Hand Ther. 10, 86–95.

Goel, V., Clark, C., McGowan, D., et al., 1984. An in vitro study of the kinematics of the normal, injured and stabilised cervical spine. J. Biomech. 17 (5), 336–376.

Goel, V., Clark, C., Gallaes, K., et al., 1988. Moment-rotation relationships of the ligamentous occipito-atlanto-axial complex. J. Biomech. 21 (8), 673–680.

Goel, V., Winterbottom, J., Schulte, K., et al., 1990. Ligamentous laxity across C0-C1-C2 complex. Axial torque-rotation characteristics until failure. Spine 15 (10), 990–996.

Goel, V., Clausen, J., 1998. Prediction of load sharing among spinal components of a C5–6 motion segment using the finite element approach. Spine 23 (6), 684–691.

Greening, J., Lynn, B., 1998. Minor peripheral nerve injuries: an underestimated source of pain? Man. Ther. 3 (4), 187–194.

Hallgren, R., Greenman, P., Rechtien, J., 1994. Atrophy of sub-occipital muscles in patients with chronic pain: a pilot study. Journal of American Osteopathic Association 94 (12), 1032–1038.

Harris, M., Duval, M., Davies, J., et al., 1993. Anatomical and roentgenographic features of atlantooccipital instability. J. Spinal Disord. 6, 5–10.

Hino, H., Abumi, K., Kanayama, M., et al., 1999. Dynamic motion analysis of normal and unstable cervical spines using cineradiography. An in vivo study. Spine 24 (2), 163–168.

Iai, H., Moriya, H., Goto, S., et al., 1993. Three-dimensional motion analysis of the upper cervical spine during axial rotation. Spine 18 (16), 2388–2392.

Ishii, T., Mukai, Y., Hosono, N., et al., 2004. Kinematics of the cervical spine in rotation in vivo three-dimensional analysis. Spine 29 (7), E139–E144.

Ishii, T., Mukai, Y., Hosono, N., et al., 2006. Kinematics of the cervical spine in lateral bending in vivo three-dimensional analysis. Spine 31 (2), 155–160.

Johnson, G., 2004. The sensory and sympathetic nerve supply within the cervical spine; review of recent observations. Man. Ther. 9, 71–76.

Jull, G., 2000. Deep cervical flexor muscle dysfunction in whiplash. Journal of Musculoskeletal Pain 8, 143–154.

Jull, G., Sterling, M., Falla, D., et al., 2008. Whiplash, headache and neck pain. Research-based direction for physical therapists. Churchill Livingstone, Edinburgh.

Jull, G., Kristjansson, E., Dall'Alba, P., 2004a. Impairment in the cervical flexors: a comparison of whiplash and insidious onset neck pain patients. Man. Ther. 9 (2), 89–94.

Jull, G., Falla, D., Treleaven, J., et al., 2004b. A therapeutic exercise approach for cervical disorders. In: Boyling, N., Palastanga, N. (Eds.), Grieves' Modern Manual Therapy. third ed. Churchill Livingstone, Edinburgh.

Kaale, B., Krakenes, J., Albreksten, G., et al., 2008. Clinical assessment techniques for detecting ligament and membrane injuries in the upper cervical spine region – a comparison with MRI results. Man. Ther. 13, 397–403.

Kaale, B., Krakenes, J., Albreksten, G., et al., 2005. Whiplash associated disorders impairment rating: neck disability index score according to severity of MR- findings of ligaments and membranes in the upper cervical spine. J. Neurotrauma 22 (4), 466–475.

Kettler, A., Hartwig, E., Schultheib, L., et al., 2002. Mechanically stimulated muscle forces strongly stabilise intact and injured upper cervical spine specimens. J. Biomech. 35, 339–346.

Kerry, R., Taylor, A., 2006. Cervical arterial dysfunction assessment and manual therapy. Man. Ther. 11 (4), 243–253.

Konig, S.A., Goldammer, A., Vitzthum, H.E., 2005. Anatomical data on the cranio-cervical junction and their correlation with degenerative changes in 30 cadaveric specimens. J. Neurosurg. Spine 3 (5), 379–385.

Krakenes, J., Kaale, B., Rorvik, J., et al., 2001. MRI assessment of normal ligamentous structures in the cranioverteberal junction. Neuroradiology 43, 1089–1097.

Krakenes, J., Kaale, B., 2006. Magnetic resonance imaging assessment of craniovertebral ligaments and membranes after whiplash trauma. Spine 31 (24), 2820–2826.

Krakenes, J., Kaale, B., Moen, G., et al., 2002. MRI assessment of the alar ligaments in the late stage of whiplash injury: a study of structural abnormalities and observer agreement. Neuroradiology 38, 44–50.

Krakenes, J., Kaale, B., Nordli, H., et al., 2003a. MR analysis of the transverse ligament in the late stage of whiplash injury. Acta Radiol. 44, 637–644.

Krakenes, J., Kaale, B., Moen, G., et al., 2003b. MR analysis of the tectorial and posterior antlanto-occipital membranes in the late stage of whiplash injury. Neuroradiology 45, 585–591.

Kristjansson, 2004. The cervical spine and proprioception. In: Grieve's Modern Manual Therapy. third ed. Churchill Livingstone.

Loeser, J., Treede, R., 2008. The Kyoto protocol of IASP basic pain terminology. Pain 137, 473–477.

Lord, S., Barnsley, L., Wallis, B., et al., 1994. Third occipital nerve headache: a prevalence study. J. Neurol. Neurosurg. Psychiatry 57, 1187.

Loudon, J., Ruhl, M., Field, E., 1997. Ability to reproduce head position after whiplash injury. Spine 22, 865–868.

Maeda, T., Saito, T., Harimaya, K., et al., 2004. Atlantoaxial instability in neck retraction and protrusion positions in patients with rheumatoid arthritis. Spine 29 (7), 757–762.

McPartland, J., Brodeur, R., 1999. Rectus capitus posterior minor: a small but important suboccipital muscle. Journal of Bodywork and Movement Therapies 3 (1), 30–35.

Meadows, J., 1998. The Sharp-Purser Test: a useful clinical tool or an exercise in futility and risk? Manual Therapy Rounds 6 (2), 97–100.

Maak, T., Tominaga, Y., Panjabi, M., et al., 2006. Alar, transverse, and apical ligament strain due to head-turned rear impact. Spine 31 (6), 632–638.

Middleditch, A., Oliver, J., 2005. Functional anatomy of the spine, second ed. Elsevier Butterworth Heinnemann, Edinburgh.

Mimura, M., Moriya, H., Watanabe, T., et al., 1989. Three dimensional motion analysis of the cervical spine with special reference to axial rotation. Spine 14 (11), 1135–1139.

Moroney, S., Schultz, A., Miller, A., et al., 1988. Load-displacement properties of lower cervical spine motion segments. J. Biomech. 21 (9), 769–779.

Myers, J., Wassinger, C., Lephart, S., 2006. Sensorimotor contribution to shoulder stability: Effect of injury and rehabilitation. Man. Ther. 11, 197–201.

Nee, R., Butler, D., 2006. Management of peripheral neuropathic pain: Integrating neurobiology, neurodynamics, and clinical evidence. Physical Therapy in Sport 7, 36–49.

Nguyen, H., Ludwig, S., Silber, J., et al., 2004. Rheumatoid arthritis of the cervical spine. Spine J. 4, 329–334.

Nightingale, R., Winklestein, B., Knaub, K., et al., 2002. Comparative strengths of and structural properties of the upper cervical spine in flexion and extension. J. Biomech. 35, 752–1732.

O'Leary, S.J.G., Kim, M., Vicenzino, B., 2007. Cranio-cervical flexor muscle impairment at maximal, moderate, and low loads is a feature of neck pain. Man. Ther. 12 (1), 34–39.

Ordway, N., Seymour, R., Donelson, R., et al., 1999. Cervical flexion, extension, protrusion and retratction: a radiographic segmental analysis. Spine 24 (3), 240–247.

Oxland, T., Panjabi, M., 1992. the onset and progression of spinal injury: a demonstration of neutral zone sensitivity. J. Biomech. 25, 1165–1172.

Palastanga, N., Field, D., Soames, R., 2006. Anatomy and human movement. Structure and function, fifth ed. Butterworth Heinnemann, Elsevier, Edinburgh.

Panjabi, M., 1992a. The stabilising system of the spine. Part I. Function, dysfunction, adaptation and enhancement. J. Spinal Disord. 5 (4), 383–389.

Panjabi, M., 1992b. The stabilising system of the spine. Part II. Neutral zone and instability hypothesis. J. Spinal Disord. 5 (4), 390–397.

Panjabi, M., Dvorak, J., Duranceau, J., et al., 1988. Three-dimensional movements of the upper cervical spine. Spine 13 (7), 726–730.

Panjabi, M., Abumi, K., Duranceau, J., et al., 1989. Spinal stability and intersegmental muscle forces: A biomechanical model. Spine 14, 194–200.

Panjabi, M., Crisco, J., Oda, T., et al., 1991. Flexion, extension and lateral bending of the upper cervical spine in response to alar ligament transection. J. Spinal Disord. 4, 157–167.

Panjabi, M., Oda, T., Crisco, J., et al., 1993. Posture affects motion coupling patterns of the upper cervical spine. J. Orthop. Res. 11 (4), 525–536.

Panjabi, M., Lydon, C., Vasavada, A., et al., 1994. On the understanding of clinical instability. Spine 19 (23), 2642–2650.

Panjabi, M., Cholewicki, J., Nibu, K., et al., 1998. Critical load of the human cervical spine: an in vitro experimental study. Clin. Biomech. 13, 11–17.

Panjabi, M., Crisco, J., Vasavada, A., et al., 2001. Mechanical properties of the human cervical spine as shown by three-dimensional load displacement curves. Spine 26 (24), 2692–2700.

Pettman, 1994. Stress tests of the craniovertebral joints. In: Boyling, N., Palastanga, N. (Eds.), Grieve's Modern Manual Therapy. second ed. Churchill Livingstone, Edinburgh.

Revel, M., Minguet, M., Gergoy, P., et al., 1994. Changes in cervicocephalic kinaesthesia after a proprioceptive rehabilitation program in patients with neck pain: a randomised controlled study. Arch. Phys. Med. Rehabil. 75, 895–899.

Riemann, B.L., Lephart, S.M., 2002a. The sensorimotor system, part 1: the physiological basis of functional joint stability. Journal of Athletic Training 37 (1), 71–77.

Riemann, B.L., Lephart, S.M., 2002b. The sensorimotor system, part 2: the role of proprioception in motor control and functional joint stability. Journal of Athletic Training 37 (1), 80–84.

Roche, C., Eyes, B., Whitehouse, G., 2002. The rheumatoid cervical spine: signs of instability on plain cervical radiographs. Clin. Radiol. 57, 241–249.

Sharp, J., Purser, D., 1961. Spontaneous atlanto-axial dislocation in ankylosing spondylitis and rheumatoid arthritis. Ann. Rheum. Dis. 20, 47–77.

Sim, J., Wright, C., 2000. Research in healthcare. Concepts, designs and methods. Nelson Thornes, Cheltenham.

Sjolander, P., Michaelson, P., Jaric, S., et al., 2008. Sensorimotor disturbances in chronic neck pain – range of motion, peak velocity, smoothness of movement and repositioning acuity. Man. Ther. 13 (2), 122–131.

Standring, S., 2008. Gray's Anatomy, fortieth ed. Churchill Livingstone, Edinburgh.

Sterling, M., Jull, G., Vincenzino, B., et al., 2003. Development of motor system dysfunction following whiplash injury. Pain 103 (1–2), 65–73.

Sterling, M., Jull, G., Vincenzino, B., et al., 2004. Characterisation of acute whiplash-associated disorders. Spine 29, 182–188.

Swinkels, R., Oostendorp, R., 1996. Upper cervical instability: fact or fiction? J. Manipulative Physiol. Ther. 19 (3), 185–194.

Swinkels, R., Beeton, K., Alltree, J., 1996. Pathogenesis of upper cervical instability. Man. Ther. 1, 127–132.

Taimela, S., Takala, E., Asklof, T., et al., 2000. Active treatment of chronic neck pain: a prospective randomised intervention. Spine 25 (8), 1021–1027.

Taylor, J., Twomey, L., 2002. Functional and applied anatomy of the cervical spine. In: Grant, R. (Ed.), Physical therapy of the cervical and thoracic spine, third ed. Churchill Livingstone, New York.

Treleaven, J., Jull, G., Sterling, M., 2003. Dizziness and unsteadiness following whiplash injury: characteristic features and relationship with cervical joint position error. J. Rehabil. Med. 35, 36–43.

Treleaven, J., 2008. Sensorimotor disturbances in neck disorders affecting postural stability, head and eye movement control. Man. Ther. 13 (1), 2–11.

Tubbs, S., Grabb, P., Spooner, A., et al., 2000. The apical ligament: anatomy and functional significance. J. Neurosurg. 97, 197–200.

Tubbs, S., Kelly, D., Humphrey, R., et al., 2007. The tectorial membrane: anatomical, biomechanical and histological analysis. Clin. Anat. 20, 382–386.

Uitvlugt, G., Indenbaum, S., 1988. Clinical assessment of atlanto-axial instability using the Sharp-Purser test. Arthritis Rheum. 31 (7), 918–922.

Van Vliet, P., Heneghan, N., 2006. Motor control and the management of musculoskeletal dysfunction. Man. Ther. 11, 208–213.

Volle, E., Montazem, A., 2001. MRI video diagnosis and surgical therapy of soft tissue trauma to the cranio-cervical junction. Ear Nose Throat J. 80, 41–44 46–48.

Yoganandan, N., Kumaresan, S., Pintar, F., 2001. Biomechanics of the cervical spine. Part 2. Cervical spine soft tissue responses and biomechanical modelling. Clin. Biomech. 16, 1–27.

Zhang, Q., Teo, E., Ng, H., et al., 2006. Finite element analysis of moment-rotation relationships for human cervical spine. J. Biomech. 39, 189–193.

# Chapter Nine

# Mid and lower cervical spine

Chris McCarthy

9

## CHAPTER CONTENTS

## Clinical anatomy and biomechanics

Ioannis Paneris

## The typical cervical segments

The remaining typical vertebral levels, although morphologically different from the C2–C3 level, still share common characteristics. The cervical intervertebral joints are a saddle shape in which the inferior surface of the superior vertebra is concave in the sagittal plane and the superior surface of the inferior vertebra is concave on the transverse plane. Additionally, the orientation of the superior surface of the inferior vertebrae is oblique, sloping caudally and anteriorly, while the anterior inferior border of each vertebra forms a lip that hangs towards the anterior superior edge of the vertebrae below. Consequently, the plane of the intervertebral disc is set obliquely to the long axis of the vertebral bodies (Bogduk & Mercer, 2000) and to the plane of the apophyseal joints (Penning, 1988).

This geometry dictates that the primary motion at this level is flexion and extension around a transverse axis of rotation. Studies on the flexion–extension centres of motion revealed that their location changes from a dorso-caudal location on the body of the C3 vertebrae, moving progressively to the centre of the C7 cranial end plate, maintaining an equal distance from the mid-perpendicular apophyseal joint spaces. Consequently, the pattern of motion for flexion and extension of the cervical spine consists of gliding in the upper segments of the typical cervical spine while in the lower levels the pattern is one of tilting which is the most stable (Penning, 1988).

A literature review (White & Panjabi, 1978) concluded that the representative angle for flexion–extension for C3–C4 is 13°, 12° for C4–C5, 17° for C5–C6, 16° for C6–C7 and 9° for C7–T1. However, Panjabi et al (2001) reported the smaller average ranges of motion for flexion–extension of 7.7° for C3–C4, 10.1° for C4–C5, 9.9° for C5–C6, 7.1° for C6–C7.

A more recent study (Wu et al, 2007) reported mean flexion and extension of the cervical motion segments. More specifically, they reported a mean of 7.56° of flexion coupled with a mean of 0.98 mm of anterior translation and 9.05° of extension coupled with 1.13 mm of posterior translation at C3/C4 levels. The corresponding results were 9.86° flexion with 1.15 mm of anterior translation and 11.24° of extension with 1.26 mm of posterior translation of the C4/C5 level, 9.24° of flexion with 1.15 mm of anterior translation and 9.88° of extension with 1.19 mm of posterior translation at the C5/C6 level. For the C6/C7 level, flexion was measured at 9.73° with 0.93 mm of anterior translation and 7.91° of extension coupled with 0.29 mm of posterior translation.

The fact that the cervical intervertebral joints are saddle joints means that the vertebra is also free to move side to side in the plane of the facets around an oblique axis perpendicular to the plane of the facets, in an angle of 45° to the transverse plane (Bogduk & Mercer, 2000). However, this axis does not pass through the apophyseal joints or the discs but through the cranial vertebral body (Penning, 1988). The geometry of the articular surfaces and the movement around the oblique axis dictate that horizontal rotation and side-flexion are always coupled to the same side (Bogduk & Mercer 2000; Penning, 1988). Not surprisingly all studies reporting on the coupling motion of rotation and side-flexion of the motion segments from C3 to T1 agree that the coupling is always on the same side regardless of which of the two side-bends or rotation is the initiating movement (Cook et al, 2006). The only exception is the contralateral coupling with lateral flexion initiation reported in the study of Ishii et al (2006) at the C7/T1 level.

Further studies have determined the centre of rotational motion to be localized in the ventral contour of the vertebral body for both lateral flexion and rotation (Lysell, 1969; Penning, 1988). The position of the centre of rotation anteriorly means that during coupled rotation and side-flexion, more movement occurred at the posterior part of intervertebral joint and less at the anterior.

This characteristic movement pattern is reflected by the morphology of the intervertebral disc. The cervical intervertebral disc is distinctively different from the lumbar one in that it lacks concentric annulus fibrosus, and its core is fibrocartilaginous and has the consistency of soap (Mercer & Bogduk, 1999). The annulus fibrosus is thicker anteriorly and consists of layers of fibres that arise out of the superior surface of the inferior vertebra and insert on the inferior surface of the inferior vertebra. The outer layer of the annulus is orientated vertically at its central part and obliquely at its lateral parts from inferio-laterally at its origin from the uncinate processes to anteriorly at the inferior margin of the superior vertebra (Mercer & Bogduk, 1999). The thickness of the annulus is about 2 to 3 mm. The deeper fibres of the annulus are orientated obliquely from inferio-laterally to superio-medially and interwoven with the corresponding fibres of the opposite side, towards the midline. The deeper fibres follow the same pattern but they insert more towards the midline of the superior vertebra (Mercer & Bogduk, 1999). This arrangement is consistent with the vertebrae pivoting about its anterior end as the majority of the fibres are arranged as an inverted 'V' pointing its apex at the centre of rotation (Bogduk & Mercer, 2000).

The annulus fibrosus is largely lacking posteriorly with only a few fibres in a lamina of about 1 mm thickness, vertically orientated. However, for the larger part of the posterior disc to the uncinate processes there is no annulus (Bogduk & Mercer, 2000; Mercer & Bogduk, 1999). Another characteristic of the cervical disc is the development of transverse fissures at the posterior part of the cervical discs. The fissures first appear at the age of 9 years as clefts in the unconvertebral region and progressively extend medially to form transverse clefts in the third decade of life (Bogduk & Mercer, 2000). With age, the clefts have a tendency to break through transversely, resulting in the posterior disc being comprised of two parts (Mercer & Jull, 1996). It is not clear if the development of transverse fissures is a result of the development of the uncinate processes, an early pathological change, or the result of the shearing forces of rotation (Mercer & Jull, 1996). Whatever the explanation, their presence allows or facilitates axial rotation (Bogduk & Mercer, 2000).

The morphological and geometrical characteristics discussed above support a pattern of movement of the typical cervical intervertebral movement of coupled side-flexion and rotation of the same side, in which the superior vertebra pivots about its anterior part and slides with its posterior. Few studies have reported on the ranges of motion of the intervertebral segments. At the C3/C4 level, White and Panjabi (1978) reported representative angles of 11° of side-bending and 11° of rotation. Mimura et al (1989) reported a 5.8° rotation from right to left at this level coupled with a side-flexion of 6.2° and a 2.9° of extension at this level. Penning and Wilmink (1987) reported a mean of 3° of rotation from right to left. Ishii et al (2004a) reported 4.5° of axial rotation coupled with lateral-bending at the same side, extension, inferior translation, opposite lateral translation and posterior translation. Ishii et al (2006) found 3.5° of lateral-bending coupled with axial rotation of the same side, flexion, superior translation lateral translation to the opposite side and anterior translation of the vertebra. Similarly, Panjabi et al (2001) reported 5.1° of axial rotation from right to left and 9.1° of lateral-bending from right to left.

For the C4/C5 level, White and Panjabi (1978) reported a mean 11° of right to left side-flexion and a mean 12° of rotation from left to right and Penning and Wilmink (1987) reported a mean 6.8° of rotation from right to left while Mimura et al (1989) reported a mean of 4.2° rotation from right to left with a mean of 6.2° of lateral-bending to the same side and a mean of 2.1° of extension. For the same level, Panjabi et al (2001) reported a mean of 6.8° right to left rotation and 9.3° mean right to left side-flexion. Ishii et al (2004a) found that the C4/C5 level rotates to a mean of 4.6° and it is coupled with ipsilateral side-flexion, extension and contralateral lateral translation while Ishii et al (2006) reported a mean of 3.3° of lateral-bending coupled with ipsilateral rotation, flexion, superior translation, contralateral coupled lateral and posterior translation.

At the C5/C6 level, White and Panjabi (1978) reported a representative angle of 8° of lateral-bending and an angle of 10° of rotation, while Penning and Wilmink (1987) reported a mean of 6.9° of rotation at this level from right to left. Mimura et al (1989) state an average of 5.4° of total rotation coupled with a mean of 4° of ipsilateral lateral-bending and 2.1° of flexion, while Panjabi et al (1988) reported a mean of 5.1° of rotation and a 6.5° of lateral-flexion respectively. Ishii et al (2004b) reported a mean of 4° of rotation coupled with ipsilateral lateral-bending, flexion, superior, opposite lateral and anterior translation while side-flexion, according to Ishii et al (2006) was measured to an average 4.3° coupled with ipsilateral rotation, flexion superior, opposite lateral translations. Similarly, for the C6/C7 level the average range of side-flexion reported by White and Panjabi (1978) was 7° and 9° of rotation. An average range of 5.4° of rotation has been reported by Penning and Wilmink (1987) and a slightly higher average range of 6.4° coupled with ipsilateral lateral-bending of 2.7° and 2.5° of flexion has been reported by Mimura et al (1989). An even lower rotation range of motion has been reported by Panjabi et al (2001) at 2.9° and an average range of lateral-bending of 5.4°. Similarly, Ishii et al (2006) reported an average of 5.7° of lateral-bending coupled with ipsilateral rotation, flexion, superior and contralateral lateral translation; there was also an average range of rotation of 1.6° coupled with ipsilateral lateral-bending, flexion, superior opposite lateral and anterior translation of the vertebra.

At the C7–T1 level the average ranges, according to White and Panjabi (1978), are 4° for lateral-bending and 8° for rotation, while Penning and Wilmink (1987) reported 2.1° of rotation. Ishii et al (2004a) reported an average of 1.5° of rotation coupled with ipsilateral lateral-bending, flexion, superior, opposite lateral and anterior translation. However, Ishii and colleagues' results (Ishii et al, 2006) disagree with the results of more studies at this level as they report a mean of 4.1° of lateral-bending coupled with contralateral rotation to a mean of 0.4° also coupled with flexion, superior ipsilateral lateral translation. The results of the studies of Ishii et al (2006) and Ishii et al (2004a) reveal that regardless of which movement initiates the coupling, the range of the lateral flexion component of the movement is greater in range than the rotation component. Furthermore, there is no progressive reduction of the available range, as is expected from the top to the bottom of the typical cervical spine column.

## Clinical point

Whilst rotation and lateral flexion are coupled ipsilaterally the motion segment also undergoes a small degree of contralateral translation in the mid to upper cervical spine. It is possible that motion segments that are likely to benefit from manipulative techniques, inducing cavitation-mediated improvement in passive movement, will be those that have developed a reduction in this contralateral side glide. The perception and use of contralateral side glide is at the centre of the assessment for and the treatment with manipulative thrust techniques.

# Assessment of the mid and lower cervical spine

## Observation (Figs 9.1 and 9.2)

The emphasis of the combined movement theory (CMT) examination is placed on the response of the spine to movement. Observation of the spine statically and dynamically is focused on relative regional movement. Statically, there are clues that will allow the therapist to focus further examination. These are skin, muscle and postural changes. Frequently, patients will present with relative hypermobility in the upper and lower cervical spine and hypermobility in the mid cervical spine.

Hypomobility is often associated with local muscle spasm. Observation or palpation of local paraspinal hypertonicity is important. Hypertonicity is often

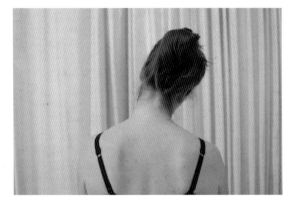

**Figure 9.1** • IN: sitting, neutral flexion. DID: active lateral flexion to the right. Note the reduced low cervical mobility and the lack of associated contralateral side glide here.

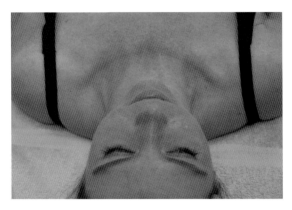

**Figure 9.2** • IN: supine, neutral flexion. DID: observation of the relative resting bulk of the anterior paraspinal muscles. Note the slightly reduced shadow under the left clavicle indicating greater bulk on this side. This is commonly associated with the palpation of hyper-tonicity of the scalenes and deeper paraspinals.

observed above and below a hypermobile segment, as the spine adopts a maladaptive mechanism to support the region. The classic poking chin posture indicates a predisposition to hypomobility of the upper and lower cervical spines and associated hypermobility of the mid cervical spine. This posture is often associated with hypertonicity of the upper fibres of trapezius, scalenes and sternocleidomastoid.

# Active movements

Before any movement of the cervical spine is undertaken, it is vital that two issues have been addressed:

- Cervical artery dysfunction has been considered
- The degree to which symptoms will be reproduced has been agreed with the patient.

## Cervical artery dysfunction

Prior to evoking movement of the cervical spine the therapist must have considered the potential likelihood of cervical artery dysfunction. Thus, the requirement to consider these issues is not specific to passive movements or particular to manipulation techniques. Chapter 6 will help you in your appreciation of cervical artery dysfunction, both theoretically and in the clinical situation. An appreciation of CAD issues will inform the therapist when making decisions over the extent of movement they wish to evoke.

## Symptom reproduction

It is imperative that before asking patients to move, or passively moving them into ranges of movement that could reproduce all or some of their symptoms, decisions are made regarding symptom reproduction. When combining movements, a process that progressively increases the stretch on tissues, it is easy to take patients into ranges of movement that can exacerbate a dysfunction. Thus, if you feel it is acceptable to reproduce only the initial degree of symptoms it is important that this degree of reproduction is produced in the combined position rather than after only one of the two or three movements you plan to use.

When a patient has severe resting pain you will be searching for combinations of movement that most reduce the resting pain and no attempt should be made to reproduce or increase pain during the examination. Only when the dysfunction has settled and no severe resting pain is present should symptom reproduction be used in assessment and treatment.

## Functional demonstration

The choice of active movements to be examined will be governed by the patient's functional demonstration. Symptoms reproduced by movement into that quadrant of dysfunction will guide the examination to include the three plane movements that take the patient into that direction. These movements will be either the combination of extension, ipsilateral lateral flexion and ipsilateral rotation **or** flexion and contralateral lateral flexion and contralateral rotation.

Active movements are ranked to establish the prime movement (most significant movement in reproducing dysfunction or easing pain in severe cases). In approximately 80% of patients the quadrant of dysfunction will be in the extension plane, as posturally our upper thoracic kyphosis and our tendency to spend our time flexed over things (keyboards, workstations, patients, etc) makes our ability to extend turn and tilt towards the side of dysfunction restricted. Approximately 20% of our patients will have pain when flexing, turning and tilting away from the side of pain with their aetiology tending to be post trauma (following whiplash) or repetitive overstrain (poor ergonomics).

Having established the prime movement and the prime combination the starting position for application of passive movements is evident. For more detail on this process see Chapter 4.

# Passive movements

## Anterior palpation of soft tissues

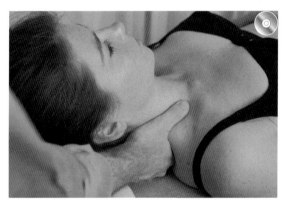

**Figure 9.3** • IN: supine. DID: soft tissue palpation of scalene and deeper paraspinal muscles. Gentle palpation of muscle tone in the posterior triangle of the neck. **See video clip number 8**

## Posterior palpation

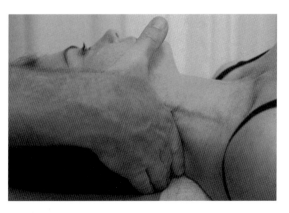

**Figure 9.4** • IN: supine, extension. DID: palpation of posterior muscles. Palpation using the radial border of the index finger.

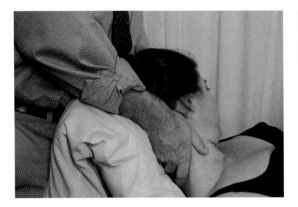

**Figure 9.5** • IN: supine, flexion. DID: palpation of posterior muscles. Palpation using the radial border of the index finger.

## Accessory movements

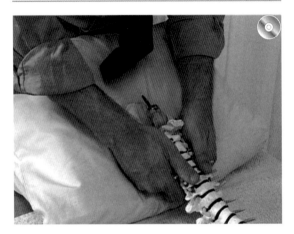

**Figure 9.6** • IN: supine, flexion. DID: key grip of the transverse process and articular pillar of C5 on the right. Pressure is distributed around the entire thumb and web space. **See video clip number 5**

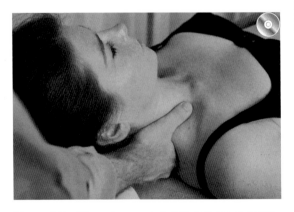

**Figure 9.7** • IN: supine, neutral. DID: anterior–posterior accessory glide of C5 on C6. Imagine you are 'shaking hands with the neck'. **See video clip number 9**

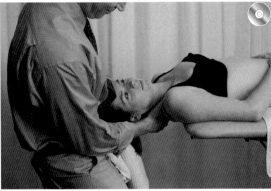

**Figure 9.8** • IN: supine, extension. DID: anterior–posterior accessory glide of C5 on C6. The angle of the AP glide is adjusted as the physiological movement that naturally occurs with the accessory pressure. **See video clip number 9**

## Passive physiological intervertebral movements

### Lateral flexion

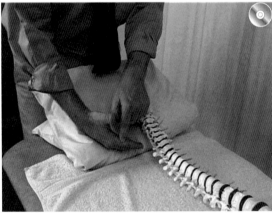

**Figure 9.9** • Illustration of the contact point for passive physiological intervertebral movement (PPIVM) (across the articular pillar running from transverse process to spinous process). **See video clip number 6**

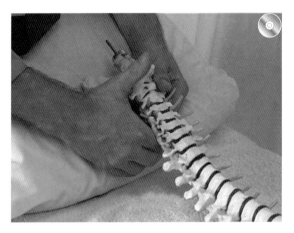

Figure 9.10 • IN: supine, extension. DID: illustration of the localized lateral flexion of the cervical spine around a fixed fulcrum of the right hand. The right hand is preventing the coupled right rotation associated with right lateral flexion. **See video clip number 7**

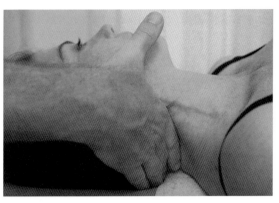

Figure 9.12 • IN: supine, extension. DID: right lateral flexion PPIVM, palpating the resistance profile of the right facet joint. The contralateral glide preventing the coupled right rotation of the lower segment.

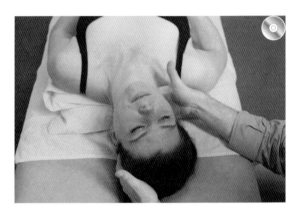

Figure 9.11 • IN: supine, extension. DID: right lateral flexion PPIVM, palpating the resistance profile of the right facet joint. Left contralateral glide applied to form a fulcrum, whilst laterally flexing the upper segments over a fixed lower segment. **See video clip number 10**

## Rotation

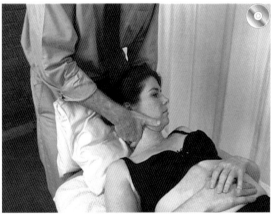

Figure 9.13 • IN: supine, flexion. DID: left rotation PPIVM, palpating the resistance profile of the right facet joint. The right upper segment is pushed to the left using the radial border of the finger against the superior segment's articular pillar. The left hand simply follows the right and scoops the upper segments into rotation. **See video clip number 58**

# Muscle assessment

## Post-isometric relaxation or reciprocal inhibition of paraspinal musculature

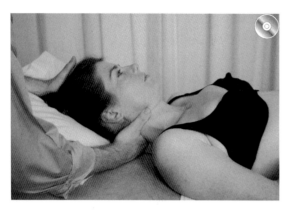

**Figure 9.14** • IN: supine. DID: isometric contraction of the right anterior paraspinals. The patient resists the AP pressure which can then be applied during the relaxation phase of the technique. **See video clip number 4**

## In sitting

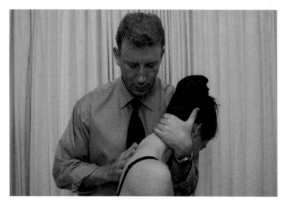

**Figure 9.15** • IN: sitting, flexion, left rotation, left lateral flexion. DID: isometric contraction of the right posterior paraspinals. The patient resists further flexion and left rotation and then allows it in the relaxation phase.

# Assessment for Grade IV−: mid-cervical manipulation

## Hand grip on spine model

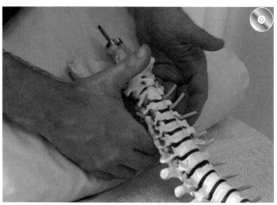

**Figure 9.16** • When assessing for manipulative thrust technique, contact must be confined to one point on the radial border of the index finger. This point both applies contralateral glide and produces the starting position for a thrust technique to be performed. **See video clip number 23**

## Step one: finding the starting position for manipulation

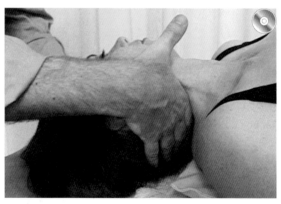

**Figure 9.17** • The starting position for application of a manipulative thrust to the right C4/C5 will be a combination of right lateral flexion and left rotation. This positioning does not follow the normal coupling for the region and results in a resistance to normal facet glide. The initiation of this resistance to normal glide is the position at which a thrust technique will cause facet gapping and thereby – cavitation. The resistance profile of both orders of applying right side-flexion and left rotation should be made, as one order will feel more suited to being the starting position than another. The order of application that evokes the 'crispest' resistance profile should be chosen. See Chapter 4. **See video clip number 12**

## Step two: establishing the direction of thrust

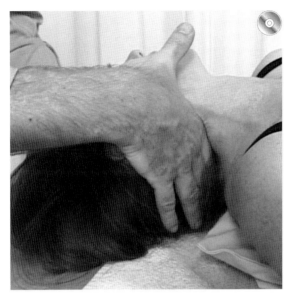

**Figure 9.18** • Having established the starting position the next decision is to decide on which thrust direction will evoke cavitation. Assess the effect on the resistance profile and choose between: (1) lateral flexion (combined contralateral translation with ipsilateral lateral flexion); (2) contralateral thrust (contralateral translation with no ipsilateral lateral flexion); (3) rotation (contralateral rotation, thrusting up and round on the ipsilateral side). The direction of thrust that makes the joint feel most likely to cavitate is the thrust to use. **See video clip number 13**

## Step three: performing the thrust technique

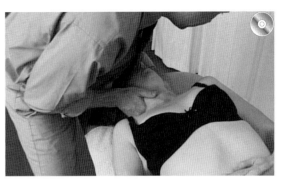

**Figure 9.19** • Having established the joint has a suitable starting position and direction of thrust the next step in the process is twofold: (1) Having already considered CAD, in your subjective examination, now undertake any physical testing of the neurovascular system you feel is valid and will help in your decision to proceed (see www.macpweb.org for up-to-date details of our understanding of this area); (2) Discuss your plan to perform a thrust technique with the patient and include a discussion of the risks (see Ch. 7) and physiological benefits (see Ch. 2). Obtain formal consent and document this process. **See video clip number 14**

## Cervical manipulation performed in flexion

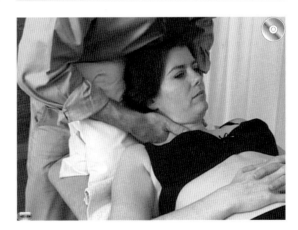

**Figure 9.20** • When wishing to avoid an extension element to the starting position, flexion can be used. An element of axial compression should be applied, through the therapist's abdomen, in order to produce the 'crisp' resistance profile suggestive of a joint that is suitable for manipulation. **See video clip number 11**

# Assessment for Grade IV—: C0/C1 manipulation

# Assessment for Grade IV—: cervico-thoracic manipulation

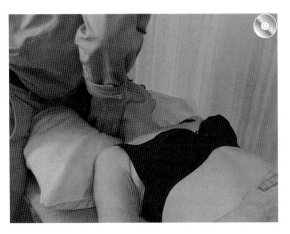

**Figure 9.21** ● IN: extension, left rotation, right lateral flexion. DID: left lateral contralateral IV— thrust C0/C1. Grade IV— thrust technique to avoid symptoms in upper cervical flexion. **See video clip number 57**

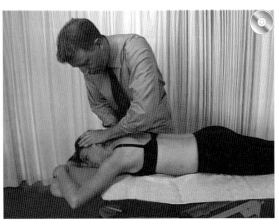

**Figure 9.23** ● IN: prone, extension, right lateral flexion, left rotation of the cervico-thoracic junction. DID: left transverse glide of the cervico-thoracic junction. Fix the head and apply a cephalad pressure. Do not rotate the head. **See video clip number 59**

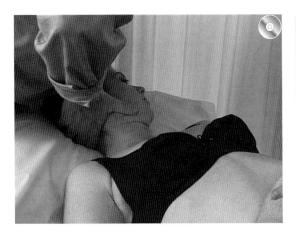

**Figure 9.22** ● IN: flexion, left rotation, right lateral flexion. DID: left lateral contralateral IV— thrust C0/C1. Grade IV— thrust technique to avoid symptoms in upper cervical extension. **See video clip number 56**

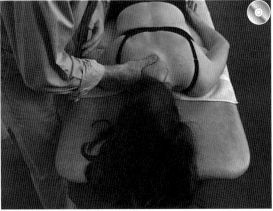

**Figure 9.24** ● IN: prone, extension, right lateral flexion, left rotation of the cervico-thoracic junction. DID: Left transverse glide of the cervico-thoracic junction (illustration of grip). Hold the first rib in your web space and distribute pressure between the thumb and the proximal interphalangeal bone of the index finger to increase comfort. **See video clip number 60**

# References

Bogduk, N., Mercer, S., 2000. Biomechanics of the cervical spine. In: Normal kinematics. Clin. Biomech. (Bristol, Avon) 15, 633–648.

Cook, C., Hegedus, E., Showalter, C., et al., 2006. Coupling behavior of the cervical spine: a systematic review of the literature. J. Manipulative Physiol. Ther. 29, 570–575.

Ishii, T., Mukai, Y., Hosono, N., et al., 2006. Kinematics of the cervical spine in lateral bending: in vivo three-dimensional analysis. Spine 31, 155–160.

Ishii, T., Mukai, Y., Hosono, N., et al., 2004a. Kinematics of the subaxial cervical spine in rotation in vivo three-dimensional analysis. Spine 29, 2826–2831.

Ishii, T., Mukai, Y., Hosono, N., et al., 2004b. Kinematics of the upper cervical spine in rotation: in vivo three-dimensional analysis. Spine 29, E139–E144.

Lysell, E., 1969. Motion in the cervical spine. An experimental study on autopsy specimens. Acta Orthopaedica Scandinavica (Suppl. 123), 121+.

Mercer, S., Bogduk, N., 1999. The ligaments and annulus fibrosus of human adult cervical intervertebral discs. Spine 24, 619–626 discussion 627–618.

Mercer, S.R., Jull, G.A., 1996. Morphology of the cervical intervertebral disc: implications for McKenzie's model of the disc derangement syndrome. Man. Ther. 1, 76–81.

Mimura, M., Moriya, H., Watanabe, T., et al., 1989. Three-dimensional motion analysis of the cervical spine with special reference to the axial rotation. Spine 14, 1135–1139.

Panjabi, M., Dvorak, J., Duranceau, J., et al., 1988. Three-dimensional movements of the upper cervical spine. Spine 13, 726–730.

Panjabi, M.M., Crisco, J.J., Vasavada, A., et al., 2001. Mechanical properties of the human cervical spine as shown by three-dimensional load-displacement curves. Spine 26, 2692–2700.

Penning, L., 1988. Differences in anatomy, motion, development and aging of the upper and lower cervical disk segments. Clin. Biomech. 3, 37–47.

Penning, L., Wilmink, J.T., 1987. Rotation of the cervical spine. A CT study in normal subjects. Spine 12, 732–738.

White 3rd, A.A., Panjabi, M.M., 1978. The basic kinematics of the human spine. A review of past and current knowledge. Spine 3, 12–20.

Wu, S.K., Kuo, L.C., Lan, H.C.H., et al., 2007. The intervertebral translations during cervical flexion and extension. J. Biomech. 40, S313.

# Thoracic spine

Chris McCarthy

## CHAPTER CONTENTS

# Clinical anatomy and biomechanics

## Ioannis Paneris

The biomechanics of the thoracic spine have been largely under-investigated, compared to the cervical or lumbar spines. This is probably due to the difficulties associated with the methodology of studying the movement analysis of the region, or the relatively low prevalence of thoracic pain in clinical practice (Edmondston & Singer, 1997). Considering the ex vivo studies of White (1969), Panjabi *et al* (1976a) and Panjabi *et al* (1981), Lee (1993) proposed a 'clinical model' of thoracic spine mechanics (Edmondston & Singer, 1997). This model was later updated (Lee, 2003, p. 44) after considering the findings of the in vivo study of Willems *et al* (1996).

In this model the mechanics of the spine are described considering the relative flexibility between the spinal column and the thoracic cage (Lee, 2003). The articulation of the superior costo-vertebral joint does not develop until about the age of 13 years (Dutton, 2004, p. 1243). Also, the ossification of the head and tubercle of the rib does not appear until puberty, and unites with the shaft of the rib soon after the 20th year (Warwick & Williams, 1973, p. 254). The delayed ossification allows for increased mobility of the thoracic spine relative to the rib cage, especially rotation and side-flexion (Dutton, 2004, p. 1243).

As the thoracic spine matures the superior costo-vertebral joint limits the degree of the rotation in all planes, while in old age, the ossification of the costal cartilages decreases the pliability of the relative flexibility of the thorax (Lee, 2003, p. 44).

Considering the above, there are three conditions for the spine. The first is the 'mobile thorax' where the rib cage is more mobile than the thoracic spine. The second is that of the 'stiff thorax' where the rib cage is less mobile than the thoracic spine and the third is that of same relative flexibility between the rib cage and thoracic spine (Lee, 2003, pp. 44–46). Furthermore, the anatomical differences between the regions of the thoracic spine dictate the differences in the biomechanical behaviour. Therefore, the following regions will be examined separately when this is necessary:

- The **vertebro-manubrial** region: T1 and T2; the first and second ribs and the manubrium
- The **vertebro-sternal** region: T3 to T7; the third to seventh ribs and the sternum
- The **vertebro-chondral** region: T8 to T10; the eighth to tenth ribs
- The **thoraco-lumbar** region: T11 and T12 and the eleventh and twelfth ribs.

## Flexion extension

Flexion and extension are relatively plane motions coupled with only slight axial rotation (Willems et al, 1996). The range of motion of flexion and extension at each motion segment increases in the cephalocaudad direction (White & Panjabi, 1978; Willems et al, 1996). Flexion is coupled with anterior translation and some compression. Furthermore, axial compression produced flexion rotation and anterior translation of the superior vertebra (Panjabi et al, 1976a). During flexion at the vertebro-sternal region, the superior vertebra flexes and translates anteriorly relative to the inferior vertebrae. The inferior facets of the superior vertebra glide superoanteriorly to the inferior one (Lee, 2003, p. 44).

The ribs rotate anteriorly along the axis of the neck of the rib, owing to the curved artricular surfaces of the costo-transverse joints (Warwick & Williams, 1973, p 418-419), with the anterior aspect of the rib travelling inferiorly and the posterior superiorly. Considering the 'mobile thorax', the ribs will continue to travel in this direction when the vertebral movement is exhausted, resulting in a coupling of superior glide and anterior roll of the tubercle at the costo-transverse joint (Lee, 2003, p. 45).

Conversely, in the 'stiff thorax' the movement of the ribs is exhausted first while the vertebrae continue to flex. This results in an inferior glide coupled with posterior roll of the tubercle of the rib at the costo-transverse joint. For the condition of 'same relative flexibility' of the thoracic spine and the rib cage there is no apparent movement between the vertebrae and the ribs (Lee, 2003, p. 46).

Extension follows a similar pattern to flexion and is coupled with posterior translation and slight distraction (Panjabi et al, 1976a). This slight distraction could be due to the resistance exerted by the approximation of the facet joints during extension that allow less motion compared to the lumbar region (Oxland et al, 1992). However, in the experimental model of Panjabi et al (1976a) when posterior translation was initially induced, the coupling changed to that of slight compression. Furthermore, the study of Panjabi et al (1976a) has shown that axial distraction produces extension rotation and posterior translation.

Lee (2003) proposes that, during extension, the ribs rotate posteriorly along the axis of the neck of the rib so that the anterior part of the rib travels superiorly and the posterior inferiorly. Similarly, for the 'mobile thorax' the ribs continue to travel in this direction after the vertebral motion is exhausted, leading to an inferior glide coupled with a posterior roll of the tubercle at the costo-transverse joints (Lee, 2003).

For the 'stiff thorax' the movement of the ribs terminates prior to the vertebral ones leading to superior glide, coupled to an anterior roll of the tubercle relative to the transverse process at the costo-transverse joint. Equally for the condition of 'equal relative flexibility' there is no apparent movement between the vertebrae and the ribs (Lee, 2003).

At the vertebro-chondral region, the facet joints and the costo-transverse joints are more flattened and face obliquely downwards medially and backwards (Warwick & Williams, 1973, p. 418–419). The ninth often fails to form joints with the tenth rib and the tenth transverse process may not present a facet for the tubercle of the tenth rib (Warwick & Williams, 1973, p. 238) Therefore, there is minimal conjunct rotation of the ribs, with minimal motion at the costo-vertebral joint (Lee, 2003, p. 54). At the vertebro-chondral region, the zygapophyseal glide superiorly during flexion and inferiorly during extension (Lee, 2003, p. 54).

At the vertebro-manubrial region, owing to the reduced relative mobility of the first two ribs, the movement pattern is similar to the 'stiff thorax' pattern on the thoraco-sternal region (Lee, 2003, p. 55). At the thoraco-lumbar region, during flexion, the inferior facets of the moving vertebra translate upwards on the superior facets of the inferior vertebra, resisted only by the joint capsule. During extension, the superior facets translate inferiorly towards the superior facet of the inferior vertebra. The extension is limited by the facet joints (Oxland et al, 1992). The motion of the 11th and 12th ribs is a pure spin (Lee, 2003, p. 55).

## Rotation and side-flexion

Regarding rotation and side-flexion of the thoracic spine the picture is somewhat less clear. The recent review of Sizer et al (2007) has revealed that 'there is poor agreement among 3-D biomechanical studies that identified coupling behaviour of the thoracic spine'. From the eight studies that Sizer et al (2007) reviewed (Gregersen & Lucas, 1967; Oxland et al, 1992; Panjabi et al, 1976a; Scholten & Veldhuizen, 1985; Schultz et al, 1973; Stewart et al, 1995; Theodoridis & Ruston, 2002; Willems et al, 1996) two were in vitro (Oxland et al, 1992; Panjabi et al, 1976a;), three were in vivo (Gregersen & Lucas, 1967; Theodoridis & Ruston, 2002; Willems et al, 1996) and two (Schultz et al, 1973; Scholten & Veldhuizen, 1985) were mathematical model analyses (Sizer et al., 2007).

Six of the above studies (Gregersen & Lucas, 1967; Oxland et al, 1992; Panjabi et al, 1976a; Scholten & Veldhuizen, 1985; Schultz et al, 1973; Willems et al, 1996) examined the thoracic motion coupling using vertebral movement initiation, while two studies (Stewart et al, 1995; Theodoridis & Ruston, 2002) examined the coupling of the thoracic spine initiated by upper extremity motion (Sizer et al, 2007).

The costo-vertebral joints and the costo-transverse joints were dissected only in the study of Oxland et al (1992) and were not represented in the studies of Schultz et al (1973) and Scholten and Veldhuizen (1985). However, Oxland et al (1992) examined only the thoraco-lumbar junction kinematics. None of the studies examined the kinematics of the costo-vertebral and costo-transverse joints.

When rotation was the initiating movement in the in vitro study of Panjabi et al (1976a) and Panjabi et al (1976b), these authors reported an ipsilateral coupling of side-flexion with left rotation and a contralateral with right rotation for all the tested motion segments. Furthermore, there was a translation to the right on the coronal plane with rotation to the left and translation to the left with right rotation. A consistently ipsilateral coupling of side-flexion with rotation initiation was also identified in the mathematical model analysis study of Schultz et al (1973) and in the in vitro study of Oxland et al (1992) for the T11–T12 and T12–L1 motion segments. Conversely, the in vivo study of Willems et al (1996) revealed variable coupling patterns with the contralateral coupling pattern being more frequent in the upper thoracic segments (T1 to T4) and ipsilateral being more frequent in the rest of the segments.

When side-flexion was the initiating movement, Panjabi et al (1976a) and Panjabi et al (1976b) reported a contralateral coupling of rotation and ipsilateral pattern of translation in the coronal plane. The coupling pattern remained the same when coronal plane translation was the initiating movement. Willems et al (1996) again reported variable coupling behaviour with 47% of their observations of the upper segments (T1–T4) to be of ipsilateral coupling. 83% of T4–T8 segments and 68% of the T8–T12 segments showed an ipsilateral coupling. The remainder of their observations were of contralateral coupling of rotation. The studies of Gregersen and Lucas (1967), Schultz et al (1973) and Scholten and Veldhuizen (1985) have all reported ipsilateral coupling patterns, while Oxland et al (1992) reported no identifiable coupling pattern of rotation with side-flexion for the T11–T12 and T12–L1 segments.

The two studies (Stewart et al, 1995; Theodoridis & Ruston, 2002) that examined the coupling behaviour of the thoracic motion with upper extremity elevation, reported variable results. However, the ipsilateral coupling of rotation and side-flexion was more dominant in the studies of Stewart et al (1995) and Theodoridis and Ruston (2002). Several reasons can be responsible for the variability of the findings of the three-dimensional biomechanical studies reported above. Although the in vitro studies may have the greatest degree of accuracy, by removing the effect of posture and muscular control, they cannot be easily extrapolated in clinical practice (Sizer et al, 2007).

Further, the preparation of the cadaveric specimens of the in vitro studies involves the resection of the whole or part of the ribs or thoracic cage, ligaments, muscles and costo-vertebral joints, which increases the neutral zone and range of motion of the thoracic spine and destabilizes the thoracic spine (Andriacchi *et al*, 1974; Oda *et al*, 1996, 2002; Panjabi *et al*, 1981).

The age of the subjects may also play a role. For their study, Stewart *et al* (1995) recruited young individuals with no severe kyphosis and found no significant pattern of coupled motion, while Theodoridis and Ruston (2002) recruited older subjects and found a predominantly ipsilateral coupling of side-flexion and rotation. Thoracic disc degeneration and disc space narrowing is common after the third decade of life. Disc degeneration will increase the flexion and rigidity of the thorax and lead to reduction of lateral flexion motion earlier and, to a greater extent, any other direction (Edmondston & Singer, 1997). The study of Scholten & Veldhuizen (1985) was the only one that examined the coupling movements of the thoracic spine in flexion and found them to be strongly ipsilateral. Perhaps the latter can explain the differences between the studies of Stewart *et al* (1995) and Theodoridis and Ruston (2002).

It is worth noting that the studies of Gregersen and Lucas (1967), Schultz *et al* (1973), Panjabi *et al* (1976a), Panjabi *et al* (1976b), Oxland *et al* (1992) and Willems *et al* (1996) investigated the coupling motions with the spine in its 'neutral' position. This may lead to variability since there is no standardized 'neutral' position amongst the investigators, especially in the in vivo studies (Sizer *et al*, 2007).

Contrary to in vitro, in vivo investigations examine the spinal motion in the presence of the extrinsic and intrinsic factors associated with the in vivo state (Willems *et al*, 1996) and therefore are clinically applicable (Sizer *et al*, 2007). However, in vivo investigations lead to challenges in controlling a number of factors such as postural control tissue adaptation, anatomical and circadian variability within and between subjects (Sizer *et al*, 2007). Furthermore, by its nature, the in vivo study allows measuring of motion in only a few specific segments (Gregersen & Lucas, 1967) or measuring of motion of the spine in space rather than measuring motion of a specific motion segment (Lee, 2003, p. 49). Furthermore, as Sizer *et al* (2007) points out, all the in vivo studies investigated the motion of healthy subjects. Therefore, their findings might not be representative of the spinal motion of symptomatic individuals since patients with spinal pain present with an altered pattern of muscle co-activation, increased

muscle activity and maladaptive postural patterns (Dankaerts *et al*, 2006).

As described above, side-flexion in the thoracic spine in the in vitro study of Panjabi *et al* (1976a) reported contralateral rotation coupling while the in vivo studies of Gregersen and Lucas (1967) and Willems *et al* (1996) and the mathematical model analyses of Schultz *et al* (1973) and Scholten and Veldhuizen (1985) reported ipsilateral rotation coupling. Lee (2003, pp 50–51) proposes a model that accommodates for these findings.

## Side-flexion

During side-flexion of the vertebro-sternal region, the ribs of the concave side approximate, while on the convex side they separate. In both the 'mobile' and 'stiff' thorax, the ribs appear to stop moving before the vertebrae. This movement causes a relative superior glide of the tubercle of the rib at the costo-transverse joint on the concave side and an inferior glide of the tubercle on the left side. Due to the covexo-concavity of the costo-transverse joint at this level the superior glide of the ribs at the concave side of the spine produce an anterior role of the neck of the rib relative to the transverse process. Equally, the inferior glide of the rib of the convex produces a posterior roll of the rib relative to the transverse process. Consequently, as the vertebra side flexes, it has to move posteriorly and inferiorly on the concave side and anteriorly and superiorly on the convex side, which produces an ipsilateral rotation of the vertebra in space relative to its starting position (Lee, 2003, p. 50). This model is in agreement with the findings of Willems *et al* (1996) in relation to ipsilateral rotation.

However, when considering the rotation of two adjacent vertebrae of a motion segment, the inferior vertebra rotates and side-flexes ipsilateraly. The superior vertebra follows the same movement pattern. However, the rotation of the superior vertebra is limited by the position of the ribs of the inferior vertebra. The end result is that the rotation of the superior vertebra is less than the rotation of the inferior vertebra, leading to a relative opposite rotation of the superior vertebra in relation to the inferior vertebra of the motion segment (Lee, 2003, p. 51) which is in agreement with the findings of Panjabi *et al* (1976a). The above model is only valid at the end of the range of side-flexion. At the mid range the pattern of coupling can be either ipsilateral or contralateral (Lee, 2003, p. 51).

At the vertebro-chondral region, the biomechanics of lateral flexion depend on the position of the apex of the curve that is produced by the side-bending. If the apex of the curve is located at the level of the greater trochanter, then all the vertebro-chondral region side flexes in the same direction. As the spine side-flexes the rib cage compresses at the side of the concavity while separating at the convexity. The ribs stop moving before the vertebrae. Due to the sequence of the movements and the relative flatness of the costo-vertebral joints, there is a 'postero-medio-superior' glide of the ribs at the costo-transverse joints on the side of concavity and 'antero-latero-inferior' at the side of convexity of the spine with minimal or no rotation of the ribs (Lee, 2003, p. 54).

In the case of the apex of the curve being located within the thorax, the osteokinematics of the lower thoracic vertebrae change. The rib cage remains compressed at the side of the concavity of the side-flexion and separated at the side of the convexity. However, the vertebrae below the apex of the curve side-flex to the opposite side of the side-flexion of the spine. The ribs move in an 'antero-latero-inferior' direction on the side of the concavity of the spine at the costo-transverse joint and a 'postero-medio-superior' direction on the side of convexity with minimal or no rotation of the ribs (Lee, 2003, p. 55). Therefore, for both the above conditions, the superior vertebra is not directed in relative opposite rotation to the inferior one (as in the vertebro-sternal region) allowing the vertebrae to 'follow the movement that is congruent with the levels above and below' (Lee, 2003, pp. 54–55).

At the vertebro-manubrial region, Lee (2003) claims that side-flexion is coupled with ipsilateral rotation. This is in agreement with the majority of the studies that investigated the coupling at this level (Gregersen & Lucas, 1967; Scholten & Veldhuizen, 1985; Schultz *et al*, 1973). During lateral flexion of the neck the transverse processes glide inferiorly relative to the rib on the side of the concavity and superiorly at the side of the convexity (Lee, 2003, p. 56). At the thoraco-lumbar region there is no costo-transverse joint and the costo-vertebral is an unmodified ovoid-shaped joint allowing pure side-flexion of the vertebrae between two fixed ribs (Lee, 2003, p. 56). This statement is in agreement with the observation of Oxland *et al* (1992) who reported no observed coupling with side-flexion initiation at this level.

## Rotation

Lee, (2003, pp. 52–53) proposed the following osteokinematics in the vertebro-sternal region of the thoracic spine during rotation. They suggested that when the superior vertebra rotates to the right it translates to the left. The left rib of the inferior vertebra rotates anteriorly and glides postero-laterally relative to the transverse process at the costo-transverse joint while the right rib rotates posteriorly and translates antero-medially. At the end of the motion the costo-transverse and costo-vertebral ligaments are tensed. Further attempt to rotate causes the superior vertebra to tilt leading to side-flexion. During rotation to the right, the left zygapophyseal joint translates supero-laterally and the right infero-medially (Lee, 2003, pp. 52–53). At the vertebro-chondral region Lee (2003, p. 55) suggests that the anatomy of the region, with the coronal orientation of the facets and minimal restriction from costal elements, allows for minimal restriction and either ipsilateral or contralateral coupling pattern.

At the vertebro-manubrial region, Lee (2003, p. 56) proposes a coupling motion of ipsilateral side-flexion with rotation. The transverse process on the side of the rotation translates inferiorly relative to the transverse process and superiorly on the opposite side.

## Respiration

According to Lee (2003, p. 57), during inspiration, the lower ribs (vertebro-chondral region) rotate posteriorly and translate antero-latero-inferiorly at the costo-vertebral joints, thus creating a lateral and antero-posterior expansion of the rib cage. Further inspiration causes the ribs of the vertebro-sternal region to posteriorly rotate by gliding inferiorly and rolling posteriorly at the costo-transverse joint. The opposite pattern takes place during expiration. At the vertebro-chondral region the ribs rotate anteriorly and glide postero-medio-superiorly at the costo-transverse joints while at the vertebro-sternal region they glide anteriorly and roll anteriorly at the costo-transverse joints.

## Conclusion

The review of Sizer *et al* (2007) has revealed a limited number of in vitro, in vivo and mathematical model studies that, in general, provide contradicting patterns of coupling motions of the thoracic vertebrae. None of the studies examined the ostokinematic behaviour of the ribs at costo-transverse and costo-vertebral joints. Although the in vivo studies (Gregersen & Lucas, 1967; Willems *et al*, 1996) point, in general, towards an ipsilateral coupling pattern in agreement with the early observations of Lovett (1903).

The model of Lee (1993, 2003) may lack an extensive research base; it is, however, a fine attempt to describe the osteokinematics of the thoracic spine bringing together anatomical facts, research evidence and clinical observation.

## Clinical note

**Kinematics of the upper and lower thoracic ribs – biomechanics as for the facet joints**

- Flexion   Anterior rotation of the ribs
- Extension   Posterior rotation of the ribs
- Right lateral flexion   Posterior rotation of the right rib, anterior rotation of the left rib
- Right rotation   Posterior rotation of the right rib, anterior rotation of the left rib

For the maximum posterior rotation of the rib on the right = E, RR, RLF + INSPIRATION

For maximum anterior rotation of the ribs on the right = F, LR, LLF + EXPIRATION

# Assessment of the upper thoracic spine

## Observation

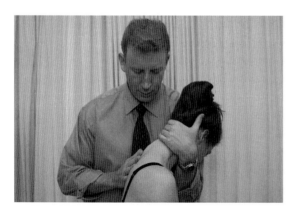

**Figure 10.1** • IN: sitting, cervical flexion. DID: localized active left rotation of the upper thoracic spine. Observation of the upper thoracic rotation/lateral flexion that occurs with movement of the neck.

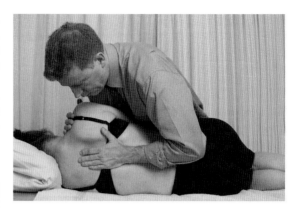

**Figure 10.2** • IN: left side-lying, flexion, neutral. DID: observation and palpation of upper thoracic muscle tone. In patients with resting pain, side-lying may allow pain-free palpation and assessment of muscle tone.

# Active movements

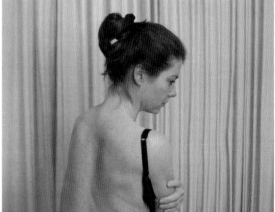

**Figure 10.3** • IN: sitting, DID: active, right rotation. Note the hypomobile region between the scapulae.

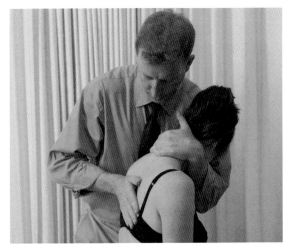

**Figure 10.4** • IN: sitting. DID: active left rotation of the thoracic spine. Fixation of the mid-thoracic spine, ensuring movement of the upper thoracic spine.

# Palpation

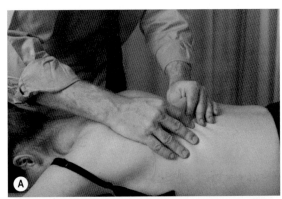

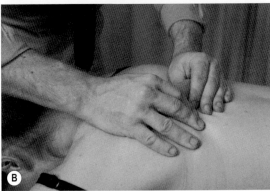

**Figure 10.5** • IN: prone. DID: palpation of resistance to stretch of paraspinal muscles. Hypertonicity will be palpable as 'bands' of resistance to the travel of the fingers perpendicularly to the muscle fibres.

# Passive movements

## Passive accessory movements

### Anterior stretch

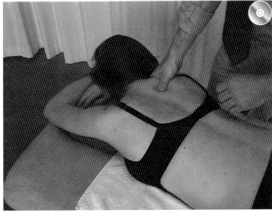

**Figure 10.6** • IN: prone, right side-flexion. DID: unilateral posterior–anterior accessory movement on T3. **See video clip number 16**

### Posterior stretch

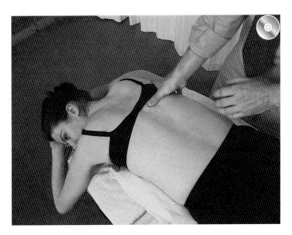

**Figure 10.7** • IN: prone, left rotation, flexed over a pillow. DID: PA pressure on T6. **See video clip number 18**

## Passive physiological movements

### Rotation

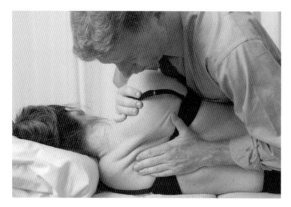

**Figure 10.8** • IN: left side-lying, extension. DID: right rotation of T3 on T4. By leaning down onto the thorax and pushing back on the clavicle, local upper thoracic rotation can be induced.

### Lateral flexion

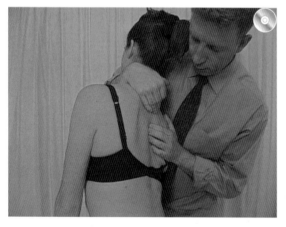

**Figure 10.9** • IN: left side-flexion, extension. DID: right lateral flexion of T3 on a fixed T4. See video clip 17

# Assessment of the mid-thoracic spine

## Active movements

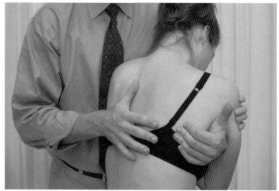

**Figure 10.10** • IN: sitting, flexion. DID: localized left rotation of the mid-thoracic spine .

## Passive movements

### Passive accessory movements

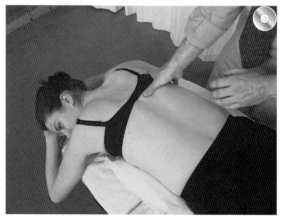

**Figure 10.11** • IN: prone, left side-flexion. DID: unilateral posterior–anterior accessory movement on T6. PA on T6 accessory, angled cephalad, inducing posterior stretch of T6/T7. See video clip number 18

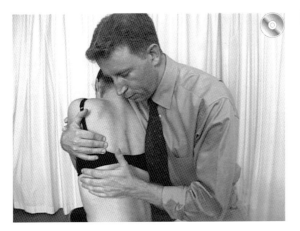

**Figure 10.12** • IN: sitting, flexion, right rotation. DID: unilateral posterior–anterior pressure on the left Rib 7. PA pressure and encouragement of the anterior rotation that occurs in this starting position. **See video clip number 19**

## Passive physiological movements

### Lateral flexion

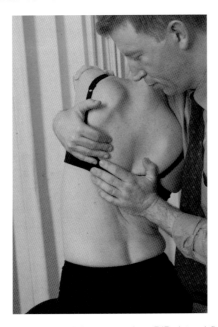

**Figure 10.13** • IN: sitting, extension. DID: lateral flexion T6 on T7. By applying contralateral lateral flexion, the technique is localized and will allow the assessment of suitability for manipulative thrust technique.

## Rotation

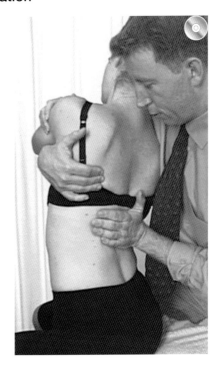

**Figure 10.14** • IN: sitting, extension. DID: right lateral flexion of T9 on T10. **See video clip number 20**

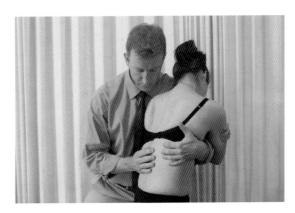

**Figure 10.15** • IN: sitting, flexion. DID: left lateral flexion, rotation of T10 on T11.

# Assessment of the low thoracic spine

## Active movements

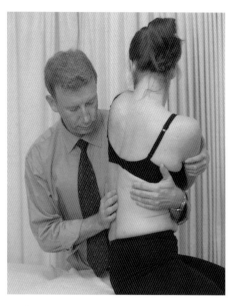

**Figure 10.16** • IN: sitting, neutral. DID: localized active rotation of low thoracic spine.

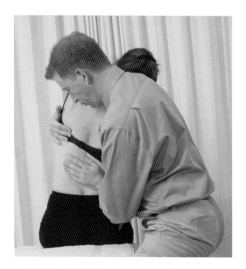

**Figure 10.17** • IN: sitting, extension, right lateral flexion. DID: guided low thoracic lateral flexion. Ensuring movement happens in the region of dysfunction, during examination, may require guidance of movement.

# Passive movements

## Passive accessory movements

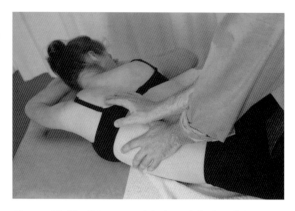

**Figure 10.18** • IN: prone, right lateral flexion. DID: unilateral posterior–anterior pressure on left T10. Emphasis is placed on angling the pressure cephalad.

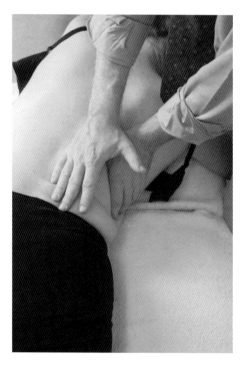

**Figure 10.19** • IN: prone, extension, right lateral flexion. DID: unilateral posterior–anterior pressure on the right T12. Emphasis is placed on angling the pressure caudad.

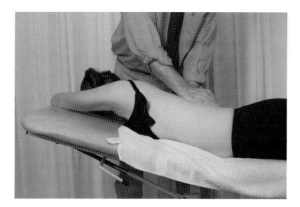

**Figure 10.20** • IN: prone, extension, right lateral flexion. DID: Unilateral posterior–anterior pressure on the right T12 (side view). Illustration of the caudad nature of the posterior–anterior.

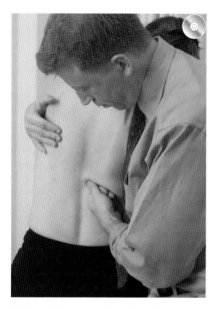

**Figure 10.21** • IN: sitting, extension, right rotation. DID: unilateral posterior–anterior T11. **See video clip number 27**

# Passive physiological movements

## Lateral flexion

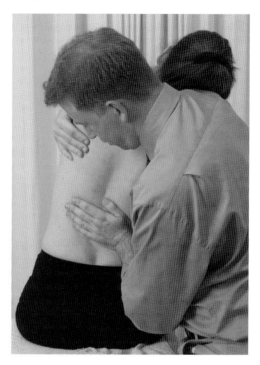

**Figure 10.22** • IN: sitting, right lateral flexion. DID: right lateral flexion of T11 on T12. Using a wide stance, the therapist can lean firmly through the fixing hand and encourage movement over this.

## Rotation

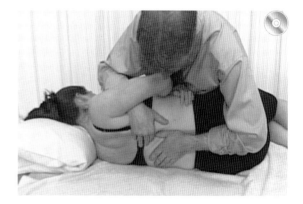

**Figure 10.23** • IN: left side-lying, extension. DID: right rotation of T10 on T11. The lumbar spine and lower thoracic spine are fixed with the left arm and combined rotation and extension induced with the right arm. **See video clip number 29**

# Assessment for Grade IV−: manipulative thrust technique

## Butterfly technique

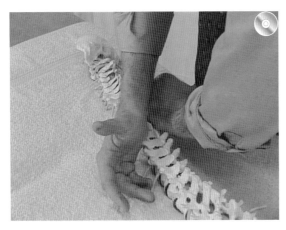

**Figure 10.24** • IN: prone, neutral flexion/extension. DID: simultaneous unilateral posterior–anterior pressure on the left T6 and right T5, using the hypothenar eminence. **See video clip number 24**

## In flexion

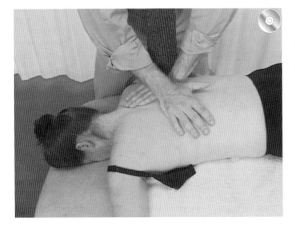

**Figure 10.25** • IN: resistance free range of flexion. DID: simultaneous unilateral posterior–anterior pressure on the left T6 and right T5, using the hypothenar eminence. A starting position of flexion can be used when avoiding a dysfunction in extension. **See video clip number 22**

## In extension

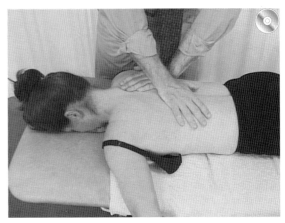

**Figure 10.26** • IN: resistance-free range of extension. DID: simultaneous unilateral posterior–anterior pressure on the left T6 and right T5, using the hypothenar eminence. A starting position of minimal extension can be used when avoiding a dysfunction in flexion. **See video clip number 23**

## Posterior–anterior thrust

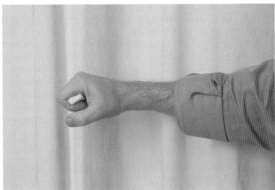

**Figure 10.27** • Prior to undertaking this manipulation, you may wish to hold a small paper block in your fingers to prevent excessive flexion of your proximal interphalangeal joints.

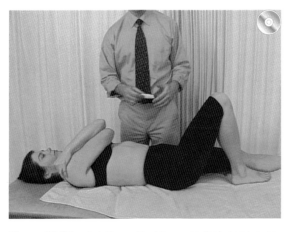

**Figure 10.28** • Ask the patient to cross their arms over their chest. Place one elbow on top of another as you will push down on them. **See video clip number 61**

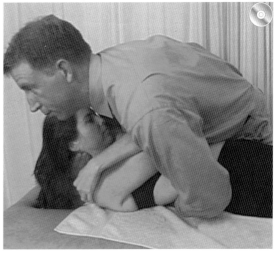

**Figure 10.29** • IN: enough flexion to push the inferior segment into your grip with the left hand. DID: anterior–posterior, cephalad pressure through the sternum via the arms. Leading to a gapping of the superior level away from the inferior level. **See video clip number 61**

# References

Andriacchi, T., Schultz, A., Belytschko, T., et al., 1974. A model for studies of mechanical interactions between the human spine and rib cage. J. Biomech. 7, 497–507.

Dankaerts, W., O'Sullivan, P., Burnett, L., et al., 2006. Altered patterns of superficial trunk muscle activation during sitting in nonspecific chronic low back pain patients: importance of subclassification. Spine 31, 2017–2023.

Dutton, M., 2004. Orthopaedic examination, evaluation and intervention. McGraw-Hill Companies, Inc.

Edmondston, S.J., Singer, K.P., 1997. Thoracic spine: anatomical and biomechanical considerations for manual therapy. Man. Ther. 2, 132–143.

Gregersen, G.G., Lucas, D.B., 1967. An in vivo study of the axial rotation of the human thoracolumbar spine. J. Bone Joint Surg. 49, 247–262.

Lee, D., 1993. Biomechanics of the thorax: a clinical model of in vivo function. Journal of Manual & Manipulative Therapy 1, 9.

Lee, D.G., 2003. The thorax: An integrated approach. Orthopedic Physical Therapy, White Rock, British Columbia, Canada.

Lovett, R.W., 1903. A contribution to the study of the mechanics of the spine. Am. J. Anat. 2, 457–462.

Oda, I., Abumi, K., Cunningham, B.W., et al., 2002. An in vitro human cadaveric study investigating the biomechanical properties of the thoracic spine. Spine 27, E64–E70.

Oda, I., Abumi, K., Lu, D., et al., 1996. Biomechanical role of the posterior elements, costovertebral joints, and rib cage in the stability of the thoracic spine. Spine 21, 1423–1429.

Oxland, T.R., Lin, R.M., Panjabi, M.M., 1992. Three-dimensional mechanical properties of the thoracolumbar junction. J. Orthop. Res. 10, 573–580.

Panjabi, M.M., Brand Jr., R.A., White 3rd, A.A., 1976a. Mechanical properties of the human thoracic spine as shown by three-dimensional load-displacement curves. J. Bone Joint Surg. 58, 642–652.

Panjabi, M.M., Brand Jr., R.A., White 3rd, A.A., 1976b. Three-dimensional flexibility and stiffness properties of the human thoracic spine. J. Biomech. 9, 185–192.

Panjabi, M.M., Hausfeld, J.N., White 3rd, A.A., 1981. A biomechanical study of the ligamentous stability of the thoracic spine in man. Acta Orthop. Scand. 52, 315–326.

Scholten, P.J., Veldhuizen, A.G., 1985. The influence of spine geometry on the coupling between lateral bending and axial rotation. Eng. Med. 14, 167–171.

Schultz, A.B., Belytschko, T.B., Andriacchi, T.P., et al., 1973. Analog studies of forces in the human spine: mechanical properties and motion segment behavior. J. Biomech. 6, 373–383.

Sizer Jr., P.S., Brismee, J.M., Cook, C., 2007. Coupling behavior of the thoracic spine: a systematic review of the literature. J. Manipulative Physiol. Ther. 30, 390–399.

Stewart, S.G., Jull, G.A., Ng, J.K., et al., 1995. An initial analysis of thoracic spine movement during unilateral arm elevation. Journal of Manual and Manipulative Therapy 3, 15–20.

Theodoridis, D., Ruston, S., 2002. The effect of shoulder movements on thoracic spine 3D motion. Clin. Biomech. (Bristol, Avon) 17, 418–421.

Warwick, R., Williams, P. (Eds.), 1973. Gray's anatomy. Longman Group Ltd, Edinburgh.

White 3rd, A.A., 1969. Analysis of the mechanics of the thoracic spine in man. An experimental study of autopsy specimens. Acta Orthop. Scand. Suppl. 127, 1–105.

White 3rd, A.A., Panjabi, M.M., 1978. The basic kinematics of the human spine. A review of past and current knowledge. Spine 3, 12–20.

Willems, J.M., Jull, G.A., Ng, J.K.F., 1996. An in vivo study of the primary and coupled rotations of the thoracic spine. Clin. Biomech. (Bristol, Avon) 11, 311–316.

# 11

# Lumbo-sacral spine

Chris McCarthy

## CHAPTER CONTENTS

# Clinical anatomy and biomechanics

## Ioannis Panneris

The association of segmental rotation and lateral-bending of the human spine has been observed and studied since at least the end of the 19th century. In 1903, Lovett referred to the observed phenomenon of rotation that appears when any patient's spine develops a degree of side-bending (Lovett, 1903). Panjabi *et al* (1974) described movement in three axes of motion: X for flexion–extension, Y for rotations, and Z for side-bending. White and Panjabi (1978) defined coupling motion as 'motion in which rotation or translation of a rigid body about one axis is consistently associated with rotation and translation of the same rigid body about another axis'.

A spine motion segment has 6° of freedom, and therefore, there are theoretically 21 coupling coefficients. However, owing to the geometrical and ligamentous symmetry about the sagittal plane the coupling coefficients for flexion and extension are zero, and only coupling between rotation, lateral-bending and translation is observed (Panjabi *et al*, 1974). The early observations of segmental motion were developed by Fryette who, in 1954, undertook experiments upon 'a spine mounted in soft rubber' and subsequently published three laws of coupling motion (Gibbons & Tehan, 1998). The first law stipulates that with the spine neutral, side-bending produces rotation to the opposite side. The second law refers to the condition of flexion or extension of the vertebrae where the rotation and side-bending are both directed to the same side. The third law indicates that motion of a vertebral joint in one plane automatically reduces its mobility to the other two planes (Gibbons & Tehan 1998, 2000).

Contrary to Fryette's laws, several textbooks report that in the lumbar spine there is contralateral rotation side-bending in extension and ipsilateral rotation side-bending in flexion (Huijbregts, 2004).

However, these textbooks lack support from primary references (Huijbregts, 2004). In 1978, White and Panjabi studied the coupling directions using two-dimensional imagery. They found that the direction of the coupling did not depend on the position of the spine, (flexion–extension) as Fryette's laws would predict, but on which movement would be initially engaged. Therefore, when side-bending was initially engaged the coupling would be contralateral rotation, but in the case of rotation being engaged first the coupling would be ipsilateral. However, two-dimensional radiographic methods of examining coupling behaviour have been criticized as they can lead to inaccurate and misleading results (Coleman *et al*, 1999; Evans & Lissner, 1959; Harrison *et al*, 1998).

A number of studies have been published that used three-dimensional measurement of the coupling motions, both in vivo (Hindle *et al*, 1990; Pearcy & Tibrewal, 1984) and in vitro (Cholewicki *et al*, 1996; Oxland *et al*, 1992; Panjabi *et al*, 1989, 1994; Vincenzino & Twomey, 1993) which are thought to provide more accurate readings that reflect the true motion of the spine (Harrison *et al*, 1998; Rab & Chao, 1977). All the above studies used non-pathological, asymptomatic subjects.

## Coupled motion with side-bend initiation with the spine in neutral

The study of Pearcy and Tibrewal (1984) showed no coupling rotation at the level of L1–L2 which is in agreement with the studies of Panjabi *et al* (1989, 1994) and Cholewicki *et al* (1996). However, the studies of Cholewicki *et al* (1996) indicated that there might be cases of rotation coupling in the opposite direction; in the study of Panjabi (1989) a similar tendency was indicating rotation occurring on the same side as side-bending. Although there is general agreement that the coupling rotation occurs in the opposite direction to the side-bend (Hindle *et al*, 1990, Oxland *et al*, 1992; Panjabi *et al*, 1989, 1984; Pearcy & Tibrewal, 1984), the study of Cholewicki et al (1996) reports an ipsilateral coupling of rotation to side-bending at the L4–L5 motion segment.

## Coupled motion with rotation initiation with the spine in neutral

Under this condition there seems to be more agreement amongst the researchers. The studies of

Pearcy and Tibrewal (1984), Panjabi *et al* (1989, 1994) and Cholewicki *et al* (1996) have shown the contralateral coupling of side-bend for the L1–L2, L2–L3 and L3–L4 motion segments. The same studies have shown ipsilateral side-bend coupling for the L4–L5 and L5–S1 which is in agreement with the study of Oxland *et al* (1992). It is worth mentioning though that the study of Pearcy and Tibrewal (1984) reported some subjects who exhibited coupling of side-bend to the same side as rotation at the L4–L5 level.

## Coupled motion with side-bend initiation with the spine in extension

There are two studies that explored the coupling behaviour of the lumbar spine under this condition (Panjabi *et al*, 1989, Vincenzino & Twomey, 1993). Both studies report that at the L3–L4 motion segment, the direction of coupling rotation is contralateral to the side-bend. However, the studies reach opposite conclusions for the rest of the levels of the lumbar spine with the L5–S1 segment displaying extreme variety in the study of Vincenzino and Twomey (1993) where coupled rotation was identified in both directions or none at all.

## Coupled motion with side-bend initiation with the spine in flexion

Under this condition the studies of Panjabi *et al* (1989) and Vincenzino and Twomey (1993) reported agreement for the L2–L3 and L4–L5 motion segments where the rotation was contralateral to the side-flexion. For the L1–L2 level, Panjabi reported occurrences where the rotation was ipsilateral or contralateral, while Vincenzino and Twomey reported occurrences with ipsilateral coupling or none at all. For the L3–L4 level, the coupling was found to be ipsilateral by Vincenzino and Twomey (1993) and ipsilateral or non-existent for L5–S1, whereas for Panjabi *et al* (1989) both the above levels displayed contralateral coupling.

## Coupled motion with rotation initiation with the spine in extension and flexion

The only study that explored the coupling motion of side-flexion with rotation in extension of flexed lumbar spine was that of Panjabi *et al* (1989). In the extended spine the coupled side-flexion is ipsilateral for the L1–L2, L4–L5 and L5–S1 levels and contralateral for the L2–L3. The L3–L4 level exhibited both ipsilateral and contralateral coupling. With the spine in flexion the L1–L2, L2–L3 and L3–L4 exhibited contralateral side-bend coupling while the L4–L5 and L5–S1 segments ipsilateral (Panjabi *et al*, 1989). It is worth mentioning that lateral translations were found to be in the range of 1 to 2 mm in all directions (Pearcy & Tibrewal, 1984) and when associated with lateral-bending to the same side, and to be at an average of 1.1 mm at all levels (Panjabi *et al*, 1994) and therefore of doubtful clinical significance.

Flexion and extension were found to cause minimal to negligible coupling rotation or side-flexion (Cholewicki *et al*, 1996, Hindle *et al*, 1990). However, Cholewicki *et al* (1996) have found flexion motion associated with side-bending in all lumbar levels.

Pearcy and Tibrewal (1984) have reported extension of all levels from L1 to L4 during lateral-bending. The L4–L5 level showed variable behaviour extending in general but occasionally flexing. The L5–S1 generally flexed.

In contrast to the above studies on coupling movements that studied non-pathological asymptomatic subjects, there are few studies that looked at the coupling movement of subjects with low back pain. The study of Lund *et al* (2002) showed inconsistencies of coupled motions during both axial rotation and side-bending in subjects with low back pain (LBP). Axial rotation to either side produced side-flexion to the right in some of the majority of the subjects, with the rest displaying ipsilateral side-bending and some no coupled side-flexion. During lateral-bending, axial rotation coupling was observed in 50% of the patients studied. In 8 of the 22 cases there was no coupled axial rotation and contralateral rotation in 3 cases. The results of the coupling behaviour during side-bending are of interest as they are not in agreement with the consistent pattern of contralateral axial rotation in normal subjects in the majority of the studies (Panjabi *et al*, 1989, 1994; Pearcy & Tibrewal, 1979). This can be attributed to the altered role of the neuromuscular system during LBP as it may be an important contributor to the coupling behaviour (Cholewicki *et al*, 1996; Pearcy & Tibrewal, 1984). Furthermore, the study of Oxland *et al* (1992) on cadavers showed that acute injury of the disc and facet joints altered the magnitude of the coupling motions but not the direction of the coupling.

# Conclusions

Interestingly, there is a wide variability of the coupling behaviour of the lumbar spine segments among the studies. However, there seems to be agreement in that when axial rotation produces a contralateral side-bending at the L4–L5 and L5–S1 levels and ipsilateral to the rest of the segments in neutral. However, reviewing the current studies it has become apparent that there is variance of coupling motion behaviour within the studies themselves and within the subjects of each study.

One of the reasons might be that instrumentation used for these studies is not standardized. Also, even though three-dimensional studies have small measurement error, inaccuracies still exist. Also the differences in the experimental techniques employed by some of the studies may account for some of the differences (Hindle *et al*, 1990). In their studies on dissected spine specimens, Panjabi *et al* (1989, 1994) preloaded the spine axially while Vincenzino and Twomey (1993) did not. Compressive preload could play a role in the production of coupled rotation in the presence of facet tropism (Vincenzino & Twomey, 1993).

The effects of the morphology (tropism) of the facet joints have been found not to play a significant role in the direction of the coupled rotation (Vincenzino & Twomey, 1993). Furthermore, the removal of the facet joints did not influence the direction of the conjunct rotation (Oxland *et al*, 1992; Vincenzino & Twomey, 1993). Degeneration of the facet joints seems to change the magnitude of the range of motion between males and females. Facet joint degeneration increased axial rotation but decreased lateral flexion and flexion. In males, the range of all movements increased with degeneration up to grade 3 but decreased with grade 4 degeneration (Fujiwara *et al*, 2000).

The degeneration of the intervertebral disc did not exert any influence on the direction of axial rotation coupled to side-flexion in the study of Vincenzino and Twomey (1993); however, by their own admission, the sample was too small to produce any conclusive results. Oxland *et al* (1992) report that disc injury did not influence the direction of the coupling motion on the tested L5–S1 level. Fujiwara *et al* (2000) examined the effects of intervertebral disc and facet joint degeneration in relation to gender. Disc degeneration seemed to increase the range of motion in both males and females but with grade 5 degeneration the range decreased.

Interestingly though, Oxland *et al* (1992) reported that injury to the disc increased lateral flexion coupled to lateral rotation. Conversely, removal of the facets increased axial rotation coupled to lateral flexion. This finding seems to define the roles of the intervertebral disc and facet joints in the kinematics of the intervertebral segment. Despite the differences in gender or age, these do not seem to affect the coupling behaviour of the lumbar spine (Hindle *et al*, 1990). However, Fujiwara *et al* (2000) reported that female subjects displayed more range than males which is not in agreement with Gatton and Pearcy (1999) and Hindle *et al* (1990) who reported the opposite.

The role of the neuromuscular system and its influence on the lumbar spine has not been widely examined. This is probably due to the fact that in vitro studies have used cadaveric specimens. The in vitro study of low back pain subjects of Lund *et al* (2002), discussed above, has reported inconsistent coupling. This may be due to the greater spinal loads experienced by subjects with low back pain reported by Marras *et al* (2001) and subjects with increased psychological stress (Marras *et al*, 2000) that result in altered levels of guarding, muscle recruitment and altered range of motion and speed. Despite the lack of agreement on the direction of the coupled motion of the segments of the lumbar spine, a study of 369 physiotherapists, trained in a wide range of manual therapy disciplines, revealed that lumbar coupling biomechanics was important for the application and validation of manual therapy (Cook & Showalter, 2004).

Despite the variance of the coupled motions reported in the in vivo and in vitro experimental studies, this may be the reason why the osteopathic profession has developed a convention of naming the coupled movements as 'type 1' and 'type 2', where type 1 refers to side-bending and rotation occurring on the opposite sides in neutral and extension, and type 2 refers to side-bending and rotation accruing on the same side in flexion (Gibbons & Tehan, 2001). This concept seems to be in agreement with the general findings of Vincenzino and Twomey (1993) and Pearcy *et al* (1987) (Vincenzino & Twomey, 1993). However, Vincenzino and Twomey (1993) state that, clinically, their results can be considered when choosing a general passive movement technique.

Additionally, the studies of Tsung *et al* (2005) and Lee (2001) found that during passive rotations of the lumbar spine, as described by Maitland (1986), there was always side-bending to the opposite direction. It should be noted that at the starting point of the manoeuvre the spines were already in flexion, rotation, and opposite side-flexion. Furthermore the application of axial rotation produced movement in all anatomical planes. Despite the above, when considering segmental lumbar passive movement technique, lumbar axial rotation initiated coupling has yielded the more consistent results.

# Assessment of the lumbar spine

## Observation

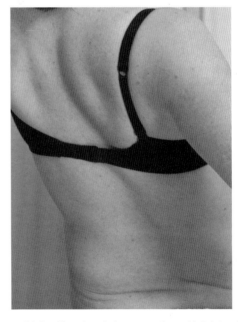

**Figure 11.1** • Functional demonstration of left lateral flexion and right rotation.

# Active movements

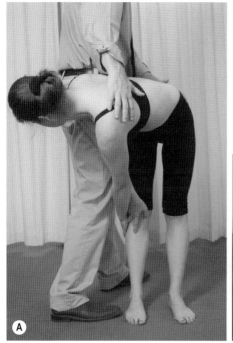
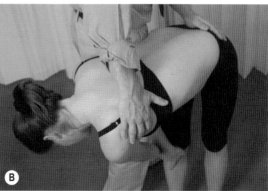

**Figure 11.2** • IN: standing, flexion. DID: right lateral flexion, guided active movement.

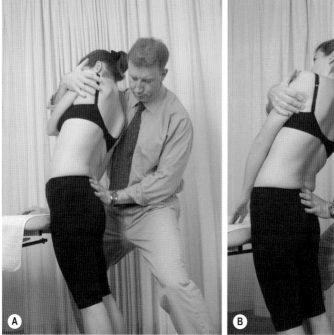
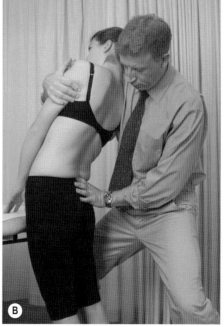

**Figure 11.3** • IN: standing, lumbar extension. DID: right lateral flexion, guided active movement of the low lumbar spine.

# Palpation

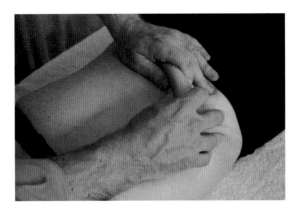

**Figure 11.4 •** IN: prone lying, neutral. DID: assessment of superficial muscle tone of lumbar spine.

# Passive movements

## Passive accessory movements

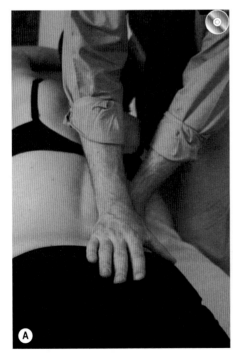

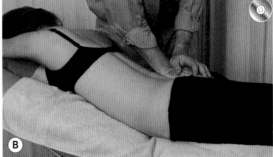

**Figure 11.5 •** IN: prone, extension, right lateral flexion. DID: unilateral posterior anterior accessory glide of L4 (caudad emphasis). **See video clip numbers 32 and 33**

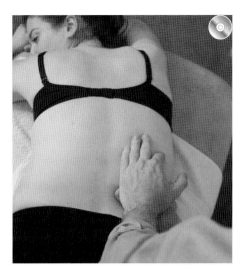

**Figure 11.6** • IN: prone, flexion, left lateral flexion. DID: unilateral posterior anterior accessory glide of L3 (cephalad emphasis). **See video clip number 34**

## Passive physiological movements

### Rotation

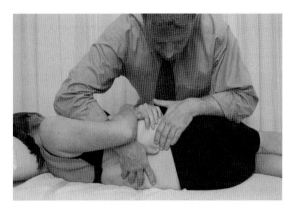

**Figure 11.8** • IN: left side-lying, extension, right lateral flexion. DID: left rotation of L3 on L4.

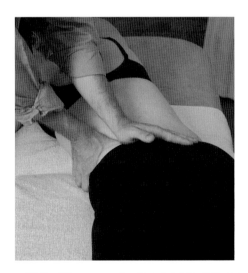

**Figure 11.7** • IN: prone, extension, left lateral flexion. DID: unilateral posterior anterior accessory glide of L5. Note the medial angulation and the localization with the inferior hand.

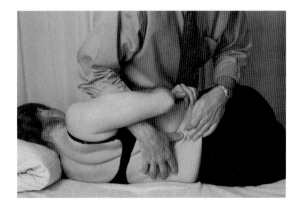

**Figure 11.9** • IN: left side-lying, flexion. DID: left rotation of L4 on L3 (movement initiated with right iliac crest). This technique involves movement of the inferior segment – therefore it can be confusing!

## Lateral flexion

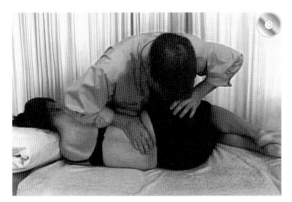

**Figure 11.10** • IN: left side-lying. DID: right lateral flexion of L3 on L4. Note the caudo-medial pressure of the right hand to fix L3. See video clip number 35

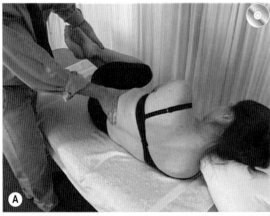

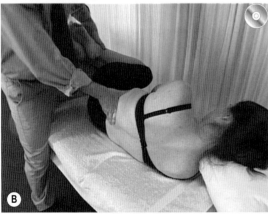

**Figure 11.11** • IN: right side-lying, left lateral flexion, neutral flexion. DID: left lateral flexion of L3 on L4 (end of range, patient's feet on therapist's knee, lateral flexion encouraged with pressure on iliac crest). See video clip number 36

# Assessment for Grade IV−: manipulative technique

## Upper body fixation – patient grip

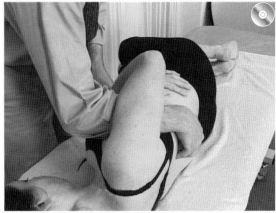

**Figure 11.12** • IN: left side-lying. Ask the patient to reach down and grasp their under forearm. This process 'locks' the thoracic spine and helps to localize movement to the lumbar spine. See video clip number 39

## Therapist grip

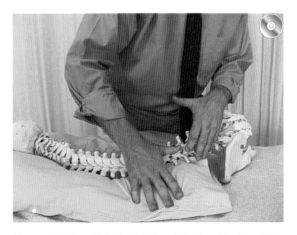

**Figure 11.13** • IN: left side-lying, left lateral flexion. DID: right rotation of L3 on L4 (thumb on the upper side of the spinous process with index finger flexed under the L4 spinous process). See video clip number 40

## In flexion

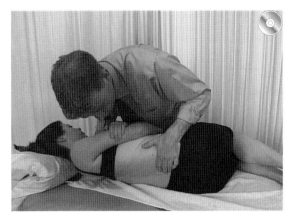

**Figure 11.14** • IN: left side-lying, left lateral flexion. DID: right rotation of L3 on L4 (pulling the upper body into right rotation and flexion until movement is perceived at L4). See video clip numbers 30 and 37

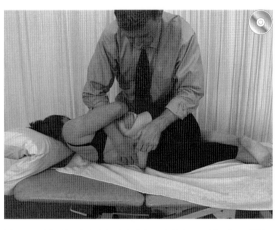

**Figure 11.16** • IN: left side-lying, left lateral flexion. DID: roll the patient under your sternum and fix the thoracic spine by leaning down on the ribs. See video clip number 37

## In extension

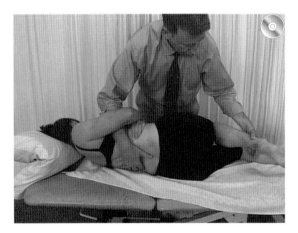

**Figure 11.15** • Ask the patient to extend their hip to move the underside knee from under the upper knee. Stop the patient from extending the hip too far (keep the lumbar spine in flexion).

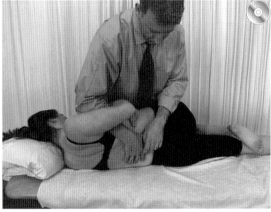

**Figure 11.17** • IN: left side-lying, left lateral flexion, extension. DID: right rotation of the upper segment by pushing the thorax and upper level back into rotation in a combined manner. See video clip numbers 31 and 38

# References

Cholewicki, J., Crisco, J.J., Oxland, T.R., et al., 1996. Effects of posture and structure on three-dimensional coupled rotations in the lumbar spine. A biomechanical analysis. Spine 21 (21), 2421–2428.

Coleman, R.R., Bernard, B.B., Harrison, D.E., et al., 1999.

Correlation and quantification of projected 2-dimensional radiographic images with actual 3-dimentional Y-axis vertebral rotations. Journal of Manual and Physiological Therapeutics 22 (1), 21–25.

Cook, C., Showalter, C., 2004. A survey on the importance of lumbar

coupling biomechanics in physiotherapy practice. Man. Ther. 9 (3), 164–172.

Evans, G.F., Lissner, H.R., 1959. Biomechanical studies on the lumbar spine and pelvis. J. Bone Joint Surg. 41-A (2), 278–290.

Fujiwara, A., Lim, T., An, H.S., et al., 2000. The effect of disc degeneration and facet joint osteoarthritis on the segmental flexibility of the lumbar spine. Spine 25 (23), 3036–3044.

Gatton, M.L., Pearcy, M.J., 1999. Kinematics and movement sequencing during flexion of the lumbar spine. Clin. Biomech. 14, 376–383.

Gibbons, P., Tehan, P., 1998. Muscle energy concepts and coupled motion of the spine. Man. Ther. 3 (2), 95–101.

Gibbons, P., Tehan, P., 2000. Manipulation of the spine thorax and pelvis. An osteopathic perspective. Churchill Livingstone, Edinburgh.

Gibbons, P., Tehan, P., 2001. Patient positioning and spinal locking for lumbar spine rotation manipulation. Man. Ther. 6 (3), 130–138.

Harrison, D.E., Harrison, D.D., Troyanovich, S.J., 1998. Three-dimensional spinal coupling mechanics: part I. A review of the literature. J. Manipulative Physiol. Ther. 21 (2), 101–113.

Hindle, R.J., Pearcy, M.J., Cross, A.T., 1990. Three-dimensional kinematics of the human back. Clin. Biomech. 5, 218–228.

Huijbregts, P., 2004. Lumbar spine coupled motions: A literature review with clinical implications. Orthopaedic Division Review (Sep/Oct), 21–25.

Lee, R.Y.W., 2001. Kinematics of rotational mobilisation of the lumbar spine. Clin. Biomech. 16, 481–488.

Lovett, R., 1903. A contribution to the study of the mechanics of the spine. Am. J. Anat. 2, 457–462.

Lund, T., Nydegger, T., Schlenzka, D., et al., 2002. Three-dimensional motion patterns during active bending in patients with chronic low back pain. Spine 27, 1865–1874.

Maitland, G.D., 1986. Vertebral manipulation, fifth ed. Butterworth Heinemann, Oxford.

Marras, W.S., Davis, G.K., Heaney, C.A., et al., 2000. The influence of psychological stress, gender and personality on mechanical loading of the lumbar spine. Spine 25 (23), 3045–3054.

Marras, W.S., Davis, K.G., Ferguson, S.A., et al., 2001. Spine loading characteristics of patients with low back pain compared with asymptomatic individuals. Spine 26 (23), 2566–2574.

Oxland, T.R., Crisco, J.J., Panjabi, M.M., 1992. The effect of injury in rotational coupling at the lumbosacral joint. Spine 17 (1), 74–80.

Panjabi, M.M., White, A.A., Brand Jr., R.A., 1974. A note on defining body parts configurations. J. Biomech. 7, 385–387.

Panjabi, M.M., Oxland, T.R., Yamamoto, I., et al., 1989. How does posture affect the coupling in the lumbar spine? Spine 14 (9), 1003–1011.

Panjabi, M.M., Oxland, T.R., Yamamoto, I., et al., 1994. Mechanical behaviour of the lumbar spine as shown by three-dimensional load-displacement curves. J. Bone Joint Surg. 76-A (3), 413–424.

Pearcy, M.J., Gill, J.M., Whittle, M.W., et al., 1987. Dynamic back movement measured using a three-dimensional television system. J. Biomech. 20 (10), 943–949.

Pearcy, M.J., Tibrewal, S.B., 1984. Axial rotation and lateral bending in the normal lumbar spine measurement by three dimensional radiography. Spine 9 (6), 582–587.

Rab, G.T., Chao, E.Y., 1977. Verification of roentgenographic landmarks in the lumbar spine. Spine 2 (4), 287–293.

Tsung, B.Y.S., Evans, J., Tong, P., et al., 2005. Measurement of lumbar spine loads and motions during rotational mobilization. J. Manipulative Physiol. Ther. 28 (4), 238–244.

Vincenzino, G., Twomey, L., 1993. Sideflexion induced lumbar spine conjunct rotation and its influencing factors. Aust. J. Physiother. 39 (4), 299–306.

White, A.A., Panjabi, M.P., 1978. The basic kinematics of the human spine. Spine 3 (1), 12–20.

# Chapter Twelve

12

# Sacroiliac joint

Chris McCarthy

## CHAPTER CONTENTS

## Clinical anatomy and biomechanics

### Ioannis Paneris

The sacroiliac joints (SIJs) are designed mainly for stability, with their function being to transmit and dissipate load from the trunk to the lower extremities and vice versa during weight-bearing activities (Cohen, 2005). Although, for many decades, clinicians considered the SIJ to be immobile, this notion has been overturned over the recent years (Forst et al, 2006; Pool-Goudzwaard et al, 1998). Research has shown that the SIJ is a synovial joint where motion occurs as coupling with 6° of freedom. In fact, the advantage of a mobile SIJ is that it is more efficient as a shock absorber and as a provider of proprioception (Pool-Goudzwaard et al, 1998). The amount and direction of movement of the SIJ is not clearly agreed amongst researchers owing to the employment of different methodological approaches. Recently, the development of Roentgen Stereophotogrammetric Analysis (RSA) has led to more robust studies in the small movements of the SIJ (Goode et al, 2008).

## Standing and sitting

In the normal bipedal standing posture, the line of gravity from the upper body falls posteriorly to the centre of the acetabula. In return the ground reaction force, transferred through the hip joints falls anteriorly to the SIJ. The interaction of these forces rotates the ilia posteriorly on the SIJs (DonTigny, 1985, 1990). This anterior rotation of the sacrum has been shown in both cadaveric (Wang & Dumas, 1998) and in vivo (Sturesson et al, 2000a) studies. In addition to the posterior rotation, the ilia rotate laterally, opening the superior part of the joint, and translate anteriorly and to a lot lesser degree inferiorly (Wang & Dumas, 1998).

The forward motion of the sacral promontory into the pelvis about a coronal axis is called 'nutation' (Lee, 1999, p. 49). Nutation increases the tension of the interosseous and short dorsal sacroiliac ligaments as well as the sacrotuberous ligament which increase compression of the SIJ and thus contribute to the stability of the joint (Pool-Goudzwaard et al, 1998).

Further to the ligamentous tension, the shape and morphology of the joint is a significant factor that contributes to stability. During the second and third decades of life, the articular surfaces become irregular and uneven with duller and rougher cartilage (Bowen & Cassidy, 1981). These changes reflect the dynamic development of the joint and allow for reduced load to be exerted on the ligaments when bearing the upper body (Vleeming et al, 1990). DonTigny (1990) states that in the lordotic posture of the spine, as well as in lifting, the line of gravity falls anteriorly to the centre of the acetabula which leads to posterior rotation of sacrum. This posterior sacral rotation is termed 'counter-nutation' and is a 'position of vulnerability' as the joint is less stable (Lee, 1999, p. 62). However, DonTigny (1990) claims that counter-nutation limits the caudal glide of the sacrum. This could possibly be due to the effect of the long dorsal sacroiliac ligament that limits counter-nutation and due to its attachments working together with the sacrotuberous ligament to stabilize the SIJ (Pool-Goudzwaard et al, 1998).

Similarly to standing, sitting upright should also result in nutation of the sacrum. A study (Snijders et al, 2004) has shown that in sitting conditions, where there is lumbar flexion and posterior rotation of the pelvis, counter-nutation of the sacrum is the result. In contrast, maintaining and/or supporting the lumbar lordosis in sitting results in nutation of the sacrum.

## Lumbar flexion/extension

Lee (1999, p. 62) states that during the first 60° of forward bending of the trunk the nutation of the sacrum can be felt to increase. However, in some subjects, slight counter-nutation occurs towards the end of the range (Lee, 1999, pp. 62–63). The study of Jacob and Kissling (1995) mixed results of the rotation of the sacrum leading to the conclusion that 'during forward flexion, the sacrum is as likely to nutate as to counter-nutate' (Jacob & Kissling, 1995). An explanation for this phenomenon is offered by Lee (1999, p. 62) who states that when during forward flexion, the extensibility of the biceps femoris, sacrotuberous ligament and the deep lamina of the posterior layer of the thoracodorsal fascia has been reached, the relative flexibility of the sacrum becomes less than one of the innominates. Continuation of anterior rotation of the innominates on the femoral heads, after this point,

leads to relative posterior rotation of the sacrum on the innominates and thus counter-nutationutation. Lee (1999, p. 63) claims that during extension, the thoraco-lumbar spine extends while the innominates posteriorly rotate at the hip joints, thus the nutation of the sacrum should not reverse.

## Gait

During ambulation the innominates follow the direction of motion of the femurs causing intra-pelvic torsion between the innominates and the sacrum (DonTigny, 1990; Lee, 1999, p. 64; Smidt et al, 1997). The right innominate rotates posteriorly while the left rotates anteriorly following the extended right femur. The opposite motion of the innominates causes rotation of the sacrum to the right which is counteracted by the contralateral rotation of the trunk (DonTigny, 1990; Lee, 1999, p. 64). The intra-pelvic torsion causes nutation on the heel strike side and counter-nutationutation on the toe off side.

This arrangement seems to be theoretically sound as the nutation on the one side is essential to prepare the low limb for heel strike. However, the study of Smidt et al (1995) produced results that do not agree with the above assumption, in that only 10 out of their 32 healthy subjects demonstrated the expected pattern on reciprocal straddle position while 8 subjects demonstrated the internominate position changed in the same direction in both straddle positions.

The findings of the study of Smidt et al (1995) were not replicated by the later study of Sturesson et al (2000b) which experimentally confirmed the patterns of movement expected theoretically. In the Sturesson et al study, 6 subjects with posterior pelvic pain showed a uniform pattern in which changing from left leg extension to flexion, with parallel right leg flexion to extension, produced left innominate nutation and right counter-nutation with sacral rotation to the left around a vertical axis (with the exception of one person) and, in some subjects, rotation of the sacrum towards the left innominate on a sagittal axis where there was compression of the upper part of the left SIJ.

There is also a lack of agreement between the above studies regarding the magnitude of the motions observed, with the values reported by Smidt et al (1995) to be five times higher than the results of Sturesson *et al* (2000b). In fact, the results of Smidt *et al* (1995) imply that movements of the symphysis pubis range from 2.5 to 8 cm (Sturesson *et al*, 2000b). Perhaps the differences between the studies is that Smidt *et al* (1995) used bony landmark palpation and marking which is likely to lead to errors in determining the range of motion (Hungerford *et al*, 2004). In contrast, the study of Sturesson *et al* (2000b) utilized Roentgen stereophotogrammetric analysis (RSA) (radiosteriomatic analysis) which is regarded as the gold standard in evaluating small joint and tendon mobility (Goode *et al*, 2008). During the swing phase, the non-weight-bearing innominate is moving with the lower limb from anterior rotation to posterior rotation. In other words, the innominate moves from a position of counter-nutation to a position of nutation ready to accept the ground reaction force on heel strike while, at the weight-bearing side, the innominate rotates anteriorly to a position of counter-nutation (Lee, 1999, p. 70).

Studies on the mobility of the SIJs during standing hip flexion have shown that both innominates rotate posteriorly (with few exceptions) while the sacrum rotates slightly to the side of hip flexion and rotates slightly on a sagittal axis gapping the top part of the SIJ on the side of hip flexion (Sturesson *et al*, 2000a). Similar findings were reported in the study of Hungerford *et al* (2004) where, during single leg flexion in standing, the non-weight-bearing innominate rotated posteriorly, there was gapping of the superior part of the joint and rotation of the anterior part of the innominate medially. Additionally, the innominate translated superiorly, anteriorly and laterally. This motion pattern was observed consistently in subjects with or without SIJ dysfunction and irrespective of side of hip flexion.

On the weight-bearing asymptomatic side, there was posterior rotation of the innominate, gapping of the superior part of the SIJ and rotation of the anterior innominate medially. The innominate rotated posteriorly, superiorly and medially (Hungerford *et al*, 2004). This pattern of translation can be attributed to the action of the multifidus and transversus abdominis whose action has been found to increase the stiffness of the SIJ (Richardson *et al*, 2002). On the weight-bearing symptomatic side the innominate rotated anteriorly and translated inferiorly and posteriorly, which is a pattern associated with inefficient intra-pelvic compression (Hungerford *et al*, 2004). The study of Mens *et al* (1999) reported

that symptomatic SIJs have the tendency to exhibit excessive anterior rotation when the leg is hanging down with weight bearing on the asymptomatic leg over a block. Further, anterior rotation of the symptomatic SIJ is exhibited during supine active straight leg raising of the ipsilateral leg which is an indication of impaired stability of the joint.

## The sacroiliac joints' range of motion

There is some controversy regarding the nature but more importantly the magnitude of the motion that occurs at these joints (Harrison *et al*, 1997). Furthermore, clinicians claim that they can detect motion by palpation or two-dimensional radiography (Harrison *et al*, 1997). Studies that used skin markers (Smidt *et al*, 1995; Hungerford *et al*, 2004) reported SIJ motions ranging between a mean value of 9° and 10° respectively. However, as it is stated above, such ranges of rotation inevitably lead to excessive symphysis pubis translation which, for 10° would span to 2.5 cm. The review of Walker (1992) reports results that range up to 20° but uses measurements of no reported reliability. However the mean values of the rotatory motion averaged less than 4°.

A more recent review (Goode *et al*, 2008) of experimental studies of more robust methodology, using two-dimensional motion analysis such as RSA, found that rotational and translational movements of the SIJs are minute, ranging between −1.1° and 2.2° of sagittal rotation, −0.8° and 4.0° of transverse rotation of the sacrum and between −0.5° and 8.0° of frontal plane rotation of the sacrum. Translation ranged between −0.3° and 8.0°. Additionally, the reviewed studies that demonstrated highest levels of quality and lowest levels of error in measurements reported the lowest values of range available at the SIJs. Further, even in the presence of SIJ dysfunction, motions available at the SIJs are not greater (Goode *et al*, 2008). As a result, the ability of clinicians to manually palpate and evaluate changes in range of motion and position is disputed (Goode *et al*, 2008; Sturesson *et al*, 2000a). Perhaps it is not surprising that a great body of studies evaluating clinical tests and manual assessments of the SIJ found them to be short in specificity, sensitivity and reliability (Dreyfuss *et al*, 1994; Freburger & Riddle, 1999; Levangie, 1999; Riddle & Freburger, 2002).

## Clinical note

- Flexion – induces nutation then counter-nutation at end of range
- Flexion and left lateral flexion (in standing) – induces counter-nutation of right SIJ
- Extension – induces neutral movement then nutation at end of range
- Extension and right lateral flexion (in standing) – induces nutation of right SIJ

Positions that induce maximum stretch of the ipsilateral, anterior muscles and superior capsule also induce maximum ipsilateral nutation.

Positions that induce maximum stretch of the ipsilateral posterior muscles and inferior capsule also induce maximum ipsilateral counter-nutation.

When differentiating between the lumbar spine and SIJ use the same starting position to assess both regions.

# Assessment of the sacroiliac joints

## Nutation

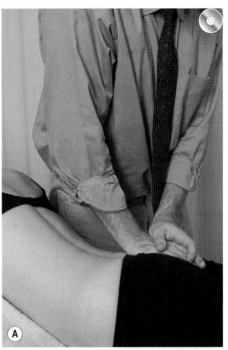

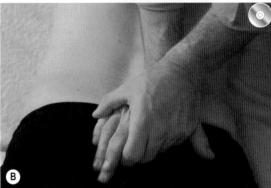

**Figure 12.2** • IN: prone, right lateral flexion, extension. DID: caudad pressure on the left sacral base. **See video clip number 41**

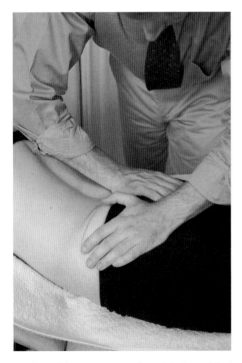

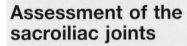

**Figure 12.1** • IN: prone, extension, right lateral flexion. DID: caudad pressure on the right sacral base.

# Counter-nutation

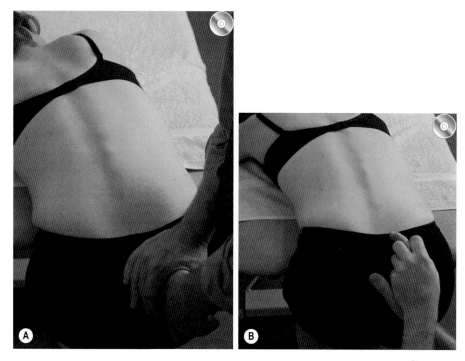

**Figure 12.3** • IN: standing, prone, over the couch, left lateral flexion. DID: cephalad angled pressure on the right inferior lateral angle, using a reinforced thumb or hypothenar eminence. See video clip number 42

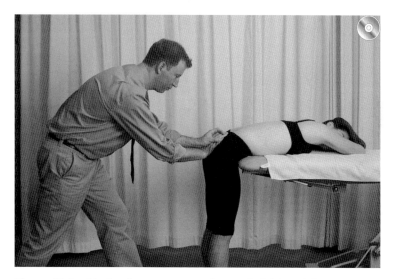

**Figure 12.4** • IN: standing, prone, over the couch, left lateral flexion. DID: cephalad angled pressure on the right inferior lateral angle, using the hypothenar eminence (showing the operator's stance). See video clip number 42

# Assessment for Grade IV−: manipulative technique

## In flexion (the 'adapted Chicago' technique)

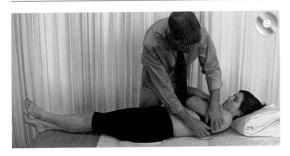

**Figure 12.5** • IN: supine, lateral flexion, flexion. DID: cross the patient's arms and hold onto the low thorax. This technique places the lumbar spine in a regular pattern (following its normal couples) and thus when cavitation occurs it is likely to have occurred at the SIJ. See video clip number 43

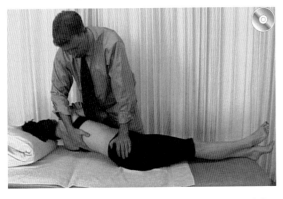

**Figure 12.6** • IN: supine, left lateral flexion, flexion, left rotation. DID: fix on the right ASIS, direct thrust caudad and outward. See video clip number 43

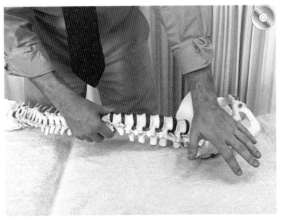

**Figure 12.7** • IN: supine, left lateral flexion, flexion, left rotation. DID: fix on the right ASIS, direct thrust caudad and outward (grip shown). See video clip number 62

## In extension

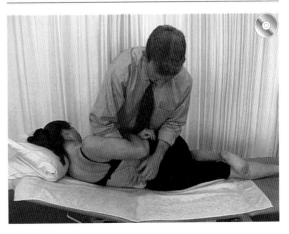

**Figure 12.8** • IN: left side-lying, right rotation, right lateral flexion. DID: right rotation with downward thrust. See video clip number 44

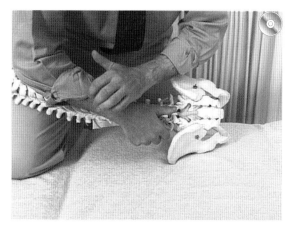

**Figure 12.9** • IN: left side-lying, right rotation, right lateral flexion, fixed with the right arm. DID: thrust using the forearm on the iliac crest (grip shown). **See video clip number 62**

# References

Bowen, V., Cassidy, J.D., 1981. Macroscopic and microscopic anatomy of the sacroiliac joint from embryonic life until the eighth decade. Spine 6, 620–628.

Cohen, S.P., 2005. Sacroiliac joint pain: a comprehensive review of anatomy, diagnosis, and treatment. Anesth. Analg. 101, 1440–1453.

DonTigny, R.L., 1985. Function and pathomechanics of the sacroiliac joint. A review. Phys. Ther. 65, 35–44.

DonTigny, R.L., 1990. Anterior dysfunction of the sacroiliac joint as a major factor in the etiology of idiopathic low back pain syndrome. Phys. Ther. 70, 250–265; discussion 262–264.

Dreyfuss, P., Dryer, S., Griffin, J., et al., 1994. Positive sacroiliac screening tests in asymptomatic adults. Spine 19, 1138–1143.

Forst, S.L., Wheeler, M.T., Fortin, J.D., et al., 2006. The sacroiliac joint: anatomy, physiology and clinical significance. Pain Physician 9, 61–67.

Freburger, J.K., Riddle, D.L., 1999. Measurement of sacroiliac joint dysfunction: a multicenter intertester reliability study. Phys. Ther. 79, 1134–1141.

Goode, A., Hegedus, E.J., Sizer, P., et al., 2008. Three-dimensional movements of the sacroiliac joint: a systematic review of the literature and assessment of clinical utility. Journal of Manual & Manipulative Therapy 16, 25–38.

Harrison, D.E., Harrison, D.D., Troyanovich, S.J., 1997. The sacroiliac joint: a review of anatomy and biomechanics with clinical implications. J. Manipulative Physiol. Ther. 20, 607–617.

Hungerford, B., Gilleard, W., Lee, D., 2004. Altered patterns of pelvic bone motion determined in subjects with posterior pelvic pain using skin markers. Clin. Biomech. (Bristol, Avon) 19, 456–464.

Jacob, H.A., Kissling, R.O., 1995. The mobility of the sacroiliac joints in healthy volunteers between 20 and 50 years of age. Clin. Biomech. (Bristol, Avon) 10, 352–361.

Lee, D., 1999. The pelvic girdle. An approach to the examination and treatment of the lumbo-pelvic-hip region. Churchill Livingstone, Edinburgh.

Levangie, P.K., 1999. Four clinical tests of sacroiliac joint dysfunction: the association of test results with innominate torsion among patients with and without low back pain. Phys. Ther. 79, 1043–1057.

Mens, J.M., Vleeming, A., Snijders, C.J., et al., 1999. The active straight leg raising test and mobility of the pelvic joints. Eur. Spine J. 8, 468–473.

Pool-Goudzwaard, A.L., Vleeming, A., Stoeckart, C.J., et al., 1998. Insufficient lumbopelvic stability: a clinical, anatomical and biomechanical approach to 'a-specific' low back pain. Man. Ther. 3, 12–20.

Richardson, C.A., Snijders, C.J., Hides, J.A., et al., 2002. The relation between the transversus abdominis muscles, sacroiliac joint mechanics, and low back pain. Spine 27, 399–405.

Riddle, D.L., Freburger, J.K., 2002. Evaluation of the presence of sacroiliac joint region dysfunction using a combination of tests: a multicenter intertester reliability study. Phys. Ther. 82, 772–781.

Smidt, G.L., McQuade, K., Wei, S.H., et al., 1995. Sacroiliac kinematics for reciprocal straddle positions. Spine 20, 1047–1054.

Smidt, G.L., Wei, S.H., McQuade, K., et al., 1997. Sacroiliac motion for extreme hip positions: a fresh cadaver study. Spine 22, 2073–2082.

Snijders, C.J., Hermans, P.F., Niesing, C.W., et al., 2004. The influence of slouching and lumbar support on iliolumbar ligaments, intervertebral discs and sacroiliac joints. Clin. Biomech. (Bristol, Avon) 19, 323–329.

Sturesson, B., Uden, A., Vleeming, A., 2000a. A radiostereometric analysis of movements of the sacroiliac joints during the standing hip flexion test. Spine 25, 364–368.

Sturesson, B., Uden, A., Vleeming, A., 2000b. A radiostereometric analysis of the movements of the sacroiliac joints in the reciprocal straddle position. Spine 25, 214–217.

Vleeming, A., Volkers, A.C., Snijders, C.J., et al., 1990. Relation between form and function in the sacroiliac joint. Part II: Biomechanical aspects. Spine 15, 133–136.

Walker, J.M., 1992. The sacroiliac joint: a critical review. Phys. Ther. 72, 903–916.

Wang, M., Dumas, G.A., 1998. Mechanical behavior of the female sacroiliac joint and influence of the anterior and posterior sacroiliac ligaments under sagittal loads. Clin. Biomech. (Bristol, Avon) 13, 293–299.

# Home treatment programmes

Chris McCarthy

## CHAPTER CONTENTS

## General principles

 **Clinical point**

### Exercise Programme Tips

- **Mimic treatment at home**

Home treatment should, as far as is possible, mimic your treatment techniques. It is useful to emphasize the short term effect on pain and movement that most passive movement techniques actually cause. It is useful to ensure that the patient understands that prolonged (weeks or months) regular movement and stretching will lead to permanent change and that they must regularly mimic what you did with them.

- **Check the stretch has helped**

The patient should assess their functional demonstration (painful movement combination): do their prescribed stretch until they feel the problem getting less painful and freer and then reassess their functional demonstration. This gives them immediate feedback regarding their stretch. If their functional demonstration has not changed they need to do more stretching until it does! This approach encourages adherence as the benefit of doing the stretch is immediately reinforced.

- **Do enough to help but not too much**

If you train the patient to develop an awareness of what the stretch should do in reducing their hypertonicity and regional hypomobility they can then perform the number of stretches they need to improve their symptoms at the time. Rather than routinely asking patients to do a set number of movements, encourage the patient to do the number of sets and number of repetitions that actually changes their symptoms immediately. Also ask them to reflect on how often, hard, fast and vigorously they are doing their stretches every couple of days. Engaging them in an active approach to their own treatment combats the development of a maladaptive passive coping style. They will be actively treating themselves with the locus of control being firmly with them.

- **Goal set**

Consider asking your patient to set the goal of 'I will keep doing this until it has improved as much as it has now'. After successfully improving a patient's dysfunction with CMT engage the patient with the notion that they can evoke the same response using the same movements. If they are encouraged to meet this goal they will adhere to the programme more readily than being sent off to perform some exercises that are not obviously benefitting them.

- **Don't overload them**

Try to keep the home programme to as minimum as possible. Overloading patients with numerous exercises and stretches reduces adherence to any of them. It is worth considering that the patient needs to see the benefit of each component of a home programme or they will not do it.

## Active stretching

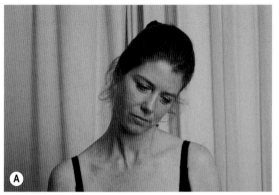

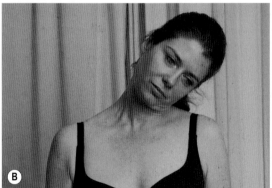

**Figure 13.1** • IN: corrected posture sitting, with the patient holding a full inspiration. DID: Active lateral flexion, followed by exhalation – stretch of the scalene muscles.

## Passive stretching

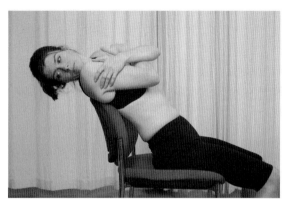

**Figure 13.2** • IN: sitting with chair back across the upper thoracic spine. DID: active right rotation down to the back of the chair, using inspiration to offload the scalenes.

# Cervical

## C0/C1 anterior stretch

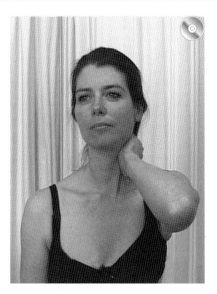

**Figure 13.3** • IN: Sitting, upper cervical extension with the patient fixing C1 with their hypothenar eminence. DID: active right rotation of C0/C1. **See video clip number 45**

## C0/C1 posterior stretch

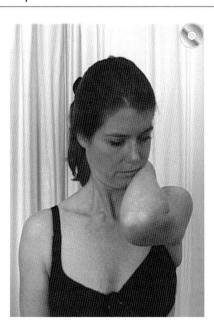

**Figure 13.4** • IN: sitting, upper cervical flexion with the patient fixing C1 with their hypothenar eminence. DID: active left rotation. **See video clip number 46**

# Thoracic

## Anterior stretch

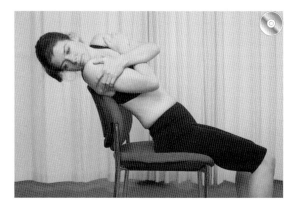

**Figure 13.5** • IN: sitting with chair back across the mid thoracic spine. DID: active right rotation and extension down to the back of the chair, using inspiration to offload the scalenes. **See video clip numbers 47 and 49**

## Posterior stretch

### Rotation

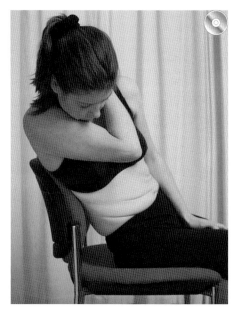

**Figure 13.6** • IN: sitting with chair back across the upper thoracic spine. DID: active right rotation and flexion down to the back of the chair. **See video clip number 48**

*Lateral flexion*

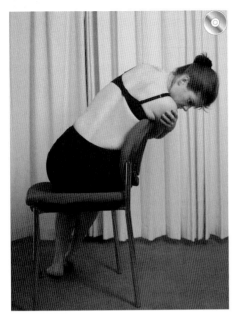

**Figure 13.7** • IN: sitting with chair back across the mid thoracic ribs. DID: active right lateral flexion and flexion down to the back of the chair. **See video clip number 50**

## Lumbar spine

### Lumbar spine superior capsule/ anterior musculature

*Anterior stretch*

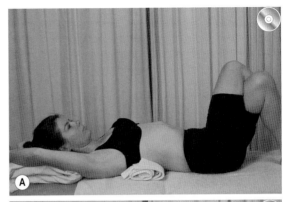

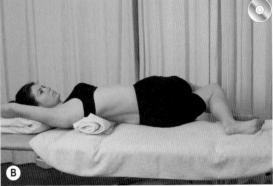

**Figure 13.8** • IN: supine, extended over a rolled towel, using the weight of the arms to extend. DID: right rotation in extension using the weight of the legs to stretch the thoracic spine. **See video clip number 55**

### In lying

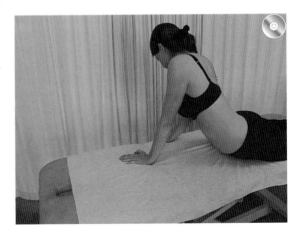

**Figure 13.9** • IN: prone doing a half press-up. DID: active assisted right lateral flexion in extension. **See video clip number 54**

**In standing**

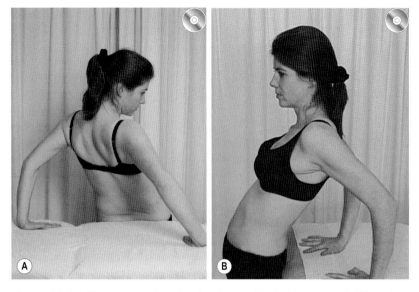

**Figure 13.10** • IN: standing with a fixed surface to block ilial movement. DID: active assisted left lateral flexion in extension, encouraging left nutation. **See video clip numbers 51 and 52**

## Lumbar spine inferior capsule/ posterior musculature

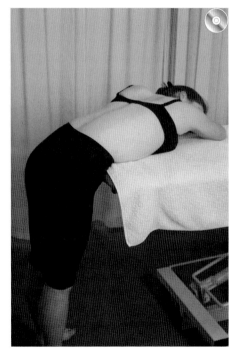

**Figure 13.11** • IN: standing, flexed over a surface to fix the ilia (feet on the floor). DID: active left lateral flexion. See video clip number 53

# Sacroiliac joint

## Nutation

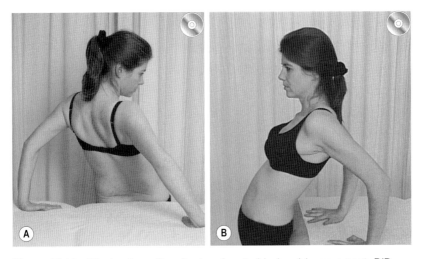

**Figure 13.12** • IN: standing with a fixed surface to block pelvic movement. DID: active assisted left lateral flexion in extension. **See video clip number 51**

## Counter-nutation

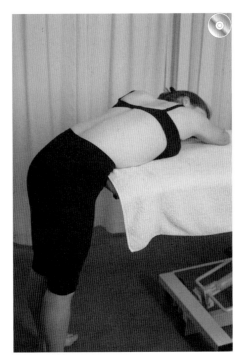

**Figure 13.13** • IN: standing, flexed over a surface to fix the ilia (feet on the floor). DID: active left lateral flexion encouraging counter-nutation. **See video clip number 53**

# Index